Angiogenesis: Physiology and Pathology

Angiogenesis: Physiology and Pathology

Edited by Vincent Wesley

hayle
medical

New York

Hayle Medical,
750 Third Avenue, 9th Floor,
New York, NY 10017, USA

Visit us on the World Wide Web at:
www.haylemedical.com

ISBN: 978-1-63241-551-6

Cataloging-in-Publication Data

Angiogenesis : physiology and pathology / edited by Vincent Wesley.
p. cm.
Includes bibliographical references and index.
ISBN 978-1-63241-551-6
1. Neovascularization. 2. Blood-vessels--Growth.
3. Blood-vessels--Pathophysiology. 4. Cardiology. I. Wesley, Vincent.
QP106.6 .A54 2019
612.13--dc23

Table of Contents

Preface

This book has been an outcome of determined endeavour from a group of educationists in the field. The primary objective was to involve a broad spectrum of professionals from diverse cultural background involved in the field for developing new researches. The book not only targets students but also scholars pursuing higher research for further enhancement of the theoretical and practical applications of the subject.

Angiogenesis is the process through which new blood vessels develop from pre-existing ones. It is an important process of growth and development and aids in wound healing and formation of granulation tissue. Angiogenesis may be stimulated mechanically and chemically. Though mechanical stimulation is not well characterized, chemical stimulation is done using angiogenic proteins such as integrins and prostaglandins, and growth factors like vascular endothelial growth factor (VEGF), fibroblast growth factor (FGF), etc. The application of angiogenesis in medicine is as a therapeutic target for the management of abnormal vasculature or poor vascularization and cardiovascular disease. This book brings forth some of the most innovative concepts and elucidates the unexplored aspects of angiogenesis. It aims to give a general view of the physiology and pathology of angiogenesis. The extensive content of this book provides the readers with a thorough understanding of the subject.

It was an honour to edit such a profound book and also a challenging task to compile and examine all the relevant data for accuracy and originality. I wish to acknowledge the efforts of the contributors for submitting such brilliant and diverse chapters in the field and for endlessly working for the completion of the book. Last, but not the least; I thank my family for being a constant source of support in all my research endeavours.

Editor

Tumor Angiogenesis: A Focus on the Role of Cancer Stem Cells

Keiko Fujita and Masumi Akita

Abstract

Angiogenesis is the process of growth of new blood vessels. Tumor angiogenesis plays pivotal roles in tumor development, progression, and metastasis. The conventional notion of tumor vasculature is that new tumor blood vessels sprout from preexisting vasculature near the tumor; hence, tumor endothelial cells are derived from normal endothelial cells. However, recent evidence suggests that CD133-positive cancer stem cells (CSCs) in glioblastomas generate tumor endothelial progenitor cells, which further differentiate into tumor endothelial cells. This chapter offers an overview of current knowledge on the role of CSCs in tumor angiogenesis. Furthermore, we discuss our recent discoveries related to human hepatoblastoma stem cells. Future efforts to elucidate the characteristics of tumor angiogenesis should enable the development of effective new anti-angiogenic therapies.

Keywords: tumor angiogenesis, cancer stem cells, hepatoblastoma, cell culture

1. Introduction

Angiogenesis is an essential process by which new blood vessels are formed. In malignancies, tumor growth and metastasis are angiogenesis dependent. It is widely accepted that new tumor blood vessels sprout from preexisting vasculature. Therefore, tumor endothelial cells are considered to be derived from normal endothelial cells. However, over the last few years, different processes by which tumor vascularization occurs have been documented. It has been shown that endothelial cells in the tumor vasculature arise from a small population of tumor cells known as cancer stem cells (CSCs) or tumor-initiating cells. Since John Dick and others identified leukemia cells in 1994 [1], the presence of CSCs with similar properties to normal stem cells has been discovered. CSCs have the ability to undergo self-renewal and differentiation into diverse cancer cells and are capable of becoming malignant. CD133 (or

Prominin1), a cell surface glycoprotein used widely as a marker for normal stem cells, is additionally recognized as a marker for CSCs. Recent reports suggest that CD133-positive CSCs in glioblastomas generate tumor endothelial progenitor cells, which further differentiate into tumor endothelial cells [2–4].

What is the origin of endothelial cells and pericytes lining tumor blood vessels? Can CSCs give rise to tumor endothelial cells? The origin of tumor endothelial cells is the main focus of this chapter. We will provide an overview of current studies and discuss the role of CSCs in tumor angiogenesis. We have investigated the relationship between tumor endothelial cells and CSCs in human hepatoblastoma, which is the most frequent type of malignant tumor to occur in the pediatric liver. Our findings are reported in this chapter.

2. Characteristics of tumor blood vessels

The field of angiogenesis research arose following a publication by Folkman in 1971. The future of anticancer therapy was emphasized in that the potential utility of angiogenesis inhibitors against cancer was identified. The term "anti-angiogenesis" was proposed by Folkman's research group to refer to the inhibition of new vessel sprouts from penetrating into an early tumor implant [5].

Tumor endothelial cells lining the inner layer of blood vessels are the main targets of anti-angiogenic therapy. It is believed that new tumor vessels generally sprout from preexisting vasculature; accordingly, new tumor vessels are considered structurally and functionally normal. However, recent studies have reported that tumor blood vessels differ morphologically and phenotypically from normal blood vessels [6]. A common feature in the architecture of the normal vasculature is a hierarchical and regular branching pattern. In contrast, tumor blood vessels are structurally distinct from normal blood vessels. Tumor endothelial cells, which are not comprised of regular monolayers, do not function as a normal barrier [7]. The pericytes form abnormally loose associations with these cells and extend cytoplasmic processes deep into the tumor tissue [8]. An inner layer of tumor blood vessels is composed of a specific phenotype of tumor-associated blood endothelial cells. Furthermore, the tumor endothelial cells are heterogeneous according to the malignancy status of tumor [9].

3. Tumor-specific angiogenesis

3.1. Cancer stem cells (CSCs) or tumor-initiating cells

The American Association for Cancer Research (AACR) defined CSCs as subpopulations of cells within a tumor that possess the capacity for self-renewal and generation of heterogeneous lineages of cancer cells that constitute the tumor [10].

The cancer stem cell theory provides an attractive explanation for tumor proliferation and progression. According to this theory, tumors retain subsets of cells with functional heterogeneity. However, the putative relationship between CSCs and tumor angiogenesis remains poorly understood [11].

3.2. The origin of the endothelial cells in the tumor vasculature

The origin of endothelial cells in the tumor vasculature is not yet known [12]. Some studies suggest that CSCs play an important role in tumor vascularization. The tumor stem cells defined as CSCs or tumor-initiating cells are considered the source of tumor cells. Moreover, novel findings, which suggest that CSCs also give rise to endothelial cells in the tumor vasculature, have been described in recent reports [2–4]. A proportion of endothelial cells that contribute to blood vessels in glioblastomas originate from the tumor itself, having differentiated from CSCs. A subset of endothelial cells that constitute tumor vessels carries genetic aberrations found in the tumor cells themselves. It has been shown that a glioblastoma cell population that could differentiate into endothelial cells and form blood vessels was enriched in cells expressing the tumor stem cell marker CD133.

3.3. The origin of pericytes in the tumor vasculature

Pericytes are mural cells that wrap around the endothelial cells of capillaries and venules. Vascular pericytes play important roles in supporting vascular structure and function. As communication between pericytes and endothelial cells has been demonstrated to occur, it is considered that pericytes may prove a novel target for tumor therapy [13]. A recent study has reported that glioblastoma stem cells give rise to vascular pericytes that support vessel function and tumor growth. These results suggest that CSCs from glioblastomas generate the majority of vascular pericytes [14].

4. Tumor angiogenesis via endothelial differentiation of human hepatoblastoma stem cells

We have investigated the relationship between tumor endothelial cells and CSCs in human hepatoblastoma, which is the most frequent type of malignant tumor that occurs in the pediatric liver.

4.1. Characteristics of human hepatoblastoma cells

4.1.1. CD133

CSCs exhibit specific cell membrane markers; CD133 is considered a stem-like cell marker in various cancers [15–17]. In human hepatocellular carcinoma (HCC) and HCC cell lines, CD133 is expressed by only a minority of the tumor cell population. CD133+ cells exhibit the ability to self-renew, produce differentiated progenies, and form new tumors [18, 19].

4.1.2. Cell culture

Human hepatoblastoma cell line (HuH-6 clone 5, well-differentiated type, JCRB0401) was procured from the Health Science Research Resources Bank (Osaka, Japan) and cultured in Dulbecco's modified Eagle's medium (DMEM) containing 10% fetal bovine serum (FBS) and 50 μg/mL gentamicin, according to a previously described protocol [20].

4.1.3. SEM and TEM

For SEM observation, the samples were fixed in 0.1 M phosphate buffer (pH 7.2) containing 2.5% glutaraldehyde for 1 h and subsequently fixed in 0.1 M phosphate buffer (pH 7.2) containing 1% OsO_4 for 1 h, dehydrated in graded ethanol, and critical-point air-dried after treatment with isoamyl acetate. The samples were sputter-coated with OsO_4 and observed under a SEM (Hitachi, S-4800; Tokyo, Japan) [21].

For TEM, the cells were fixed in 0.1 M phosphate buffer (pH 7.2) containing 2.5% glutaraldehyde for 1 h, followed by fixation in 0.1 M phosphate buffer (pH 7.2) containing 1% OsO_4 for another hour. The specimens were dehydrated in graded ethanol, embedded in epoxy resin, cut into ultrathin sections, and stained with uranyl acetate and lead citrate. The stained ultrathin sections were observed under a TEM (JEM-1010; Tokyo, Japan) [21].

4.1.4. Distribution of CD133 in human hepatoblastoma cells

We investigated CD133 distribution in human hepatoblastoma cells. CD133 was mainly localized in membrane ruffles in the peripheral regions of the cell. Examination of the CD133-positive sites using SEM revealed that they coincided with filopodia and lamellipodia. TEM revealed that CD133 was preferentially concentrated in a complex structure formed by filopodia and lamellipodia [21] (**Figure 1**).

4.2. Isolation and identification of human hepatoblastoma stem cells

A key challenge in the study of CSCs is the development of reproducible and reliable methods for CSC isolation and identification. The side population (SP) assay identifies the fraction of cells that efflux Hoechst dye through ATP-binding cassette (ABC) transporters. We identified hepatoblastoma stem cells based on their ability to efflux Hoechst 33342 dye using flow cytometry, as described in Hayashi et al. [22]. A fraction of SP cells was analyzed by flow cytometry (FACS Vantage SE, BD, Tokyo, Japan) (**Figure 2**). SP cells were injected subcutaneously into immunodeficient NOD/SCID mice (male, 4-week-old: Charles River Japan Inc.), and tumor growth was evaluated. All animal experiments were approved by the Institutional Animal Care and Use Committee of Saitama Medical University.

4.3. Sphere formation assay and three-dimensional collagen gel culture system

Digested xenograft tumor fragments were cultured, and tumor sphere assay was carried out. The spheres were cultivated using three-dimensional collagen gel culture methods, referring to the previous reports [23–25]. The spheres were fixed with 4% paraformaldehyde/phosphate buffer saline (PBS) and then embedded in Technovit 8100 (T8100, Heraeus Kulzer, Wehrheim, Germany) according to the manufacturer's instructions.

4.4. Immunohistochemical detection of CD133

The location of CD133 expression was examined in Technovit-embedded sections (**Figure 3**). Some spheres were observed to form capillary-like structures (**Figure 4**).

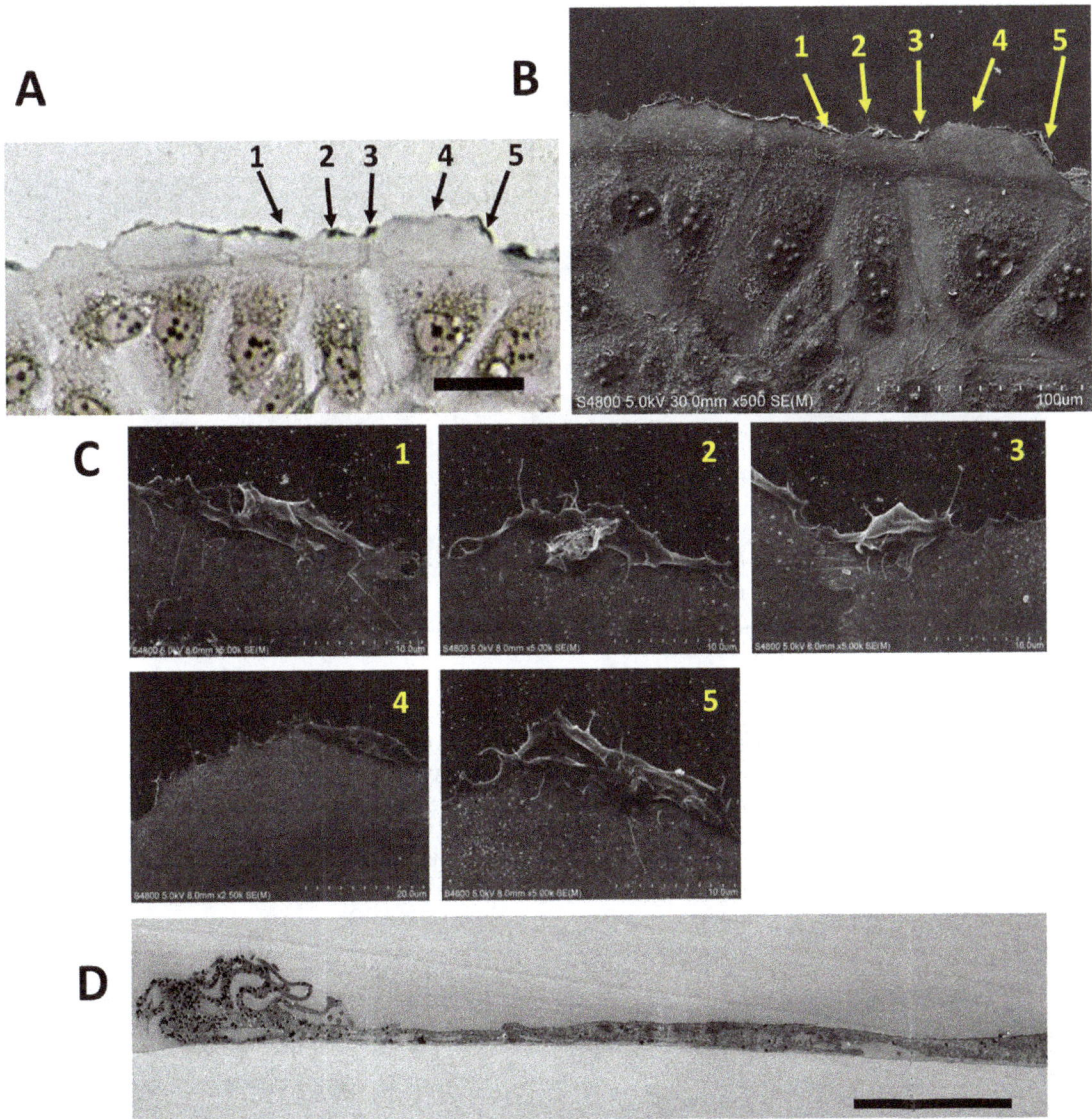

Figure 1. Immunohistochemical analyses of CD133 in hepatoblastoma cells by light microscopy, scanning electron microscopy (SEM), and transmission electron microscopy (TEM). (**A**) Intense immunolabeling of CD133 was observed at the peripheral regions of cells (arrow numbers 1, 2, 3, and 5) by light microscopy. Nanogold labeling was followed by gold enhancement for 20 min. Arrow number 4 indicated a negative site; scale bar: 50 μm. (**B**) SEM image of the sample shown in **A**; the peripheral region of cells (arrow numbers 1, 2, 3, and 5) coincided with the positive sites observed in **A**. (**C**) Higher magnification of SEM images of the positive sites shown in **B**; the positive sites were composed of a complex structure of filopodia and lamellipodia. (**D**) TEM analysis: CD133 was preferentially concentrated in the complex filopodial structure and at the leading edge of lamellipodia. The clustered particles form black spots; scale bar: 5 μm. (Modified from Akita et al. [21]).

Immunostaining for correlative observation by light microscopy and electron microscopy was performed, according to previously described methods [21], to detect the expression of CD133 in these capillary-like structures. The spheres were incubated with primary anti-CD133 antibody (Santa Cruz Biotechnology, CA). Alexa Fluor 488- and 1.4-nm nanogold-conjugated goat

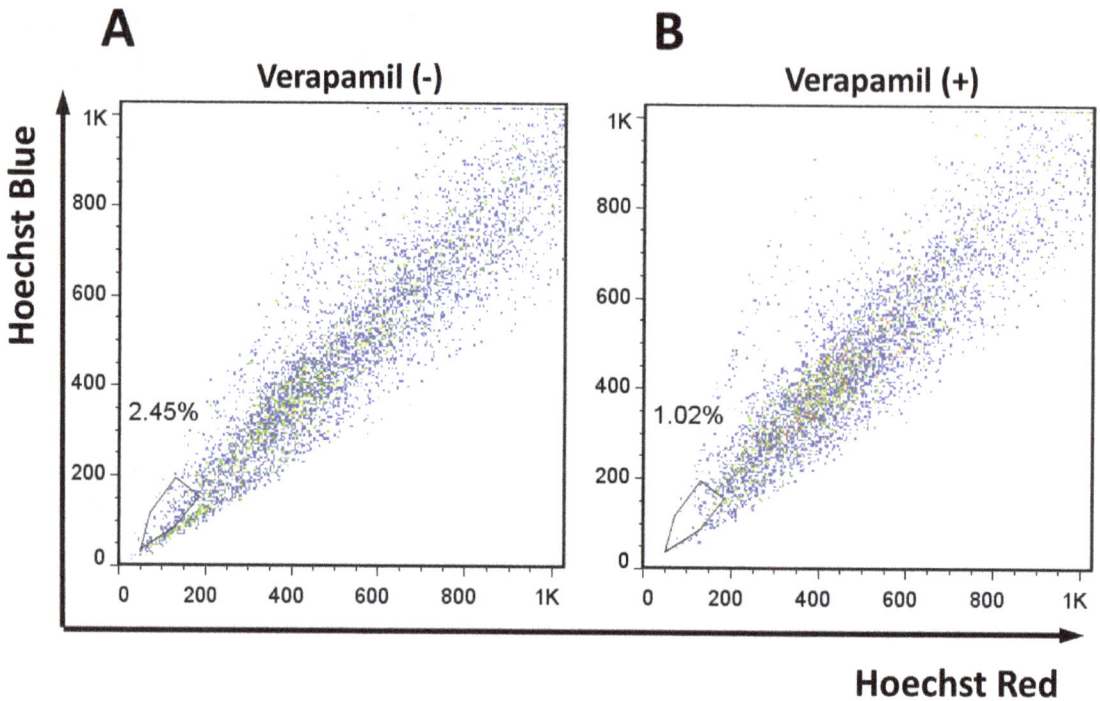

Figure 2. Identification and characterization of side population (SP) cells from a hepatoblastoma cell line. The SP cells in hepatoblastoma cells were identified by flow cytometry using a Hoechst33342-based staining procedure. (**A**) The SP cells displayed in plots show a tail-like subpopulation close to the G0/G1 phase (on the left). Representative images of dot plot analysis by FACS demonstrating the presence of 2.45% SP cells. (**B**) The ABC transporter inhibitor verapamil effectively blocks the export of the Hoechst dye, thus leading to the disappearance of the SP subpopulation. SP cells were reduced to 1.02% upon treatment with verapamil.

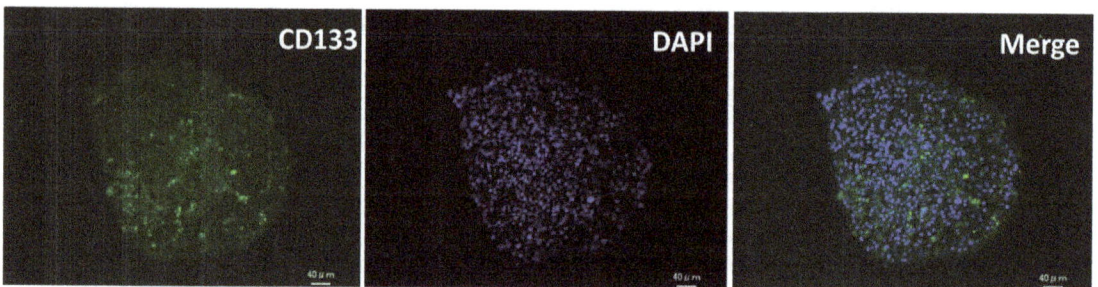

Figure 3. Immunofluorescence of hepatoblastoma tumor sphere. Immunofluorescence of tumor sphere labeled with anti-CD133 antibody (green); nuclei stained with DAPI (blue). The overlaid image is shown in the right panel (merge); scale bar: 40 μm.

anti-rabbit IgG (Nanoprobes, Yaphank, NY, USA) were used as secondary antibodies. The nanogold signal was enhanced using GoldEnhance EM (Nanoprobes) for 20 min. The spheres were analyzed by light microscopy (**Figure 5**, inset). The spheres of interest were subjected to the gold-enlargement procedure using GoldEnhance EM (Nanoprobes, Yaphank, NY, USA) to an appropriate size for TEM analysis, according to the manufacturer's instructions. Some spheres formed CD133-positive capillary-like structures. TEM imaging of these structures confirmed the presence of identifiable lumens (**Figure 5**, bottom).

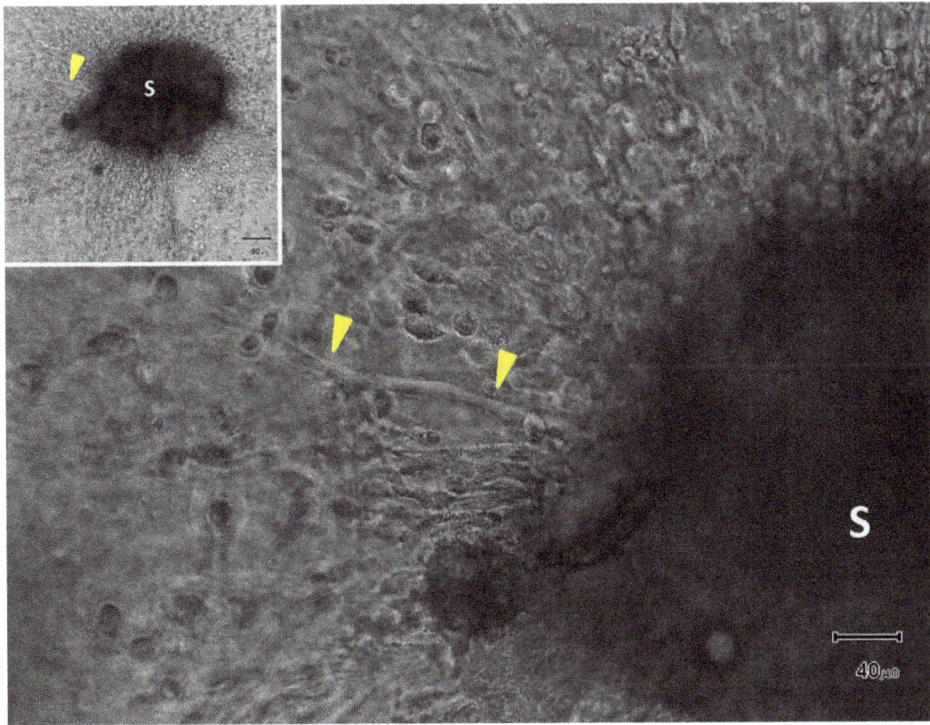

Figure 4. Tube formation assay of hepatoblastoma tumor sphere. Phase-contrast microscopy shows a tubular structure sprouting (arrowheads) from hepatoblastoma tumor sphere (S) in a three-dimensional collagen gel. Higher magnification of the inset indicated bottom; scale bar: 90 μm (inset), 40 μm (bottom).

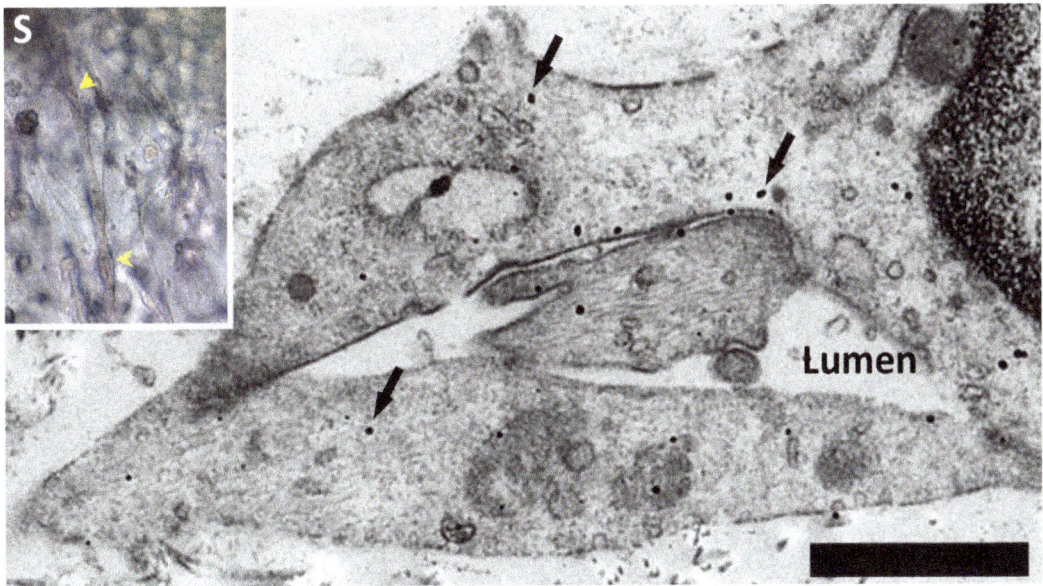

Figure 5. Immunohistochemical detection of CD133 in capillary tubes. (**Inset**) Light microscopy showed that the capillary tube formed from the hepatoblastoma tumor sphere (S) in the collagen gel was positive for CD133 (arrowheads). Nanogold labeling was followed by gold enhancement for 20 min. (**Bottom**) Transmission electron microscopy (TEM) image of the sample shown in the inset; the cross section of this tube is shown. CD133 was detected in the capillary tube. The clustered particles form black spots (arrows); scale bar: 1 μm.

5. Conclusions and perspectives

Tumor angiogenesis has been widely mentioned as a process that new blood vessels are developed from preexisting host blood vessels surrounding the tumors. However, we propose a paradigm change. Our results suggest that CD133-positive CSCs differentiate into tumor vascular endothelial cells and might be able to form tumor vessels.

Since Folkman hypothesized the notion of targeting tumor endothelial cells with anti-angiogenic therapy, numerous anti-angiogenic drugs have been discovered. Previously, we reported that CD133-positive capillary tubes were formed in vitro. Statins, which are widely used as cholesterol-lowering agents, strongly inhibited the capillary tube formation [26]. Statin diminished intraplaque angiogenesis [27] and reduced the growth and spread of many cancers [28, 29]. Khaidakov et al. suggested that statin had anti-angiogenic effects [30]. We propose that the anti-angiogenic effects of statins can be considered for the cancer therapy.

Acknowledgements

This work was supported in part by JSPS KAKENHI Grant Numbers JP25462779 and JP16K11353.

Author details

Keiko Fujita[1]* and Masumi Akita[2]

*Address all correspondence to: kfujita@saitama-med.ac.jp

1 Department of Anatomy, Faculty of Medicine, Saitama Medical University, Saitama, Japan

2 Division of Morphological Science, Faculty of Medicine, Biomedical Research Center, Saitama Medical University, Saitama, Japan

References

[1] Lapidot T, Sirard C, Vormoor J, Murdoch B, Hoang T, Caceres-Cortes J, Minden M, Paterson B, Caligiuri MA, Dick JE. A cell initiating human acute myeloid leukemia after transplantation into SCID mice. Nature. 1994;367:645–648. doi:10.1038/367645a0

[2] Bautch VL. Cancer: Tumour stem cells switch sides. Nature. 2010;468:770–771. doi:10.1038/468770a

[3] Ricci-Vitiani L, Pallini R, Biffoni M, Todaro M, Invernici G, Cenci T, Maira G, Parati EA, Stassi G, Larocca LM, De Maria R. Tumour vascularization via endothelial differentiation of glioblastoma stem-like cells. Nature. 2010;468:824–828. doi:10.1038/nature09557

[4] Wang R, Chadalavada K, Wilshire J, Kowalik U, Hovinga KE, Geber A, Fligelman B, Leversha M, Brennan C, Tabar V. Glioblastoma stem-like cells give rise to tumour endothelium. Nature. 2010;468:829–833. doi:10.1038/nature09624

[5] Folkman J. Tumor angiogenesis: therapeutic implications. N Engl J Med. 1971;285:1182–1186. doi:10.1056/NEJM197111182852108

[6] Hida K, Maishi N, Torii C, Hida Y. Tumor angiogenesis—characteristics of tumor endothelial cells. Int J Clin Oncol. 2016;21:206–212. doi:10.1007/s10147-016-0957-1

[7] Hashizume H, Baluk P, Morikawa S, McLean JW, Thurston G, Roberge S, Jain RK, McDonald DM. Openings between defective endothelial cells explain tumor vessel leakiness. Am J Pathol. 2000;156:1363–1380. doi:10.1016/S0002-9440(10)65006-7

[8] Baluk P, Hashizume H, McDonald DM. Cellular abnormalities of blood vessels as targets in cancer. Curr Opin Genet Dev. 2005;15:102–111. doi:10.1016/j.gde.2004.12.005

[9] Hida K, Maishi N, Sakurai Y, Hida Y, Harashima H. Heterogeneity of tumor endothelial cells and drug delivery. Adv Drug Deliv Rev. 2016;99:140–147. doi:10.1016/j.addr.2015.11.008

[10] Clarke MF, Dick JE, Dirks PB, Eaves CJ, Jamieson CH, Jones DL, Visvader J, Weissman IL, Wahl GM. Cancer stem cells—perspectives on current status and future directions: AACR Workshop on cancer stem cells. Cancer Res. 2006;66:9339–9344. doi:10.1158/0008-5472.CAN-06-3126

[11] Li S, Li Q. Cancer stem cells and tumor metastasis. Int J Oncol. 2014;44:1806–1812. doi:10.3892/ijo.2014.2362

[12] Krishna Priya S, Nagare RP, Sneha VS, Sidhanth C, Bindhya S, Manasa P, Ganesan TS. Tumour angiogenesis-Origin of blood vessels. Int J Cancer. 2016;139:729–735. doi:10.1002/ijc.30067

[13] Kang E, Shin JW. Pericyte-targeting drug delivery and tissue engineering. Int J Nanomedicine. 2016;11:2397–2406. doi:10.2147/IJN.S105274

[14] Cheng L, Huang Z, Zhou W, Wu Q, Donnola S, Liu JK, Fang X, Sloan AE, Mao Y, Lathia JD, Min W, McLendon RE, Rich JN, Bao S. Glioblastoma stem cells generate vascular pericytes to support vessel function and tumor growth. Cell. 2013;153:139–152. doi:10.1016/j.cell.2013.02.021

[15] Ricci-Vitiani L, Lombardi DG, Pilozzi E, Biffoni M, Todaro M, Peschle C, De Maria R. Identification and expansion of human colon-cancer-initiating cells. Nature. 2007;445:111–115. doi:10.1038/nature05384

[16] Brungs D, Aghmesheh M, Vine KL, Becker TM, Carolan MG, Ranson M. Gastric cancer stem cells: evidence, potential markers, and clinical implications. J Gastroenterol. 2016;51:313–326. doi:10.1007/s00535-015-1125-5

[17] Konishi H, Asano N, Imatani A, Kimura O, Kondo Y, Jin X, Kanno T, Hatta W, Ara N, Asanuma K, Koike T, Shimosegawa T. Notch1 directly induced CD133 expression

in human diffuse type gastric cancers. Oncotarget. 2016;7:56598-56607. doi:10.18632/oncotarget.10967

[18] Suetsugu A, Nagaki M, Aoki H, Motohashi T, Kunisada T, Moriwaki H. Characterization of CD133+ hepatocellular carcinoma cells as cancer stem/progenitor cells. Biochem Biophys Res Commun. 2006;351:820–824. doi:10.1016/j.bbrc.2006.10.128

[19] Ma S, Chan KW, Hu L, Lee TK, Wo JY, Ng IO, Zheng BJ, Guan XY. Identification and characterization of tumorigenic liver cancer stem/progenitor cells. Gastroenterology. 2007;132:2542–2556. doi:10.1053/j.gastro.2007.04.025

[20] Morimura T, Fujita K, Akita M, Nagashima M, Satomi A. The proton pump inhibitor inhibits cell growth and induces apoptosis in human hepatoblastoma. Pediatr Surg Int. 2008;24:1087–1094. doi:10.1007/s00383-008-2229-2

[21] Akita M, Tanaka K, Murai N, Matsumoto S, Fujita K, Takaki T, Nishiyama H. Detection of CD133 (prominin-1) in a human hepatoblastoma cell line (HuH-6 clone 5). Microsc Res Tech. 2013;76:844–852. doi:10.1002/jemt.22237

[22] Hayashi S, Fujita K, Matsumoto S, Akita M, Satomi A. Isolation and identification of cancer stem cells from a side population of a human hepatoblastoma cell line, HuH-6 clone-5. Pediatr Surg Int. 2011;27:9–16. doi:10.1007/s00383-010-2719-x

[23] Akita M, Murata E, Merker H-J, Kaneko K. Morphology of capillary-like structures in a three-dimensional aorta/collagen gel culture. Ann Anat. 1997;179:127–136. doi:10.1016/S0940-9602(97)80087-8

[24] Akita M, Murata E, Merker H-J, Kaneko K. Formation of new capillary-like tubes in a three-dimensional in vitro model (Aorta/Collagen Gel). Ann Anat. 1997;179:137–147. doi:10.1016/S0940-9602(97)80088-X

[25] Fujita K, Asami Y, Tanaka K, Akita M, Merker H-J. Anti-angiogenic effects of thalidomide: expression of apoptosis-inducible active-caspase-3 in a three-dimensional collagen gel culture of aorta. Histochem Cell Biol. 2004;122:27–33. doi:10.1007/s00418-004-0669-x

[26] Akita M, Tanaka K, Matsumoto S, Komatsu K, Fujita K. Detection of the hematopoietic stem and progenitor cell marker CD133 during angiogenesis in three-dimensional collagen gel culture. Stem Cells Int. 2013;2013:Article ID 927403,10 pages http://dx.doi.org/10.1155/2013/927403

[27] Karthikeyan VJ, Lip GY. Statins and intra-plaque angiogenesis in carotid artery disease. Atherosclerosis. 2007;192:455–456. doi:10.1016/j.atherosclerosis.2007.01.018

[28] Poynter JN, Gruber SB, Higgins PD, Almog R, Bonner JD, Rennert HS, Low M, Greenson JK, Rennert G. Statins and the risk of colorectal cancer. N Engl J Med. 2005;352:2184–2192. doi:10.1056/NEJMoa043792

[29] Friis S, Poulsen AH, Johnsen SP, McLaughlin JK, Fryzek JP, Dalton SO, Sørensen HT, Olsen JH. Cancer risk among statin users: a population-based cohort study. Int J Cancer. 2005;114:643–647. doi:10.1002/ijc.20758

[30] Khaidakov M, Wang W, Khan JA, Kang BY, Hermonat PL, Mehta JL. Statins and angiogenesis: is it about connections? Biochem Biophys Res Commun. 2009;387:543–547. doi:10.1016/j.bbrc.2009.07.057

2

MCAM and its Isoforms as Novel Targets in Angiogenesis Research and Therapy

Jimmy Stalin, Lucie Vivancos, Nathalie Bardin,
Françoise Dignat-George and Marcel Blot-Chabaud

Abstract

Melanoma cell adhesion molecule (MCAM) (CD146) is a membrane glycoprotein of the mucin family. It is one of the numerous proteins composing the junction of the vascular endothelium, and it is expressed in other cell types such as cancer cells, smooth muscle cells, and pericytes. Some recent works were designed to highlight its structural features, its location in the endothelium, and its role in angiogenesis, vascular permeability, and monocyte transmigration, but also in the maintenance of endothelial junctions and tumor development. MCAM exists in different splice variants and is shedded from the vascular membrane by metalloproteases. Studies about MCAM spliced and cleaved variant on human angiogenic physiological and pathological models permit a better understanding on the roles initially described for this protein. Furthermore, this knowledge will help in the future to develop therapeutic and diagnostic tools targeting specifically the different MCAM variant. Recent advances in research on angiogenesis and in the implication of MCAM in this process are discussed in this chapter.

Keywords: angiogenesis, MCAM (CD146), melanoma, physiology, pathology

1. Introduction

Angiogenesis is the process of new blood vessel formation from preexisting vessels. It contributes to physiological processes such as development and wound healing, but also to pathological processes, such as tumor angiogenesis. The identification of new targets involved in angiogenesis remains an important challenge to fully understand the involved mechanisms and to generate new therapeutic tools. Recent studies have highlighted CD146, an endothelial junctional molecule, as a key factor in angiogenesis. This molecule that displays different isoforms and that is present on different cell types could hence constitute a novel target for therapy. Different reviews have underlined its structural features, localization, and functions in the endothelium. This chapter thus mainly addresses the differences in CD146 isoforms with a special focus on their role in angiogenesis and the therapeutic tools targeting the molecule.

Historically, CD146 was discovered in 1987 by Professor J.P. Jonhson for the first time. It was identified as a marker of melanoma progression. These data were obtained by using an antibody generated by mouse immunization with a cell lysate of metastasizing melanoma. This antibody (MUC18) allowed the identification of a 113 kDa transmembrane protein. MCAM (melanoma cell adhesion molecule) described as a marker of metastasizing melanoma [1].

In 1991, the team of Professor. F. Dignat-George identified Sendo-1 antigen as a marker of circulating endothelial cells in the blood by flow cytometry. This was made possible through the generation of a mouse monoclonal antibody named Sendo -1 [2] obtained by mice immunization with a HUVEC cell lysate. Sendo-1 was able to stain the human endothelium whatever the vessel size and its anatomical location within the vascular tree [3, 4]. Gicerin and HEMCAM refer both to the avian homologues of the molecule [5].

As reported in Kobé in 1997, CD146 (cluster of differentiation 146) is now the official name grouping Sendo-1/MUC18/MCAM/gicerin/HEMCAM (Sendo-MUC18 preCD, Workshop Report).

2. Structure and characteristics of CD146

2.1. Genomic description

The specific location of the CD146 gene is on the arm q23.3 of the chromosome 11 in humans and on the chromosome 9 in mice (www.ensembl.org). The gene encoding the CD146 protein extends over 14 kb. It consists of five immunoglobulin-like domains, two variable domains, and three constant domains of C2 type, as well as a transmembrane domain and an intracytoplasmic portion [6]. The extracellular part of the molecule, including the five immunoglobulin domains, is encoded by 13 exons; the transmembrane domain and the intracellular domain are encoded by three exons.

The promoter of CD146 presents different putative binding sites and motifs including AP1, AP-2, CRE, SP1, CArG, and c-myb. Analysis of this DNA segments suggests that the four SP-1 sites, the two AP-2 domains, and one response element to AMPc-(CRE) form the minimal promotor of CD146 [7]. Specific sites play a role in CD146 expression. The AP-2 sites, which are located at −131 and −302 by relative to the initial ATG, inhibit the expression of CD146 by 70 and 44%, respectively. Moreover, when mutated, the CRE site inhibits by 70% the transcription of the genes. Therefore, AP-2 [8] and CRE sites [9] have been described to modulate CD146 expression in melanoma cells, leading to an increase in tumor growth and metastatic potential in these cancers. In fact, the AP-2 binding site located in the promoter (located at −23 bp) is an inhibitor of the transcription of CD146 while the other AP-2 sites (located at −131 and −302, respectively) are transcription activators [8].

The size of CD146 mRNA is around 3.3 kb and has been first identified in human mela-noma cancer cells [10]. Its encoding region is about 1940 bp. A large homology in the mRNA sequences exists between human and mouse, but differences can be noted. Thus, in humans, there is a lengthening of the 3′ and 5′ UTR region as wells as a loss of 6 pb in exon 2. The encoding regions and 5′UTR have a homology of about 80 and 72%, respectively, between the murine and human genes and there is only 31% of homology for the 3′UTR fragment. Finally, the protein sequence shares about 76% of homology between these two species [1, 10, 11].

2.2. Proteic structure and isoforms

The proteic structure of CD146 is composed of a signal peptide of 28 amino acids (AA), five immunoglobulin domains (including two variable domains and three constant domains), a hydrophobic transmembrane region (AA 561–585), and an intracellular region. The protein sequence derived from the coding region of CD146 has a theoretical molecular weight of about 72 kDa. However, CD146 has a molecular weight of about 113 kDa. This difference is due to the glycosylation sites present on the protein sequence. Indeed, glycosylations repre-sent about 35% of the total molecular weight of CD146 with mainly N-glycosylations. The presence of sialylation has also been shown [12].

CD146 has many similarities with other immunoglobulin family members such as BCAM (B-cell adhesion molecule) and ALCAM (activated leukocyte cell adhesion molecule), includ-ing the same number of immunoglobulin-like domains, similarity of functions and expression on tumor and endothelial cells. Thus, the ALCAM protein plays a role in CD4+ T lymphocytes and in tumor invasion [13, 14].

A short and a long isoform generated by alternative splicing have been identified as the two iso-forms of membrane CD146. They have not been identified simultaneously. The long isoform was the first discovered in human melanocytes in 1987 and the short isoform was identified as a com-plementary DNA from chicken more recently [15]. In addition, a soluble form of CD146 was also identified in endothelial cell culture supernatant (HUVEC) and in bloodstream in patient [16].

Concerning the extracellular sequence, it is common to both isoforms. The difference is located in the intracytoplasmic portion [15]. The two isoforms are the result of an alternative splicing on exon 15 causing a reading frame shift. The short isoform displays a shorter intracytoplas-mic domain containing a phosphorylation site for protein kinase C (PKC) and an interaction site for the protein with PDZ domain while the long isoform displays two domains for phos-phorylation by PKC and an endocytosis signal sequence [15].

The intracytoplasmic domain sequence is similar to mice and human at 95 and 93% for the short isoform and long isoform, respectively. This conservation across species is in accor-dance with the important functions carried by the intracytoplasmic domain of CD146.

Finally, a soluble CD146 isoform with a molecular mass around 100 kDa, was identified for the first time in 1998 [16]. This isoform is detectable in human plasma and serum [17] and is generated by a metalloprotease-dependant shedding of the extracellular domain of CD146. The use of nonspecific inhibitors of metalloproteinase (GM6001) inhibits the formation of soluble CD146 [18].

3. CD146 localization

All the data concerning the expression of the different isoforms of CD146 and their functions are summarized in **Figures 1** and **2**.

3.1. Localization in cancer cells

CD146 has been identified for the first time in melanoma where it plays an important role in disease progression. Thereafter, CD146 has been shown to be expressed in various cancers, such as pancreatic/breast/prostate/ovarian/lung/kidney cancers, osteosarcoma, Kaposi sarcoma, angiosarcoma, Schwann cell tumors, or leiomyosarcoma (**Figure 1**). The mechanism of this neo-expression is still largely unknown but, in prostate cancer, it was reported that high expression of CD146 resulted from hypermethylation at the promoter of the CD146 gene [19].

However, almost nothing is known on the differential expressions and localizations of the different isoforms of CD146 in these cells. A recent study has shown that many cancer cells expressing CD146 were able to secrete soluble CD146 through a metalloprotease-dependant shedding [20].

Tissue/Organs/Cell lines	CD146 isoform expression	Effects/roles	Pathology	References
Human endothelial cell and cell lines HUVEC/EPC	CD146	Interaction endothelial-stromal cells / angiogenesis	Tumor angiogenesis	22, 33, 37, 59, 64
	short CD146	Angiogenesis	nd	23, 39
	long CD146	Stabilization of new vascular structure	nd	23
	soluble CD146	Pro-angiogenic factor-chemotactic properties	nd	16,17, 33, 39, 41
Zebrafish endothelial cells	CD146	Involved in VEGF-a signalization / regulate blood flow rate and vessel lumen size	nd	33, 34
Central Nervous System	CD146	Increases neurite extension / involved in optic tectum process extension	nd	30, 31, 32, 55
Bone marrow stroma	CD146	Able to generate bone tissue and hematopoietic environment	nd	29
Mesenchymal cells	CD146	Increases differenciation capacity	nd	28
Intermediate trophoblast	CD146	Regulates embryon implantation	Obstetric complication	70, 71
	soluble CD146	Decreases EVT migration	Obstetric complication	72
Human B lymphocyte	CD146	Increases adhesion	Rheumatoid arthritis	25
Human T lymphocyte	CD146	Increases adhesion	Rheumatoid arthritis	25, 26, 34,36
	long CD146	Increases adhesion	nd	26
Human Natural Killer cells	CD146	Increases adhesion	Rheumatoid arthritis	25
Mesengial/tubular cells	CD146	Endocapillary proliferation/proteinuria/inflammatory syndrome	Nephropathy	73
	soluble CD146	Increased in blood patient with chronic renal failure	Type 2 diabetic nephropathy patient	74
Non Small Cell Lung Cancer	soluble CD146	Increases in plasma	Poor prognosis factor	51
Gastric cancer	CD146	Increases metastasis/EMT inducer	Cancer development	49
	soluble CD146	nd	nd	74
Breast cancer	CD146	Increased cell motility	Poor prognosis factor	46, 47, 48, 50
Osteosarcoma	CD146	Increases metastatic dissemination	Cancer development	44, 45
Ovarian cancer	CD146	Increases metastatic dissemination and cancer cell survival	Cancer development	43
Prostate cancer	CD146	Increases invasiveness and metastatic potential	Cancer development/poor prognosis marker	19, 42
	soluble CD146	nd	nd	74
Human melanoma cancer	CD146	Increases metastatic dissemination	Poor prognosis marker	8, 9, 10, 61, 62, 63
	soluble CD146	Increases tumor angiogenesis and cancer cell survival	nd	20
Murin melanoma cell line	CD146	Increases metastatic dissemination	nd	11
Suprabasal Keratinocyte	CD146	nd	Kaposi's sarcoma/acute chronic dermatitis	75

Figure 1. Summary table for the different isoforms of CD146 expressed in several organs and cells related to their functions, pathologies, and references associated.

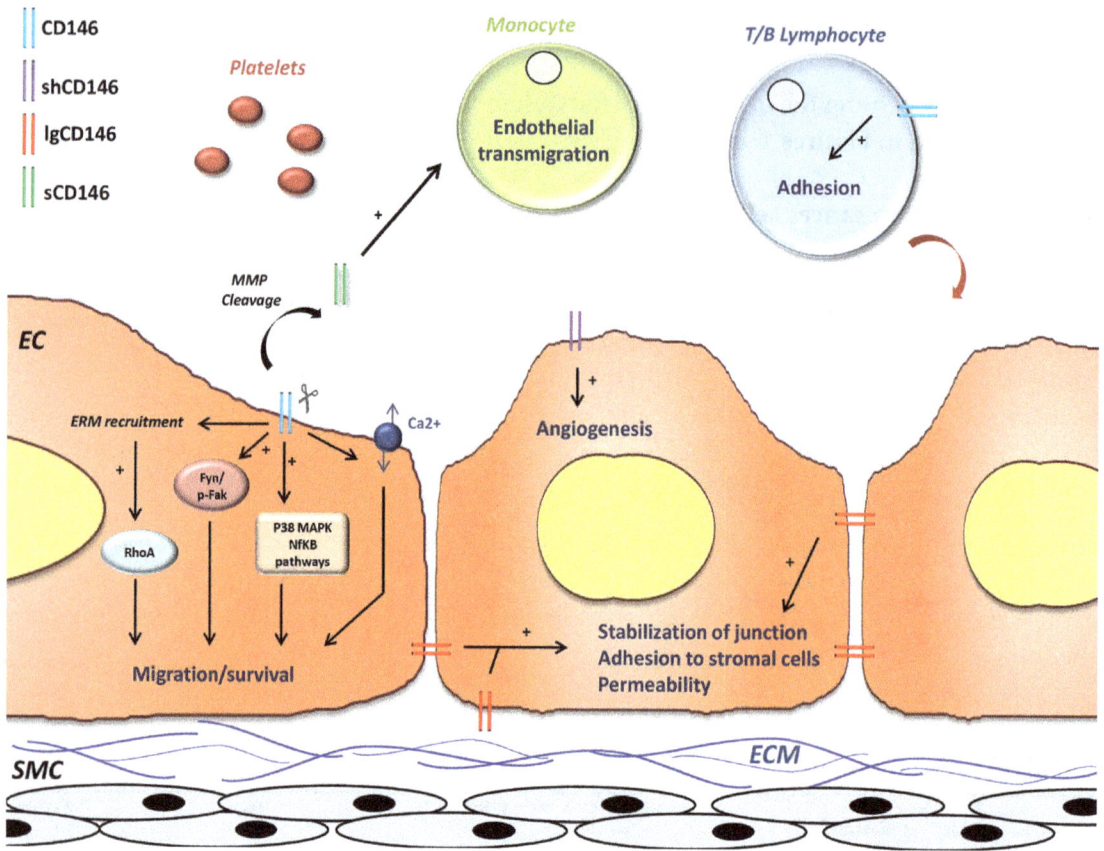

Figure 2. Expression, cell localization, and functions of the different isoforms of CD146 by endothelial cells (EC) and blood circulating cells.

3.2. Vascular localization

CD146 is expressed on the whole vascular tree whatever the vessel anatomical location and caliber. The localization of the long and short isoforms of CD146 is different. The induction of long CD146 expression in the CHO cell line (which does not constitutively express CD146) results in the expression of the protein at the intercellular junctions. Costaining of CD146 with VE-cadherin, focal adhesion kinase (FAK), PECAM, and the complex catenin/cadherin shows no colocalization, suggesting that CD146 is not located in the adherent junctions, tight junctions, or focal adhesions sites [21, 22].

Overexpression of the long form of CD146 in the MDCK cell line (Madin-Darby canine kidney) leads to a basolateral localization of the protein. A dileucine motif on its intracytoplasmic peptide sequence is necessary for this localization [21]. An immunohistochemical staining of long CD146 in endothelial colony-forming cells (ECFC) confirmed this junctional localization of the protein. In addition, the presence of a cytoplasmic pool of long CD146 that can be redistributed to the cell membrane was also described in Ref. [23].

The short isoform of CD146 does not share the same cellular localization. Transfection shows an apical localization of the protein in MDCK cells [21] that was confirmed in ECFC in a culture with a specific antibody generated against this isoform [23].

The confluence state of endothelial cells appears to regulate the spatial distribution of the two isoforms. Indeed, the long CD146 isoform was not detected at the junction in nonconfluent endothelial cells. Under this condition, the long CD146 isoform was intracytoplasmic and the short CD146 isoform was essentially nuclear and at the migration front [23]. In other experiments performed in chickens, it was shown a preferential localization of the long isoform of CD146 in the microvilli where the protein plays a role in their formation. Overexpression of CD146 increased the size of these microvilli [24].

3.3. Localization on immune cells

On peripheral blood of healthy patients approximately 1% of blood mononuclear cells express CD146. An analysis by flow cytometry of different lymphocyte populations showed an expression of CD146 on B and T lymphocytes in humans [25].

Research has shown that about 1% of B lymphocytes cells express CD146 and its expression is upregulated by a factor 5 following stimulation with IL-4 and CD40. Moreover, CD146 can be neo-expressed on some cell populations after stimulation [25]. The generation of two antibodies by rat immunization using cells from the T lymphocytic cell line HUT102 deepened these studies and shown that 2% of CD3+, CD3+/CD4+, and CD3+/CD8+ lymphocytes express CD146.

Moreover, stimulations with IL-2 [25] and PHA (phytohemagglutinin) [26] increases the amount of CD146+ T lymphocytes. The cells are also found *in vivo* in the synovial fluid of patients with rheumatoid arthritis [26].

In mice, a leucocytes screening was carried out which demonstrated that CD146 is not detectable on T/B lymphocyte populations, monocytes, and dendritic cells while 30% of neutrophils and 60% of NK cells express CD146. CD146 expression was correlated with an increased expression of CD11b and CD27 reflecting the maturity of NK. These CD146+ NK cells have a decreased cytotoxicity and produce gamma interferon in smaller quantities [27].

3.4. Bone marrow environment

In adults, hematopoiesis takes place in the bone marrow located in long bones of the human body. It is composed of a dense network of discontinuous capillaries allowing easy passage of cells produced in the bone marrow into the blood. A vascular sinus network which is mainly composed of stromal cells (reticular, endothelial, adipocyte, and osteoblast) serves to support the hematopoiesis process.

In one particular study, a subpopulation of bone marrow stroma cells was shown to express CD146 and to display characteristics of mural cells. They were characterized as a subpopulation of advential reticular cells which are abundant in the bone marrow and are able to generate bone tissue and a hematopoietic environment after isolation and implantation into an immunodeficient mouse [28].

Furthermore, angiopoietin -1 is regulated by CD146+ stromal cells. A decrease in the expression of CD146 by siRNA or FGF-2 (CD146 and Ang-1 regulator) reduces the capacity of these cells to participate in the remodeling and the assembly of pseudovascular structures *in vitro* and to form hematopoietic microenvironment *in vivo*. From data on the spatial location of adventitial reticular cells and the expression of Tie-2 (the angiopoietin-1 receptor), it was suggested that CD146 and angiopoietin-1 are involved in the interaction between endothelial and stromal cells [29].

3.5. Localization in the central nervous system (CNS)

CD146 is found in the central nervous system (CNS). It is expressed during fetal development of the embryo but decreases after birth. Studies performed in chickens and rats have shown an expression of CD146 in the cerebellum, hippocampus, Purkinje cells, and sensorimotor cells of the spinal cord [30]. In chickens, CD146 binds NOF (neurite outgrowth factor), causing neurite extension [31], and increases the extension of the optic tectum process [32].

4. The different functions of CD146

CD146 was reported to be involved in many physiological processes. It has been described to play a role during the vascular development but also during the angiogenic process. As others junction molecules, it was described to be an actor during inflammation by modulating the migration of leucocytes through vascular endothelium.

4.1. CD146 during the vascular development

The role of CD146 was studied during vascular development. To this end, a model of CD146 inactivation by antisense morpholino-oligonucleotides was developed in zebrafish. Authors observed a decrease in intersomitic vessels followed by a decrease in blood flow and a reduction in vessel lumen observed by microangiography after CD146 inactivation [33]. It was also shown an inhibition of the VEGF-dependent angiogenesis [34].

4.2. Permeability and leucocytes migration

CD146 has been shown to be involved in endothelial permeability [33]. Using both a monocyte cell line, THP-1, and freshly isolated monocytes, it was also showed that it modulates monocytes transmigration. Junctional CD146 was shown to bind monocytes through a heterophilic interaction to increase their transmigration. In addition, an increased transmigration was observed following the binding of soluble CD146 on monocytes [33]. Another study showed that neo-expression of CD146 on lymphocytes induced new cellular properties. Indeed, an increase in the adhesion of CD146+ T lymphocytes effectors was observed after stimulation with IL-1 beta. This effect was blocked by the addition of anti-CD146 blocking antibodies [34]. An increase in the adhesion of CD4+/CD146+ T lymphocytes on endothelium was also observed after an inflammatory stimulus. In this study, *in vitro* transfection of the long isoform of CD146 in NKL.1 cell line induced a reduction of rolling cells and an increased adhesion to the endothelial monolayer. Moreover, these phenomena were accompanied by an increase in microvilli in T lymphocyte cell membrane. Another study showed an increased permeability of HMVEC (human microvascular endothelial cells) following incubation with an anti-CD146 antibody (P1H12) [35]. Finally, CD146 is coexpressed with CCR6 on a population of TH17 lymphocytic cells [36].

4.3. Angiogenesis

Angiogenesis is an important mechanism, both in fetal life and at adulthood. Endothelial cells with angiogenic capacities are able to proliferate, migrate, adhere, and generate new capillaries from a preexisting one.

The injection of an anti-CD146 antibody (AA98) led to a decrease of 70% in the number of vessels in a membrane model, chorioallantoic membrane model, in chicken. Furthermore, in mice, this antibody reduced the number of vessels in different models of xenografted tumors (hepatocellular carcinoma, pancreatic, and leiomyosarcoma) [37], demonstrating a role of CD146 in tumor angiogenesis.

The recent discovery of the existence of two isoforms of CD146 and the description of a soluble form of CD146 led to study their implications in the angiogenic process. Specific siRNA directed against these two isoforms has shown that the absence of the short CD146 decreased the proliferation, migration, and adhesion of endothelial cells, whereas its overexpression led to the reverse phenomena. These experiments showed that the long CD146 was also necessary to generate pseudocapillaries in Matrigel *in vitro* by stabilizing the junctions of neovessels. It thus appears that both the short and long isoforms of CD146 display complementary effects to generate neovessels. The effects of the short CD146 were confirmed *in vivo* by the transplantation of endothelial colony-forming cells (ECFC) overexpressing this isoform in a mouse model of hind limb ischemia. Indeed, it increased the incorporation of ECFC in ischemic muscle and favored the generation of neovessels [23]. A study of the mechanism showed that the short CD146 is associated with VEGF-R2 [38], but also angiomotin and VEGF-R1 at the endothelial cell surface [39, 40]. This association is essential for these different pathways. Indeed, the absence of the short CD146 isoform decreases the phosphorylation of VEGF-R2 in endothelial cells and prevents the proangiogenic effect of vascular endothelial growth factor (VEGF).

Soluble CD146 is also able to increase the formation of pseudocapillaries *in vitro* and to induce neovascularization in a rat model of hindlimb ischemia. In addition, subcutaneous injection of Matrigel containing soluble CD146 in mice increased the recruitment of both mature and immature endothelial cells, as well as smooth muscle cells, resulting in the formation of capillary-like structures [41]. Of interest, it was reported that soluble CD146 stimulates the short CD146 isoform through its binding on angiomotin [39] and that the angiogenic properties of soluble CD146 are additive to those of VEGF [41]. The roles of the different forms of CD146 are summarized in **Figure 2**.

4.4. Cancer cell growth and dissemination

CD146, which is neo-expressed on cancer cells, modulates their growth and dissemination. In prostate cancer, CD146 expression was observed in different cell lines. CD146 overexpression increased their invasiveness and metastatic potential [42]. CD146 overexpression was also observed in biopsies of patients. Its expression was correlated with a poor prognosis. In ovarian carcinomas, CD146 expression was also correlated with the increase of the metastatic potential. In addition, inhibition of CD146 protein expression in ovarian cancer cell lines led to inhibition of invasiveness, tumor spread and induced cancer cell apoptosis. This was explained by the fact that a lack of CD146 induced a decreased activity of Rho GTPase [43] involved in the invasion, proliferation, and metastatic spread of cancer cells.

It was also demonstrated that CD146 expression is increased in osteosarcomas as compared to nonpathological osteoblasts [44]. Injection of antibodies against CD146 decreased the amount of lung metastases in an immunodeficient mouse model injected with cells derived from human osteosarcoma [45].

In breast cancer, it was reported that CD146 would act as a tumor suppressor [46] while other studies have described CD146 as a poor prognosis marker [47]. Indeed, CD146 overexpression in a breast cancer cell line induced an increased motility and tumorigenicity [48]. Recent studies have also shown that CD146 induces the epithelial-mesenchymal transition (EMT) in so far as its expression is correlated with markers of EMT in gastric cancer [49]. Moreover, in triple negative breast cancers, an increase of CD146 expression in epithelial cells correlates with a loss of epithelial markers in favor of mesenchymal markers, increasing their invasiveness, migration, and the number of mammospheres. In addition CD44 expression increases and CD24 expression decreases on the cell surface suggesting that cells acquire phenotypic characteristics of cancer stem cells [50].

At present, there is no data on the differential expression and roles of the two membrane isoforms of CD146 on cancer cells. However, recent studies have shown an important role of soluble CD146 in tumor development. First, an increase of soluble CD146 concentration was described in blood of cancer patients with nonsmall cell lung cancer as compared to patients with respiratory inflammatory disease and healthy subjects [51]. In this chapter, we showed that association between an increased soluble CD146 concentration and an increased number of circulating endothelial cells (CEC) constitute a poor prognostic factor [51].

Recently, a study showed that human cancer cells that express membrane CD146 on their surface have also the ability to secrete the soluble form of CD146 [20]. This was described in melanoma, colorectal and pancreatic cancer cell lines. The authors demonstrated that soluble CD146 secreted by cancer cells could display autocrine effects on cancer cells and paracrine effects on vascular endothelial cells. Indeed, *in vitro* stimulation of cancer cells with recombinant soluble CD146 increased their proliferation and the production of protumorigenic factor such as VEGF. They also demonstrated that this stimulation protected cancer cells from apoptosis induced by H_2O_2 and decreased cancer cell senescence. In particular, the c-myc signaling pathway appeared to be upregulated by soluble CD146. Soluble CD146 secreted by cancer cells also increased the proliferation of surrounding endothelial cells, stimulating tumor angiogenesis. These effects were confirmed *in vivo* in different models of xenografted mice and an antisoluble CD146 antibody was able to block these effects. Thus, soluble CD146 was described as a proangiogenic factor and seems to have a major role in tumor development.

5. Ligand and cell signalization

Historically, the first molecule interacting with the extracellular portion of CD146 is NOF (neurite outgrowth factor). A stable transfection of complementary DNA encoding for CD146 induces an adhesion of neuronal cells on a NOF matrix [32]. More recently, laminin-8 has been identified as a new vascular ligand of CD146 expressed by TH17 lymphocytes. In this study, it has been demonstrated that the laminin-411/CD146 interaction favor adhesion and tissue transmigration of these lymphocytes, leading to an increased inflammation [52]. Furthermore, one study showed that CD146 DNA transfection in the CD146-deficient melanoma cell line Mel-888 induced an increased aggregation between these cells and cells which do not express CD146 suggesting that there are other still unidentified partners [53].

The existence of a homophilic interaction for CD146 is controversial. One study showed that CD146 transfection in neuronal cells induced their aggregation, suggesting that CD146 could create homophilic bonds [32]. Another *in vitro* study demonstrated that the neurite growth of PC12 cells is increased when cells are in a chimeric CD146 protein substrate. In addition, under these conditions, the use of an anti-CD146 antibody blocks neurite growth. This inhibition would be associated with an inhibition of CD146-CD146 homophilic interaction [54]. CD146 dimerization at the cell membrane following stimulation with an activating CD146 antibody (clone AA98) was also demonstrated using fluorescence resonance energy transfer (FRET) and pull-down. The use of an NFkB signaling pathway inhibitor reduced this dimerization [55]. Finally, a recent study highlighted dimerization after stimulation with VEGF [56].

Conversely, other studies could not replicate the homophilic interaction, in particular, between soluble CD146 and CD146-Fc [33].

Recently, new ligands for CD146 were identified. A direct and strong interaction between CD146 and VEGFR-2 was demonstrated in endothelial cells and this association was important for VEGFR-2 phosphorylation by VEGF. These results were confirmed in a CD146 KO mouse model where the absence of CD146 inhibited vessel formation induced by VEGF. Experiments in mouse models of pancreas and melanoma cancer cell xenograft have shown that the combined use of anti-VEGF antibody (bevacizumab) and anti-CD146 antibody (AA98) displayed a synergistic effect on tumor development [57].

Another work identified galectin 1 as a new CD146 ligand on the endothelium [58]. This protein induced apoptosis of endothelial cells and specifically bound to CD146 via extracellular glycosylations. This interaction is specific for galectin 1 since it is not found with galectin 2. Using siRNA or antibodies able to block CD146 resulted in an increased cell apoptosis, suggesting a protective role of CD146 against apoptosis.

Different factors have been shown to modulate CD146 expression:

- A stimulation with TNF-alpha increases the amount of CD146 present at the endothelial cell surface [33].

- TGF-beta administered to hepatocyte cells pretreated with an inducer of acute hepatitis (tetrachloride carbonate) increases the amount of CD146 mRNA and the regenerative capacity of these cells [59].

- HSP27 (heat shock protein 27), a chaperone molecule involved mainly in tumor differentiation and tumorigenesis, inhibits the migration and invasion of melanoma cells and thus acts on the tumor phenotype [60]. Overexpression of HSP27 has been shown to decrease the expression of CD146 and increase the expression of E-cadherin in melanoma cell lines. These variations in protein expression determine, among other, malignant phenotype of melanoma cells [61].

- AKT activation by PD98059 and Wortmannin increases CD146 expression at the cell membrane in melanoma cell lines. Conversely in these cell lines, overexpression of CD146 increases AKT which inhibits BAD (Bcl-2-associated death promoter), increasing cell survival [62].

Membrane CD146 activates multiple signaling pathways, leading to the activation of the NFkB pathway. CD146 dimerization has been described in the membrane of endothelial cells following the addition of culture medium of tumor cells (A375 cell line). Inhibition of the NFkB pathway (by BAY11-7082 compound) causes a reduction of the nuclear translocation of NFKB but also inhibits the dimerization of CD146 [63, 64]. The junctional molecules involved in adhesion such as VE-cadherin or claudins are also involved in a phenomenon of actin cytoskeleton reorganization. CD146 is also connected to the actin cytoskeleton.

Indeed, CD146 targeting with the S-ENDO1 antibody led to FAK phosphorylation and an increase in the release of intracellular calcium and extracellular calcium entry. This mechanism of action of calcium flux was mediated by the recruitment and activation of Fyn leading to the phosphorylation of PLC gamma. Calcium entry also caused the recruitment of PYK2 and p130. On the other hand, FAK activation led to signaling pathways involved in the reorganization of the actin cytoskeleton and also modulated transcription factors involved in cells survival and migration. In these studies, there was no evidence of direct interaction between CD146, paxillin, and FAK. It seems therefore important to identify the intermediate partners [65, 66].

Recently, a study confirmed the role of CD146 in the migration and induction of signals related to the actin cytoskeleton. Indeed, CD146 displays direct physical interaction with the ezrin-radixin-moesin (ERM) proteins, allowing the recruitment of ERM at the protrusions of melanoma cells. This phenomenon induces the elongation and expansion of microvilli at these protrusions [67].

Recruitment by CD146 allows the sequestration of a RhoA inhibitor (Rho guanine nucleotide dissociation inhibitory factor 1) leading to RhoA activation and an increased cell motility. Another study showed that CD146 is redistributed in a polarized structure named W-RAMP (Wnt5a-mediated actin-myosin receptor-polarity) in subconfluent melanoma cells stimulated with Wnt5a. W-RAMP is involved in membrane retraction and the direction of cell migration with an intervention of Rho-A [68].

In another study that focused on the priming of ECFC with soluble CD146 in order to improve the therapeutic potential of these cells *in vivo*, the authors showed that a priming of these cells

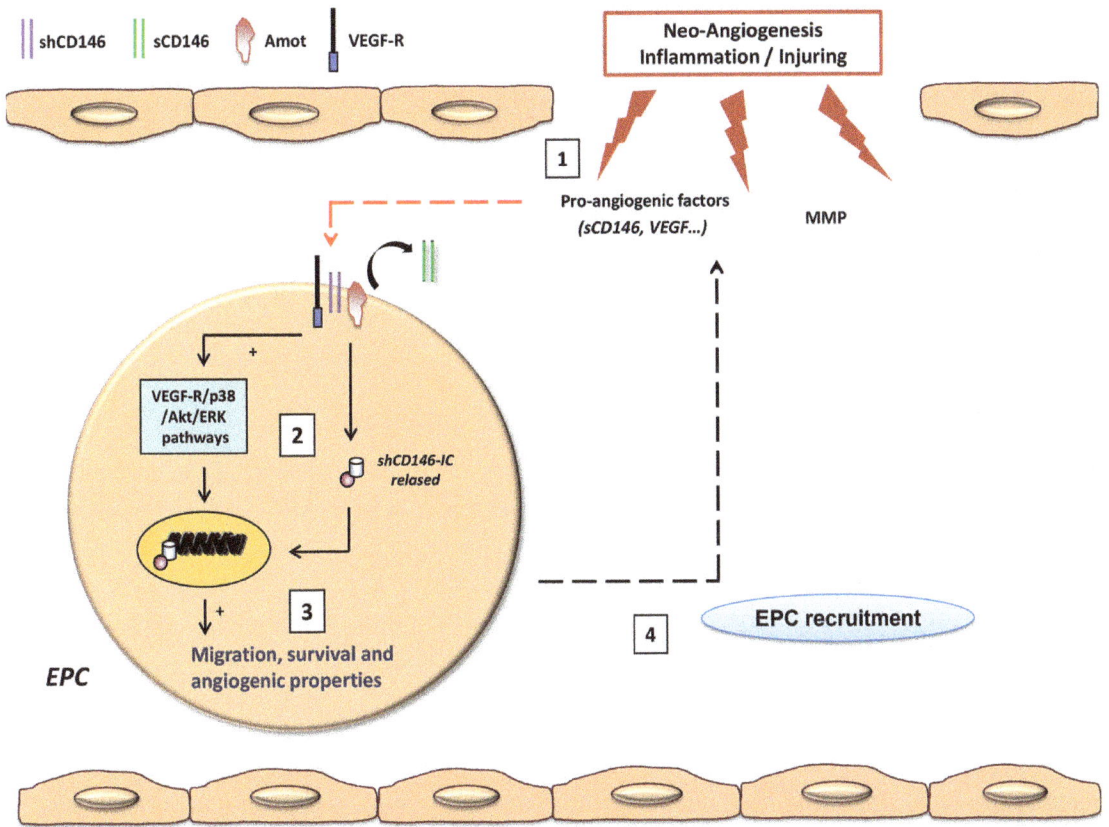

Figure 3. Mechanism of actions of endothelial progenitor cells (EPC) activation leads to their recruitment after inflammatory or angiogenic stimulation.

with soluble CD146 did not modify the number of engrafted ECFC in the ischemic muscle but improved their survival capacity leading to an enhanced revascularization [39]. They showed that in ECFC, it exists a signalosome that is located in a particular region of cell membrane called lipid rafts. This signalosome contains soluble CD146, the short isoform of CD146 (shCD146), presenilin-1 but also the two VEGF receptor called flt1 and flk1. The mechanism of action is characterized by a sequential proteolytic cleavage, induced by soluble CD146, with an extracellular shedding of the short CD146 followed by an intramembrane cleavage which is mediated by both the ADAM/matrix metalloproteases (MMP) and the gamma-secretase protein. The consequences of this shedding involved a nuclear translocation of the new intracellular peptide of shCD146 which binds to the transcription factor CSL and is associated with a modulation of gene transcription leading to angiogenesis (eNOS) and cell survival (FADD, Bcl-xl). The association between CD146 and VEGFR2 was described in a previous paper and based on these results the authors showed that the effect of soluble CD146 on EFCF is dependent on VEGFR2 but also VEGFR1 which are phosphorylated by soluble CD146. All these findings show that the stimulation of this cell by soluble CD146 and the proteolytic cleavage of shCD146 is a promising pathway to increase the regenerative properties of endothelial progenitor cells for the treatment of cardiovascular diseases (**Figure 3**).

6. CD146 in pathology

6.1. Obstetrical pathologies

About 2% of fertile women are affected by spontaneous fetal loss. The mechanism of this fetal loss is not yet understood.

One study showed that CD146 is highly expressed during the implantation window. During the following steps, the level of CD146 decreased rapidly and CD146 blocking with an antibody caused abortion [69]. CD146 is expressed by the intermediate trophoblasts (or extravillous) in humans but is not detected on the syncytiotrophoblasts and cytotrophoblasts [70].

After this work, soluble CD146 was described as a novel physiological factor with angiogenic properties involved in the regulation of placenta vascular development by acting on extravillous trophoblast (EVT). Using placenta explants, soluble CD146 was demonstrated to inhibit the growth of extravillous trophoblasts and the ability of EVT to migrate and form pseudocapillary tubes on Matrigel. A clinical study on the role of soluble CD146 in 50 pregnant women was also conducted. A physiological decrease of plasmatic soluble CD146 was observed in pregnant women as compared to nongestational women. These results inspired the authors to study the effects of prolonged administration of soluble CD146 in a pregnant rat model. Repeated systemic injection of soluble CD146 after mating caused a significant decrease in the pregnancy rate and the number of embryos. Histological studies of placenta showed a decreased migration of glycogen cells (cells that are similar to the EVT in rat) in female rat treated with soluble CD146.

In mice the use of a specific antibody blocking CD146 (AA98) caused a decrease in the blastocysts adhesion on a uterine epithelium cell monolayer and a decrease in the growth of trophoblastic cells. In addition, injection of this antibody in the uterine horn of the mouse at 3.5 dpc (days post coitum) resulted in a decrease of embryo implantation at 7.5 dpc. Histological analysis showed that the embryos were present but smaller and in poor condition [69]. Two clinical studies were in line with these observations. A first clinical study showed that the rate of membrane CD146 expression was lower on intermediate trophoblasts in the placenta of preeclamptic patients when compared to patients with nonpathological pregnancies [70]. In a second study, two populations of women have been used to compare the blood level of soluble CD146. In this study, the authors used 100 blood samples which were taken 2 months after the last obstetrical events between women with no pregnancy lost which have at least one living child and 100 blood samples from women with at least two consecutive losses at/ or before 21 weeks of gestation. They found an increase in the level of soluble CD146 in the second population compared to the first control population [71]. In this study, the two populations used are age matched.

Thus, in view of these results soluble CD146 may represent an attractive biomarker of vascular placental development as well as a therapeutic target in obstetric complications.

6.2. Inflammatory diseases

Endothelial functions are altered in inflammatory diseases.

In inflammatory kidney disease, biopsies of patients with nephropathy show an increased expression of membrane CD146 on endothelial cells, but also on the mesangial cells and a neo-expression of CD146 on tubular cells [72]. In addition, there is a correlation between CD146 expression and proteinuria, endocapillary proliferation and inflammatory syndrome. The serum level of soluble CD146 is also modulated. Thus, an increase in CD146 secretion was observed in chronic renal failure which was correlated with the severity of this disease in type 2 diabetic nephropathy patients [73].

In a second type of inflammatory disease, CD146 has also been identified in primary cultures of keratinocytes while its expression was not observed on healthy skin. An increase in the expression of CD146 has been observed in various skin diseases. For example, CD146 is expressed in suprabasals keratinocytes of psoriasis patients [74]. CD146 is also detected in Kaposi's sarcoma, lichen planus, on the skin overlying skin neoplasms or in chronic and acute chronic dermatitis [74]. On the other hand, the expression of CD146 is not increased in other skin diseases such as lupus erythematosus.

6.3. Tumor pathologies

CD146 is expressed in many cancers, such as melanoma, prostate cancer, breast cancer, pancreatic cancer, lung cancer, Kaposi sarcoma, angiosarcoma, Schwann cells tumors, or leiomyosarcoma.

The role of tumor CD146 was first studied in melanoma. A direct correlation has been demonstrated between the increase in metastasizing capacities and the increased expression of CD146 [75]. The level of expression of CD146 by human melanoma cell lines has been shown to correlate with their ability to form tumors and metastasis in a mouse xenograft model in immunodeficient nude or SCID mice [76]. In addition, CD146 increases the number of lung metastases following intravenous injection of melanoma cells in nude mice *in vivo* [77]. These observations were confirmed through the use of interfering RNA directed against CD146 leading to a decrease in migration, proliferation, and invasion *in vitro* [78].

CD146 immunohistochemistry staining was performed on human primary melanoma tissue, showing a CD146 expression on tumor-associated endothelium and on smooth muscle cells [79]. The role of CD146 in tumor angiogenesis has been described in particular thanks to the use of the AA98 antibody [37, 64] that is able to block tumor angiogenesis and decrease tumor growth of human melanoma xenograft model in immunodeficient mice.

Currently, mechanisms involved in melanoma progression are unclear. A study showed that a particular population of B lymphocyte cells, the B1 lymphocytes, has a prometastatic potential. Indeed, depletion of this population caused a decrease of tumor growth and metastasis dissemination in mice in an experimental metastasis model, following a B16 cell line injection. The decrease in metastases dissemination involved homophilic interactions between B1 and B16 cells thanks to CD146 [80]. In addition, coculture of B1 cells with melanoma cells increased the expression of CD146 at the cell membrane of cancer cells, increasing the number of metastases *in vivo*.

A clinical study was conducted on a cohort of patients with skin cancer. Patients were divided into two groups: early and late stage melanoma, in order to analyze the presence of different commonly used cancer markers including CD146. Analysis in the blood of patients showed that CD146 was the only protein correlated with the advanced stages of the disease [81]. Another study confirmed this finding by demonstrating that CD146 is a marker of poor prognosis and survival in melanoma patients. CD146 constitutes a better marker than biopsies analysis of sentinel lymph node [82].

6.4. Angiogenesis-related diseases and therapeutic approaches

Recent studies revealed that both isoforms of CD146 are involved in angiogenesis with a pro-migratory and a proproliferative role of the short CD146 and a vessel stabilization role of long CD146, which is also described in this chapter. Soluble CD146 secreted by both endothelial and cancer cells is also able to stimulate angiogenesis. These different forms are involved in physiological angiogenesis but also in pathological angiogenesis, in particular in tumor angiogenesis.

Therefore, different antibodies have been generated to block its functions. The first one was ABX-MA1, an antibody recognizing the human form of this molecule. This antibody was able to inhibit the formation of spheroids containing melanoma cells, reducing metastasis, tumorigenicity, and vascularization of the tumor *in vivo*. This reduction was related to the inhibition of MMP-2 expression which is heavily involved in metastasis formation [83].

Another team-generated monoclonal antibody specifically directed against the vascular endothelium of tumors. During the screening of these antibodies, the authors focused on the AA98 antibody. This antibody recognizes CD146 localized in the intratumoral vasculature but not recognizes CD146 expressed on blood vessels in healthy tissues [37]. This antibody inhibits both *in vitro* and *in vivo* angiogenic properties of CD146 in human tumors xenografted in immunodeficient mice. In addition, it was demonstrated that the AA98 antibody is a potential diagnostic and therapeutic agent in vascular and cancer diseases. Following this work, it was shown that AA98 antibody inhibits phosphorylation of p38/MAPK, suppresses NFkB activation, and inhibits MMP-9 and ICAM-1 expression. This suggests that deleting NFkB is a pivotal point of the inhibitory effects of the antibody on endothelial cell migration, angiogenesis, and development of tumor metastases [64].

Of interest, this antibody displays additive inhibitory effects when used in combination with the anti-VEGF antibody bevacizumab in xenografted models of human pancreatic tumors and melanoma [57]. In addition, it reduces significantly the chronic inflammation in the colon in a mouse model and prevents the development of cancer associated with this chronic inflammation [38].

Recently, a novel antibody was generated against the soluble form of CD146 [20]. The authors demonstrated that this antibody was able to decrease tumor angiogenesis and growth but to also induce apoptosis of human melanoma and pancreatic tumors xenografted in immunodeficient mice. Of interest, this antibody cannot bind membrane CD146, a property that should limit the side effects that could be observed with antibodies targeting the membrane form.

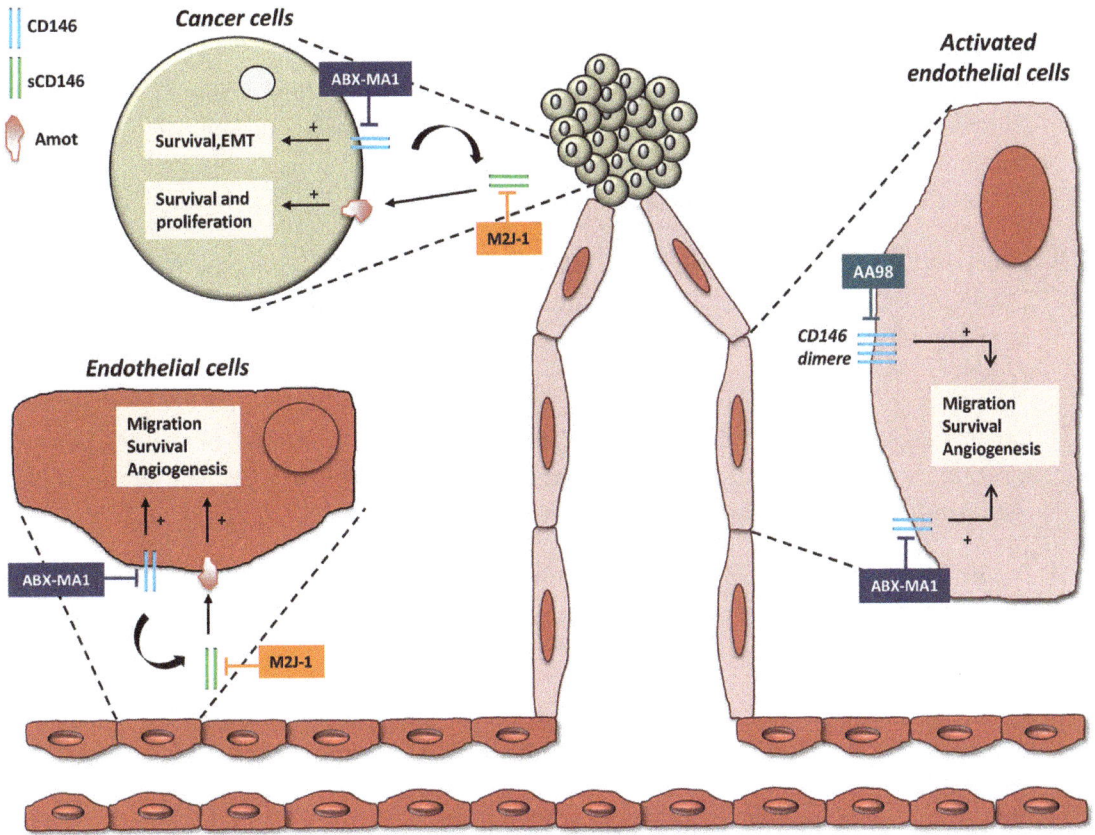

Figure 4. Functions of the different isoforms of CD146 and the inhibitory antibodies associated during tumor growth and angiogenesis.

Functions of the different CD146 isoforms and the inhibitory antibodies associated are summarized in **Figure 4**.

Author details

Jimmy Stalin[1]*, Lucie Vivancos[2], Nathalie Bardin[3], Françoise Dignat-George[3] and Marcel Blot-Chabaud[3]

*Address all correspondence to: jimmy.stalin@unige.ch

1 Department of Pathology and Immunology, University Medical Center, Geneva University, Switzerland

2 Pediatric Hematology-Oncology Research Laboratory, Pediatric Division, University Hospital CHUV, Lausanne, Switzerland

3 INSERM UMR-S 1076, Aix-Marseille University, UFR Pharmacy, Marseille, France

References

[1] Lehmann JM, Holzmann B, Breitbart EW, Schmiegelow P, Riethmüller G, Johnson JP. Discrimination between benign and malignant cells of melanocytic lineage by two novel antigens, a glycoprotein with a molecular weight of 113,000 and a protein with a molecular weight of 76,000. Cancer Res. 1987 Feb 1;47(3):841–845.

[2] George F, Poncelet P, Laurent JC, Massot O, Arnoux D, Lequeux N, Ambrosi P, Chicheportiche C, Sampol J. Cytofluorometric detection of human endothelial cells in whole blood using S-Endo 1 monoclonal antibody. J Immunol Methods. 1991 May 17;139(1):65–75.

[3] Bardin N, George F, Mutin M, Brisson C, Horschowski N, Francés V, Lesaule G, Sampol J. S-Endo 1, a pan-endothelial monoclonal antibody recognizing a novel human endothelial antigen. Tissue Antigens. 1996 Nov;48(5):531–539.

[4] Bardin N, Francès V, Lesaule G, Horschowski N, George F, Sampol J. Identification of the S-Endo 1 endothelial-associated antigen. Biochem Biophys Res Commun. 1996 Jan 5;218(1):210–216.

[5] Vainio O, Dunon D, Aïssi F, Dangy JP, McNagny KM, Imhof BA. HEMCAM, an adhesion molecule expressed by c-kit+ hemopoietic progenitors. J Cell Biol. 1996 Dec;135(6 Pt 1):1655–1668.

[6] Sers C, Kirsch K, Rothbächer U, Riethmüller G, Johnson JP. Genomic organization of the melanoma-associated glycoprotein MUC18: implications for the evolution of the immunoglobulin domains. Proc Natl Acad Sci U S A. 1993 Sep 15;90(18):8514–8518.

[7] Mintz-Weber CS, Johnson JP. Identification of the elements regulating the expression of the cell adhesion molecule MCAM/MUC18. Loss of AP-2 is not required for MCAM expression in melanoma cell lines. J Biol Chem. 2000 Nov 3;275(44):34672–34680.

[8] Jean D, Gershenwald JE, Huang S, Luca M, Hudson MJ, Tainsky MA, Bar-Eli M. Loss of AP-2 results in up-regulation of MCAM/MUC18 and an increase in tumor growth and metastasis of human melanoma cells. J Biol Chem. 1998 Jun 26;273(26):16501–16508.

[9] Xie S, Price JE, Luca M, Jean D, Ronai Z, Bar-Eli M. Dominant-negative CREB inhibits tumor growth and metastasis of human melanoma cells. Oncogene. 1997 Oct 23;15(17):2069–2075.

[10] Lehmann JM, Riethmüller G, Johnson JP. MUC18, a marker of tumor progression in human melanoma, shows sequence similarity to the neural cell adhesion molecules of the immunoglobulin superfamily. Proc Natl Acad Sci U S A. 1989 Dec;86(24):9891–9895.

[11] Yang H, Wang S, Liu Z, Wu MH, McAlpine B, Ansel J, Armstrong C, Wu G. Isolation and characterization of mouse MUC18 cDNA gene, and correlation of MUC18 expression in mouse melanoma cell lines with metastatic ability. Gene. 2001 Mar 7;265(1–2):133–145.

[12] Schön M1, Kähne T, Gollnick H, Schön MP. Expression of gp130 in tumors and inflammatory disorders of the skin: formal proof of its identity as CD146 (MUC18, Mel-CAM). J Invest Dermatol. 2005 Aug;125(2):353–363.

[13] Ihnen M, Kilic E, Köhler N, Löning T, Witzel I, Hagel C, Höller S, Kersten JF, Müller V, Jänicke F, Milde-Langosch K. Protein expression analysis of ALCAM and CEACAM6 in breast cancer metastases reveals significantly increased ALCAM expression in metastases of the skin. J Clin Pathol. 2011 Feb;64(2):146–152. doi: 10.1136/jcp.2010.082602.

[14] Kijima N, Hosen N, Kagawa N, Hashimoto N, Nakano A, Fujimoto Y, Kinoshita M, Sugiyama H, Yoshimine T. CD166/activated leukocyte cell adhesion molecule is expressed on glioblastoma progenitor cells and involved in the regulation of tumor cell invasion. Neuro Oncol. 2012 Oct;14(10):1254–1264.

[15] Taira E, Nagino T, Taniura H, Takaha N, Kim CH, Kuo CH, Li BS, Higuchi H, Miki N. Expression and functional analysis of a novel isoform of gicerin, an immunoglobulin superfamily cell adhesion molecule. J Biol Chem. 1995 Dec 1;270(48):28681–28687.

[16] Bardin N, Francès V, Combes V, Sampol J, Dignat-George F. CD146: biosynthesis and production of a soluble form in human cultured endothelial cells. FEBS Lett. 1998 Jan 2;421(1):12–14.

[17] Bardin N1, Moal V, Anfosso F, Daniel L, Brunet P, Sampol J, Dignat George F. Soluble CD146, a novel endothelial marker, is increased in physiopathological settings linked to endothelial junctional alteration. Thromb Haemost. 2003 Nov;90(5):915–920.

[18] Boneberg EM, Illges H, Legler DF, Fürstenberger G. Soluble CD146 is generated by ectodomain shedding of membrane CD146 in a calcium-induced, matrix metalloprotease-dependent process. Microvasc Res. 2009 Dec;78(3):325–331. doi: 10.1016/j.mvr.2009.06.012.

[19] Liu JW, Nagpal JK, Jeronimo C, Lee JE, Henrique R, Kim MS, Ostrow KL, Yamashita K, van Criekinge V, Wu G, Moon CS, Trink B, Sidransky D. Hypermethylation of MCAM gene is associated with advanced tumor stage in prostate cancer. Prostate. 2008 Mar 1;68(4):418–426. doi: 10.1002/pros.20709.

[20] Stalin J, Nollet M, Garigue P, Fernandez S, Vivancos L, Essaadi A, Muller A, Bachelier R, Foucault-Bertaud A, Fugazza L, Leroyer AS, Bardin N, Guillet B, Dignat-George F, Blot-Chabaud M. Targeting soluble CD146 with a neutralizing antibody inhibits vascularization, growth and survival of CD146-positive tumors. Oncogene. 2016 Apr 11. doi: 10.1038/onc.2016.83.

[21] Guezguez B1, Vigneron P, Alais S, Jaffredo T, Gavard J, Mège RM, Dunon D. A dileucine motif targets MCAM-l cell adhesion molecule to the basolateral membrane in MDCK cells. FEBS Lett. 2006 Jun 26;580(15):3649–3656. Epub 2006 Jun 2.

[22] Bardin N1, Anfosso F, Massé JM, Cramer E, Sabatier F, Le Bivic A, Sampol J, Dignat-George F. Identification of CD146 as a component of the endothelial junction involved in the control of cell-cell cohesion. Blood. 2001 Dec 15;98(13):3677–3684.

[23] Kebir A, Harhouri K, Guillet B, Liu JW, Foucault-Bertaud A, Lamy E, Kaspi E, Elganfoud N, Vely F, Sabatier F, Sampol J, Pisano P, Kruithof EK, Bardin N, Dignat-George F, Blot-Chabaud M. CD146 short isoform increases the proangiogenic potential of endothelial progenitor cells *in vitro* and *in vivo*. Circ Res. 2010 Jul 9;107(1):66–75. doi: 10.1161/CIRCRESAHA.109.213827.

[24] Okumura S, Muraoka O, Tsukamoto Y, Tanaka H, Kohama K, Miki N, Taira E. Involvement of gicerin in the extension of microvilli. Exp Cell Res. 2001 Dec 10;271(2):269–276.

[25] Elshal MF, Khan SS, Takahashi Y, Solomon MA, McCoy JP Jr. CD146 (Mel-CAM), an adhesion marker of endothelial cells, is a novel marker of lymphocyte subset activation in normal peripheral blood. Blood. 2005 Oct 15;106(8):2923–2924.

[26] Pickl WF1, Majdic O, Fischer GF, Petzelbauer P, Faé I, Waclavicek M, Stöckl J, Scheinecker C, Vidicki T, Aschauer H, Johnson JP, Knapp W. MUC18/MCAM (CD146), an activation antigen of human T lymphocytes. J Immunol. 1997 Mar 1;158(5):2107–2115.

[27] Despoix N1, Walzer T, Jouve N, Blot-Chabaud M, Bardin N, Paul P, Lyonnet L, Vivier E, Dignat-George F, Vély F. Mouse CD146/MCAM is a marker of natural killer cell maturation. Eur J Immunol. 2008 Oct;38(10):2855–2864. doi: 10.1002/eji.200838469.

[28] Sorrentino A, Ferracin M, Castelli G, Biffoni M, Tomaselli G, Baiocchi M, Fatica A, Negrini M, Peschle C, Valtieri M. Isolation and characterization of CD146+ multipotent mesenchymal stromal cells. Exp Hematol. 2008 Aug;36(8):1035–1046. doi: 10.1016/j.exphem.2008.03.004.

[29] Sacchetti B1, Funari A, Michienzi S, Di Cesare S, Piersanti S, Saggio I, Tagliafico E, Ferrari S, Robey PG, Riminucci M, Bianco P. Self-renewing osteoprogenitors in bone marrow sinusoids can organize a hematopoietic microenvironment. Cell. 2007 Oct 19;131(2):324–336.

[30] Taira E1, Kohama K, Tsukamoto Y, Okumura S, Miki N. Characterization of Gicerin/MUC18/CD146 in the rat nervous system. J Cell Physiol. 2004 Mar;198(3):377–387.

[31] Taira E1, Takaha N, Taniura H, Kim CH, Miki N. Molecular cloning and functional expression of gicerin, a novel cell adhesion molecule that binds to neurite outgrowth factor. Neuron. 1994 Apr;12(4):861–872.

[32] Taira E1, Tsukamoto Y, Kohama K, Maeda M, Kiyama H, Miki N. Expression and involvement of gicerin, a cell adhesion molecule, in the development of chick optic tectum. J Neurochem. 2004 Feb;88(4):891–899.

[33] Bardin N1, Blot-Chabaud M, Despoix N, Kebir A, Harhouri K, Arsanto JP, Espinosa L, Perrin P, Robert S, Vely F, Sabatier F, Le Bivic A, Kaplanski G, Sampol J, Dignat-George F. CD146 and its soluble form regulate monocyte transendothelial migration. Arterioscler Thromb Vasc Biol. 2009 May;29(5):746–753. doi: 10.1161/ATVBAHA.108.183251.

[34] Elshal MF1, Khan SS, Raghavachari N, Takahashi Y, Barb J, Bailey JJ, Munson PJ, Solomon MA, Danner RL, McCoy JP Jr. A unique population of effector memory lymphocytes

identified by CD146 having a distinct immunophenotypic and genomic profile. BMC Immunol. 2007 Nov 13;8:29.

[35] Solovey AN1, Gui L, Chang L, Enenstein J, Browne PV, Hebbel RP. Identification and functional assessment of endothelial P1H12. J Lab Clin Med. 2001 Nov;138(5):322–331.

[36] Kamiyama T1, Watanabe H, Iijima M, Miyazaki A, Iwamoto S. Coexpression of CCR6 and CD146 (MCAM) is a marker of effector memory T-helper 17 cells. J Dermatol. 2012 Oct;39(10):838–842. doi: 10.1111/j.1346-8138.2012.01544.x.

[37] Yan X1, Lin Y, Yang D, Shen Y, Yuan M, Zhang Z, Li P, Xia H, Li L, Luo D, Liu Q, Mann K, Bader BL. A novel anti-CD146 monoclonal antibody, AA98, inhibits angiogenesis and tumor growth. Blood. 2003 Jul 1;102(1):184–191.

[38] Wellbrock J1, Fiedler W. CD146: a new partner for VEGFR2. Blood. 2012 Sep 13;120(11):2164–2165. doi: 10.1182/blood-2012-07-439646.

[39] Stalin J1, Harhouri K1, Hubert L1, Garrigue P2, Nollet M1, Essaadi A1, Muller A1, Foucault-Bertaud A1, Bachelier R1, Sabatier F3, Pisano P1, Peiretti F4, Leroyer AS1, Guillet B2, Bardin N1, Dignat-George F1, Blot-Chabaud M5. Soluble CD146 boosts therapeutic effect of endothelial progenitors through proteolytic processing of short CD146 isoform. Cardiovasc Res. 2016 Aug 1;111(3):240–251. doi: 10.1093/cvr/cvw096.

[40] Stalin J1, Harhouri K, Hubert L, Subrini C, Lafitte D, Lissitzky JC, Elganfoud N, Robert S, Foucault-Bertaud A, Kaspi E, Sabatier F, Aurrand-Lions M, Bardin N, Holmgren L, Dignat-George F, Blot-Chabaud M. Soluble melanoma cell adhesion molecule (sMCAM/sCD146) promotes angiogenic effects on endothelial progenitor cells through angiomotin. J Biol Chem. 2013 Mar 29;288(13):8991–9000. doi: 10.1074/jbc.M112.446518.

[41] Harhouri K1, Kebir A, Guillet B, Foucault-Bertaud A, Voytenko S, Piercecchi-Marti MD, Berenguer C, Lamy E, Vely F, Pisano P, Ouafik L, Sabatier F, Sampol J, Bardin N, Dignat-George F, Blot-Chabaud M. Soluble CD146 displays angiogenic properties and promotes neovascularization in experimental hind-limb ischemia. Blood. 2010 May 6;115(18):3843–3851. doi: 10.1182/blood-2009-06-229591.

[42] Wu GJ1, Peng Q, Fu P, Wang SW, Chiang CF, Dillehay DL, Wu MW. Ectopical expression of human MUC18 increases metastasis of human prostate cancer cells. Gene. 2004 Mar 3;327(2):201–213.

[43] Wu Z1, Wu Z, Li J, Yang X, Wang Y, Yu Y, Ye J, Xu C, Qin W, Zhang Z. MCAM is a novel metastasis marker and regulates spreading, apoptosis and invasion of ovarian cancer cells. Tumour Biol. 2012 Oct;33(5):1619–1628. doi: 10.1007/s13277-012-0417-0.

[44] Schiano C1, Grimaldi V, Casamassimi A, Infante T, Esposito A, Giovane A, Napoli C. Different expression of CD146 in human normal and osteosarcoma cell lines. Med Oncol. 2012 Dec;29(4):2998–3002. doi: 10.1007/s12032-012-0158-3.

[45] McGary EC1, Heimberger A, Mills L, Weber K, Thomas GW, Shtivelband M, Lev DC, Bar-Eli M. A fully human antimelanoma cellular adhesion molecule/MUC18 antibody

inhibits spontaneous pulmonary metastasis of osteosarcoma cells in vivo. Clin Cancer Res. 2003 Dec 15;9(17):6560–6566.

[46] Shih LM1, Hsu MY, Palazzo JP, Herlyn M. The cell-cell adhesion receptor Mel-CAM acts as a tumor suppressor in breast carcinoma. Am J Pathol. 1997 Sep;151(3):745–751.

[47] Zabouo G, Imbert AM, Jacquemier J, Finetti P, Moreau T, Esterni B, Birnbaum D, Bertucci F, Chabannon C. CD146 expression is associated with a poor prognosis in human breast tumors and with enhanced motility in breast cancer cell lines. Breast Cancer Res. 2009;11(1):R1. doi: 10.1186/bcr2215.

[48] Zeng G1, Cai S, Liu Y, Wu GJ. METCAM/MUC18 augments migration, invasion, and tumorigenicity of human breast cancer SK-BR-3 cells. Gene. 2012 Jan 15;492(1):229–238. doi: 10.1016/j.gene.2011.10.024.

[49] Liu WF1, Ji SR, Sun JJ, Zhang Y, Liu ZY, Liang AB, Zeng HZ. CD146 expression correlates with epithelial-mesenchymal transition markers and a poor prognosis in gastric cancer. Int J Mol Sci. 2012;13(5):6399–6406. doi: 10.3390/ijms13056399.

[50] Zeng Q, Li W, Lu D, Wu Z, Duan H, Luo Y, Feng J, Yang D, Fu L, Yan X. CD146, an epithelial-mesenchymal transition inducer, is associated with triple-negative breast cancer. Proc Natl Acad Sci U S A. 2012 Jan 24;109(4):1127–1132. doi: 10.1073/pnas.1111053108.

[51] Ilie M1, Long E1, Hofman V2, Selva E3, Bonnetaud C3, Boyer J4, Vénissac N5, Sanfiorenzo C6, Ferrua B7, Marquette CH6, Mouroux J5, Hofman P2. Clinical value of circulating endothelial cells and of soluble CD146 levels in patients undergoing surgery for non-small cell lung cancer. Br J Cancer. 2014 Mar 4;110(5):1236–1243. doi: 10.1038/bjc.2014.11.

[52] Flanagan K1, Fitzgerald K, Baker J, Regnstrom K, Gardai S, Bard F, Mocci S, Seto P, You M, Larochelle C, Prat A, Chow S, Li L, Vandevert C, Zago W, Lorenzana C, Nishioka C, Hoffman J, Botelho R, Willits C, Tanaka K, Johnston J, Yednock T. Laminin-411 is a vascular ligand for MCAM and facilitates TH17 cell entry into the CNS. PLoS One. 2012;7(7):e40443. doi: 10.1371/journal.pone.0040443.

[53] Johnson JP1, Bar-Eli M, Jansen B, Markhof E. Melanoma progression-associated glyco-protein MUC18/MCAM mediates homotypic cell adhesion through interaction with a heterophilic ligand. Int J Cancer. 1997 Nov 27;73(5):769–774.

[54] Taira E1, Kohama K, Tsukamoto Y, Okumura S, Miki N. Gicerin/CD146 is involved in neurite extension of NGF-treated PC12 cells. J Cell Physiol. 2005 Aug;204(2):632–637.

[55] Bu P1, Zhuang J, Feng J, Yang D, Shen X, Yan X. Visualization of CD146 dimerization and its regulation in living cells. Biochim Biophys Acta. 2007 Apr;1773(4):513–520.

[56] Zhuang J1, Jiang T, Lu D, Luo Y, Zheng C, Feng J, Yang D, Chen C, Yan X. NADPH oxidase 4 mediates reactive oxygen species induction of CD146 dimerization in VEGF signal transduction. Free Radic Biol Med. 2010 Jul 15;49(2):227–236. doi: 10.1016/j.freeradbiomed.2010.04.007.

[57] Jiang T1, Zhuang J, Duan H, Luo Y, Zeng Q, Fan K, Yan H, Lu D, Ye Z, Hao J, Feng J, Yang D, Yan X. CD146 is a coreceptor for VEGFR-2 in tumor angiogenesis. Blood. 2012 Sep 13;120(11):2330–2339. doi: 10.1182/blood-2012-01-406108.

[58] Jouve N1, Despoix N, Espeli M, Gauthier L, Cypowyj S, Fallague K, Schiff C, Dignat-George F, Vély F, Leroyer AS. The involvement of CD146 and its novel ligand Galectin-1 in apoptotic regulation of endothelial cells. J Biol Chem. 2013 Jan 25;288(4):2571–2579. doi: 10.1074/jbc.M112.418848.

[59] Tsuchiya S1, Tsukamoto Y, Taira E, LaMarre J. Involvement of transforming growth factor-beta in the expression of gicerin, a cell adhesion molecule, in the regeneration of hepatocytes. Int J Mol Med. 2007 Mar;19(3):381–386.

[60] Aldrian S1, Trautinger F, Fröhlich I, Berger W, Micksche M, Kindas-Mügge I. Overexpression of Hsp27 affects the metastatic phenotype of human melanoma cells in vitro. Cell Stress Chaperones. 2002 Apr;7(2):177–185.

[61] Aldrian S1, Kindas-Mügge I, Trautinger F, Fröhlich I, Gsur A, Herbacek I, Berger W, Micksche M. Overexpression of Hsp27 in a human melanoma cell line: regulation of E-cadherin, MUC18/MCAM, and plasminogen activator (PA) system. Cell Stress Chaperones. 2003 Fall;8(3):249–257.

[62] Li G1, Kalabis J, Xu X, Meier F, Oka M, Bogenrieder T, Herlyn M.Reciprocal regulation of MelCAM and AKT in human melanoma. Oncogene. 2003 Oct 9;22(44):6891–6899.

[63] Zheng C1, Qiu Y, Zeng Q, Zhang Y, Lu D, Yang D, Feng J, Yan X. Endothelial CD146 is required for in vitro tumor-induced angiogenesis: the role of a disulfide bond in signaling and dimerization. Int J Biochem Cell Biol. 2009 Nov;41(11):2163–2172. doi: 10.1016/j.biocel.2009.03.014.

[64] Bu P1, Gao L, Zhuang J, Feng J, Yang D, Yan X. Anti-CD146 monoclonal antibody AA98 inhibits angiogenesis via suppression of nuclear factor-kappaB activation. Mol Cancer Ther. 2006 Nov;5(11):2872–2878.

[65] Anfosso F1, Bardin N, Francès V, Vivier E, Camoin-Jau L, Sampol J, Dignat-George F. Activation of human endothelial cells via S-endo-1 antigen (CD146) stimulates the tyrosine phosphorylation of focal adhesion kinase p125(FAK). J Biol Chem. 1998 Oct 9;273(41):26852–26856.

[66] Anfosso F1, Bardin N, Vivier E, Sabatier F, Sampol J, Dignat-George F. Outside-in signaling pathway linked to CD146 engagement in human endothelial cells. J Biol Chem. 2001 Jan 12;276(2):1564–1569.

[67] Luo Y1, Zheng C, Zhang J, Lu D, Zhuang J, Xing S, Feng J, Yang D, Yan X. Recognition of CD146 as an ERM-binding protein offers novel mechanisms for melanoma cell migration. Oncogene. 2012 Jan 19;31(3):306–321. doi: 10.1038/onc.2011.244.

[68] Witze ES1, Litman ES, Argast GM, Moon RT, Ahn NG. Wnt5a control of cell polarity and directional movement by polarized redistribution of adhesion receptors. Science. 2008 Apr 18;320(5874):365–369. doi: 10.1126/science.1151250.

[69] Liu Q1, Zhang B, Zhao X, Zhang Y, Liu Y, Yan X. Blockade of adhesion molecule CD146 causes pregnancy failure in mice. J Cell Physiol. 2008 Jun;215(3):621–626. doi: 10.1002/jcp.21341.

[70] Shih IM, Kurman RJ. Expression of melanoma cell adhesion molecule in intermediate trophoblast. Lab Invest. 1996 Sep;75(3):377–388.

[71] Pasquier E1, Bardin N, De Saint Martin L, Le Martelot MT, Bohec C, Roche S, Mottier D, Dignat-George F. The first assessment of soluble CD146 in women with unexplained pregnancy loss. A new insight? Thromb Haemost. 2005 Dec;94(6):1280–1284.

[72] Daniel L1, Bardin N, Moal V, Dignat-George F, Berland Y, Figarella-Branger D. Tubular CD146 expression in nephropathies is related to chronic renal failure. Nephron Exp Nephrol. 2005;99(4):e105–111.

[73] Wang F1, Xing T, Wang N, Liu L. Clinical significance of plasma CD146 and P-selectin in patients with type 2 diabetic nephropathy. Cytokine. 2012 Jan;57(1):127–129. doi: 10.1016/j.cyto.2011.10.010.

[74] Weninger W1, Rendl M, Mildner M, Mayer C, Ban J, Geusau A, Bayer G, Tanew A, Majdic O, Tschachler E. Keratinocytes express the CD146 (Muc18/S-endo) antigen in tissue culture and during inflammatory skin diseases. J Invest Dermatol. 2000 Aug;115(2):219–224.

[75] Luca M1, Hunt B, Bucana CD, Johnson JP, Fidler IJ, Bar-Eli M. Direct correlation between MUC18 expression and metastatic potential of human melanoma cells. Melanoma Res. 1993 Feb;3(1):35–41.

[76] Schlagbauer-Wadl H1, Jansen B, Müller M, Polterauer P, Wolff K, Eichler HG, Pehamberger H, Konak E, Johnson JP. Influence of MUC18/MCAM/CD146 expression on human melanoma growth and metastasis in SCID mice. Int J Cancer. 1999 Jun 11;81(6):951–955.

[77] Xie S, Luca M, Huang S, Gutman M, Reich R, Johnson JP, Bar-Eli M. Expression of MCAM/MUC18 by human melanoma cells leads to increased tumor growth and metastasis. Cancer Res. 1997 Jun 1;57(11):2295–2303.

[78] Watson-Hurst K1, Becker D. The role of N-cadherin, MCAM and beta3 integrin in melanoma progression, proliferation, migration and invasion. Cancer Biol Ther. 2006 Oct;5(10):1375–1382.

[79] Sers C1, Riethmüller G, Johnson JP. MUC18, a melanoma-progression associated molecule, and its potential role in tumor vascularization and hematogenous spread. Cancer Res. 1994 Nov 1;54(21):5689–5694.

[80] Staquicini FI1, Tandle A, Libutti SK, Sun J, Zigler M, Bar-Eli M, Aliperti F, Pérez EC, Gershenwald JE, Mariano M, Pasqualini R, Arap W, Lopes JD. A subset of host B lymphocytes controls melanoma metastasis through a melanoma cell adhesion molecule/

MUC18-dependent interaction: evidence from mice and humans. Cancer Res. 2008 Oct 15;68(20):8419–8428. doi: 10.1158/0008-5472.CAN-08-1242.

[81] Rapanotti MC1, Bianchi L, Ricozzi I, Campione E, Pierantozzi A, Orlandi A, Chimenti S, Federici G, Bernardini S. Melanoma-associated markers expression in blood: MUC-18 is associated with advanced stages in melanoma patients. Br J Dermatol. 2009 Feb;160(2):338–344. doi: 10.1111/j.1365-2133.2008.08929.x.

[82] Pearl RA1, Pacifico MD, Richman PI, Wilson GD, Grover R. Stratification of patients by melanoma cell adhesion molecule (MCAM) expression on the basis of risk: implications for sentinel lymph node biopsy. J Plast Reconstr Aesthet Surg. 2008;61(3):265–271.

[83] Mills L1, Tellez C, Huang S, Baker C, McCarty M, Green L, Gudas JM, Feng X, Bar-Eli M. Fully human antibodies to MCAM/MUC18 inhibit tumor growth and metastasis of human melanoma. Cancer Res. 2002 Sep 1;62(17):5106–5114.

3

Angiogenesis and Cardiovascular Diseases: The Emerging Role of HDACs

Ana Moraga, Ka Hou Lao and Lingfang Zeng

Abstract

Cardiovascular diseases (CVD) continue to be the leading cause of death in the world despite recent therapeutic advances. Although many CVDs remain incurable, enormous efforts have been placed in harnessing angiogenesis as therapeutics for these diseases. Epigenetics, the modification of gene expression post-transcriptionally and post-translationally, are important in regulating many biological processes. One of the main post-translational epigenetic modifications, modification of chromatin structure by the acetylation of histone tails within the chromatin by either histone deacetylases (HDACs) or histone acetyltransferases (HATs), is important in modulating gene transcription and has emerged as an important regulatory player from pathogenesis to therapeutics in CVDs. Particularly, HDACs, which are largely involved in promoting chromatin compaction and hence inhibitions of gene transcription, have been implicated in the pathogenic signalling underlying many aspects of CVDs. Recently, histone modifications have been demonstrated to play important roles in the angiogenesis process. Pharmacological inhibitions of HDACs have displayed promising therapeutic potentials in several pre-clinical models of CVDs where angiogenesis is of paramount importance. There are many evidences proving that pro- and anti-angiogenic therapies—and the impact of epigenetics in these processes—can help to artificially reconstruct the vasculature in patients with cardiovascular diseases. Conversely, utilising knowledge of HDACs in angiogenesis might help to develop anti-angiogenic therapies in tackling diseases that are characterised with excessive pathological angiogenesis, including cancer and age-related macular degeneration. Understanding the molecular mechanisms underlying HDACs in modulating angiogenesis will undoubtedly benefit future therapeutics development. This chapter focuses on the emerging role of HDACs in angiogenesis and discuss their potentials and challenges in utilising HDAC inhibitors as therapeutics in several major cardiovascular diseases.

Keywords: angiogenesis, cardiovascular disease, atherosclerosis, histone deacetylase, epigenetics

1. Introduction

Cardiovascular diseases (CVDs) are a worldwide epidemic that have serious implication in public health and constitute a huge amount of healthcare expenditure. Although there are a number of preventable controllable risk factors, such as hypertension, hypercholesterolemia, smoking, obesity, lack of physical activity and diabetes, and others such as age, gender and family history are unmodifiable [1]. Progress in genetic sequencing has allowed the identification of numerous genetic variants associated with specific CVDs [2], but their mechanisms remain unclear. The last few years of research have been a key in understanding how epigenetic mechanisms such as histone modifications are involved in the occurrence and progression of CVDs including atherosclerosis, heart failure, myocardial infarction and cardiac hypertrophy.

Epigenetics represent a phenomenon of altered heritable gene expression without changes to the underlying DNA sequences. The epigenetic alterations can be affected by exogenous stimuli such as diabetes milieu, diets and smoking, while at other times these alterations can subsequently trigger disease initiation [3]. Thus, the impact of epigenetics in CVD is now emerging as an important regulatory key player at different levels from pathophysiology to therapeutics. For instance, histone alterations have been implicated in ECs response to hypoxia and shear stress, in angiogenesis and in endogenous recovery following myocardial infarction (MI) [4]. On the other hand, HDAC inhibitors (HDACi) have been investigated for potential protective effects in heart muscles during acute MI [4, 5].

Tissue repair is one of the main therapeutic challenges facing the scientific community. There are various approaches in improving tissue recovery depending on the pathological conditions, but most of these conditions are initiated by local ischaemia and require a rich network of blood supply for tissue regeneration. Hence, angiogenesis plays a vital part in tissue regeneration in the treatment of CVDs. At present, the promising potentials of angiogenesis therapies are in full swing.

2. Vascular system

2.1. Cardiovascular system

The cardiovascular system consists of three main components: heart, blood vessels (arteries, veins and capillaries) and blood. There are three types of anatomically and functionally distinct blood vessels: arteries, veins and capillaries. The arteries are primarily involved in the delivery of oxygenated blood and nutrients from the heart to target organs and tissues. They have thicker and more elastic vessel walls to complement the higher blood pressure for blood delivery from the heart. The veins carry deoxygenated blood, together with waste products and other factors secreted by the tissues back to the heart. They tend to have larger luminal areas and thinner vessel walls compared to the arteries, and have valves to complement the pressure changes. Connecting these two vessel systems are the capillaries that allow the direct exchanges of oxygen and nutrients with carbon dioxide and waste products between the target tissues and the blood. The walls of all vessels are generally composed of three layers: the tunica intima, tunica media and tunica adventitia. The inner-most layer is formed by the tunica intima, which is made up of a single layer of ECs and connective tissues, both of which overlie the internal elastic lamina. The tunica intima has an important function as a selective permeable barrier between the extravascular space, the vascular wall and the blood. The tunica media forms the muscular element of blood vessels that resides between the tunica intima and the tunica adventitia, and comprises circumfer-entially arranged smooth muscle cells (SMCs) enclosed by a layer of external elastic lamina. They provide supports to the vessels and regulate blood flow and pressure via controlling the luminal diameter. The outermost layer, the tunica adventitia, is made up of connective tissues and matrix-secreting fibroblasts. It is critical to maintaining vascular structure and helps to anchor vessels in place to fit into the surrounding tissues. Capillaries constitute non-muscular vessels and are only made up of an internal elastic lamina covered by a monolayer of ECs, and provide a huge surface area for exchanges of vital blood components and factors between vessels and tissues.

2.2. Endothelial cells and their impairments in CVDs

Vascular endothelial cells (ECs) have a crucial and diverse role, arraying the innermost layer of the entire circulatory system. They act as the semi-selective and non-adherent barrier between the lumen of the vessels and the underlying tissues, regulating tissue perfusion and movement of inflammatory cells between them [6]. They are involved in regulating vascular permeability, blood flow, vascular tone and blood coagulation and are essentially involved in vascular remodelling in responses to diverse physiological and pathological stimuli. Physiologically, ECs exert anti-coagulant and anti-thrombotic effects through the secretion of anti-coagulant factors such as prostacyclin, nitric oxide (NO) and prostaglandin-E_2, and inhibit inflammatory cell adhesion in order to maintain vascular homeostasis [7]. Under path-ological states, ECs are activated by vascular insults or pro-inflammatory cytokines, leading to increased permeability, encouraging extravasations of immune cells, which are followed by a series of pathological events leading to eventual vascular remodelling [7]. Decreased EC secretion of the potent vasodilator NO as a result of repressed activity of endothelial NO synthase (eNOS) also contributes to the circus of vascular pathogenesis [8]. These endothelial dysfunctions, whether environmental, genetic or a combination of both, critically contribute to the pathophysiology of many CVDs such as hypertension and atherosclerosis, and repre-sent the discernible therapeutic targets for drug development [9].

3. Angiogenesis

There are three main processes that contribute to the formation of new blood vessels that are termed globally as neovascularisation:

– Vasculogenesis is defined as the de novo formation of vascular structures by the migration of stem cells to the site of vascularisation and differentiation into ECs. Although it was originally thought to be exclusive to embryonic development, it is now widely accepted that the process can also take place in adults, which opens up a new avenue for clinical applications [10].

– Angiogenesis is the formation of new blood vessels by sprouting from pre-existing small vessels in embryonic and adult tissue or by intravascular subdivision process [11]. This process is believed to be induced by angiogenic factors including fibroblast growth factor (FGF) and vascular endothelial growth factor (VEGF).

– Arteriogenesis results from the hypertrophy and luminal distention of pre-existing collateral vessels, which involves specific remodelling of existing nascent EC tubules for greater size, elasticity and stability through the recruitment of and enclosure by SMCs and pericytes that secrete specific extracellular matrices. Therefore, these vessels have fully developed tunica media and tunica adventitia [11].

Angiogenesis is a very complex process that can be simplified into three categories: mechanical, chemical and molecular factors (see Ref. [12] for a more extensive review).

– **Cellular factors**: There are many molecules that can modulate angiogenesis. The most essential angiogenic growth factors are as follows: FGF, VEGF, placenta growth factor, angiopoietin-1 and angiopoietin-2. Several pathological conditions can also initiate angiogenesis. For example, hypoglycaemia increases the expression of critical angiogenic inductor VEGF [13]. It has also been extensively demonstrated that the presence of inflammatory cells, like macrophages and neutrophils, is sufficient to induce angiogenesis [14].

– **Environmental factors**: Angiogenesis can be induced by hypoxia and through increased EC production of NO. Hypoxia stimulates the release of several angiogenic factors including platelet-derived growth factor and FGF-1 and FGF-2 by macrophages. Hypoxia also upregulates VEGF production, which is known to induce the production and secretion of NO from ECs, while eNOS production is amplified during VEGF-induced angiogenesis [15].

– **Mechanical factors**: There are two main factors: haemodynamic and shear stress. Haemodynamic changes trigger an augmentation of blood flow and might therefore stimulate vascular sprouting, maintain patency of the newly formed collateral vessels and provide blood flow to the ischemic area [16]. Shear stress has an important influence on the development of collateral vessel networks in the ischaemic tissues.

4. Epigenetics

The nucleosome is the fundamental subunit of chromatin in eukaryotes. Each nucleosome consists of a 146-bp DNA segment wrapped around an octamer of core histone proteins that includes two molecules of histones H2A, H2B, H3 and H4 associated with a single copy of histone H1. Epigenetics is defined as the study of stable alterations of gene expression without alterations of DNA itself. These alterations include the post-translational addition or removal of methyl groups to DNA as well as methyl, acetyl, sumoyl and phospho groups to histones and other kind of proteins. These changes participate in remodelling chromatin and modifying its accessibility to transcription factors and cofactors [17]. Epigenetic control is one of the main regulatory systems contributing to phenotypic differences between cell types in multicellular organisms. Epigenetic changes may explain why subjects with similar genetic backgrounds and risk factors for particular diseases can differ greatly in clinical manifestation and therapeutic response [18]. It has been reported that epigenetic mechanisms play a critical role in regulating endothelial gene expression [19]. Among these epigenetic changes are the methylation of DNA, RNA-based mechanisms and the posttranslational modification of histone proteins.

DNA methylation

The methylation of DNA involves the covalent modification of the 5-position of cytosine to define the 'fifth base of DNA', 5-methyl-cytosine [20]. In mammals, DNA methylation is almost exclusively restricted to CpG dinucleotides. DNA methylation is catalysed by DNA methyltransferases and regulates biological processes underlying CVD, such as atherosclerosis, inflammation, hypertension, and diabetes [21].

RNA-based mechanisms

1.   miRNA therapeutics

     MicroRNAs (miRNA or miR) are short (20–22 nucleotides) non-coding RNAs modulating gene expression further by down-regulating the translation of target mRNAs through the inhibition of post-transcriptional events, through transcript degradation or through direct translational repression.

2.   Long non-coding RNAs (lncRNAs)

     Long non-coding RNAs (lncRNAs) are gaining more prominence as regulators of gene expression. The central role that lncRNAs play in heart development is only slowly being recognised [18]. Besides, understanding the function of these molecules in CVD is even further away.

Histone modification

It is well established that histone residues can undergo a wide array of modifications. At least eight different types of modification have been characterised with a range of enzymes identified for each: acetylation, methylation, phosphorylation, ubiquitination, sumoylation, ADP-ribosylation, deimination, and proline isomerisation (**Table 1**).

Histone methylation is modulated by two enzymes: histone methyltransferases and histone demethylases. The acetylation status of histone is fine-tuned by histone acetyltransferases (HATs) and HDACs. HDACs are enzymes that remove acetyl groups from histone lysine residues thereby increasing their negative charges, which lead to chromatin condensation and gene repression [17].

4.1. The HDAC family

Deacetylation of histones in nucleosomes induces chromatin compaction, which represses transcription by preventing the binding of transcription factors and other components of the

Modification type	Amino acid modification	Examples of modifying enzymes	Role
Acetylation	Lysine	Histone acetyl transferases (HATs)	Transcription Repair
		Histone deacetylases (HDACs)	Replication Condensation
Methylation	Lysine	Lysine methyltransferases	Transcription
		Lysine demethylases	Repair
	Arginine	Arginine methyltransferases	Transcription
		Arginine demethylases	
Phosphorylation	Serine	Serine/threonine kinases	Transcription
	Threonine	Dephosphorylated by phosphatases	Repair Condensation
Ubiquitination	Lysine	Ubiquinases (ubiquitin ligases)	Transcription
		Deubiquinating enzymes	Repair
SUMOylation	Lysine	Small ubiquitin-like modifier (SUMO)	Transcription
		De-SUMOylating enzymes: sentrin-specific proteases	
ADP ribosylation	Glutamate	ADP-ribosyltransferases	Transcription
Deimination	Arginine (to Citrulline)	Peptidylarginine deiminases	Transcription
Proline isomerisation	Proline	Proline isomerases	Transcription

Table 1. Types of histone modifications and the enzymes responsible (modified from Ref. [22]).

transcriptional machinery onto the gene promoter and enhancer regions. HDACs are enzymes that remove acetyl groups from hyperacetylated histones, and modification by HDACs leads to a closed chromatin structure and suppression of genes. HDACs are recruited to gene promoters by DNA-binding proteins that recognise certain DNA sequences and in this way provide specific modulation on gene expression.

There are 18 characterised members of the HDAC family in mammals, which can be grouped into four classes depending on their functional similarities and their homology with yeast HDACs. The class I and class II HDACs are considered as the 'classical' HDACs [23].

Class I HDACs comprise nuclear, ubiquitously expressed HDACs 1, 2, 3, and 8. HDAC1, 2, and 8 reside nearly exclusively in the nucleus. HDAC3 is found to shuttle between nucleus and cytoplasm. Because these are ubiquitously expressed and involved in cell proliferation and survival, aberrations in their gene expression have been implicated in a wide range of cancers [24, 25].

Class II HDACs shuttle between the cytoplasm and the nucleus depending on specific cellular signals; they share a tissue-specific expression pattern and are divided into two subgroups:

class IIa (HDACs 4, 5, 7, and 9) and class IIb (HDACs 6 and 10). Class IIa HDACs distinguish themselves with their extended N-terminal regulatory domain, whereas class IIb HDACs contain two catalytic domains. Class IIa HDACs appear to have tissue-specific roles and can shuttle between the cytosol and the nucleus. In fact, the phosphorylation status is a critical event to determine their localisation in the nucleus or cytoplasm and the ability to act as transcriptional co-repressors in the nuclear region. Conversely, class IIb is mostly found in the cytosol [26].

Class III HDACs regroup the ubiquitously expressed silent information regulator 2 (Sir2) family of nicotinamide adenine dinucleotide (NAD+)-dependent HDACs (SIRT1–7), which share structural and functional similarities with the yeast Sir2 protein. Interestingly, these have a critical role in a wide range of cellular processes such as ageing, transcription, cell survival, DNA repair, apoptosis, and inflammation. Sirtuins appear to have contradictory roles in disease. On the one hand, they control many vital functions involved in cellular protection, while on the other hand, they are also involved in several disease pathologies such as metabolic diseases, neurodegenerative disorders, and cancer [27].

Finally, class IV HDAC is the newly discovered HDAC11. HDAC11 is most closely related to class I HDACs. However, since the overall sequence similarities are low, it cannot be grouped into any of the three existing classes. HDAC11 is primarily expressed in heart, smooth muscle, kidney, and brain tissues.

Recent reports suggest that HDACs can deacetylate non-histone proteins as additional functions of HDACs (**Figure 1**). The roles of HDACs in cancer and neurological diseases have

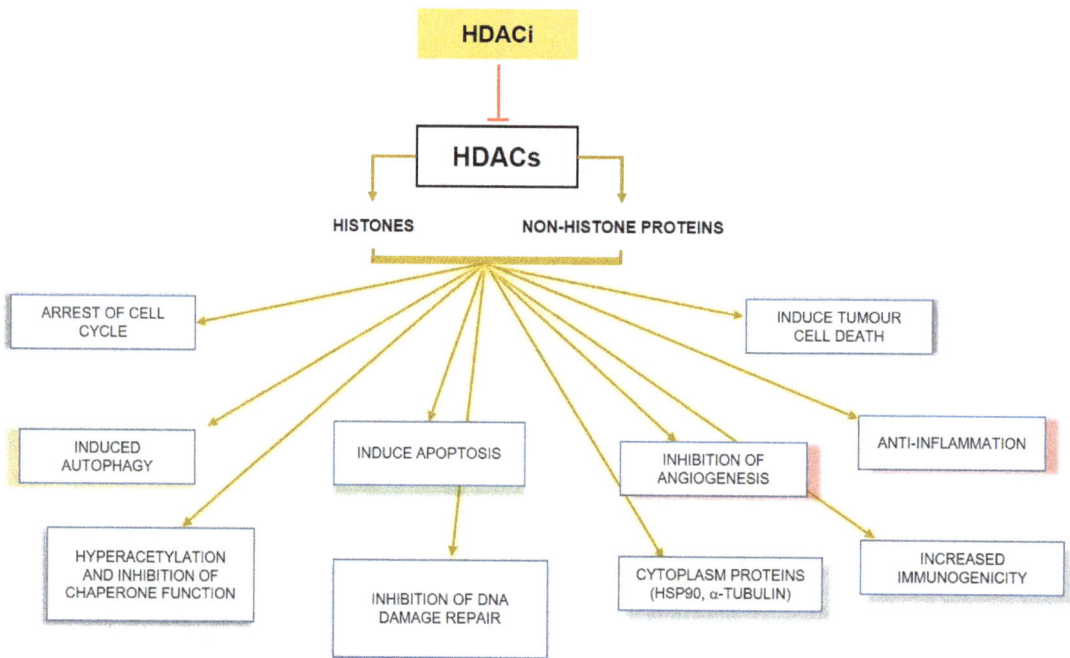

Figure 1. Schematic illustration of HDACi downstream effects. Inhibition of HDACs by HDACi induces acetylation of histone proteins as well as non-histone proteins, which leads to the alteration in various physiological and pathological processes (modified from Refs. [28–30]).

been extensively examined. However, the functions of HDACs in cardiovascular diseases and arteriosclerosis are less explored [23].

4.2. HDAC inhibitors

There has been a breakthrough in the development of HDACi. These HDACi induce acetylation of histone proteins, as well as non-histone proteins, which leads to the alteration and regulation of biological events including angiogenesis, apoptosis/autophagy, cell cycle, fibrogenesis, immune response, inflammation, and metabolism (**Figure 1**). As a result, HDAC inhibitor-based therapies have gained substantial attention as treatments for cardiovascular diseases and cancer.

In the following sections, we will describe the different exerted functions of HDACi in different physiological and pathological conditions.

5. The role of HDACs in angiogenesis: HDAC-regulated ECs functions in vitro

During development of the embryo and the physiological repairs of any tissue damages, the formation of new blood vessels plays a major role. The process can either involve vasculogenesis where ECs may be derived from the differentiation of different kinds of stem cells such as embryonic stem (ES) cells, while angiogenesis requires the proliferation, migration, and sprouting of ECs. Some of these new blood vessel formations are normal and beneficial as seen in wound healing after trauma and ischemic tissue restoration. However, pathological neovascularisation leads to many diseases such as diabetic retinopathy, tumour, and inflammation. Over the past decade, investigations into the role of HDACs in the regulations of these processes have gained some tractions. We have previously shown that the stabilisation of the class I HDAC3 plays an essential role in VEGF receptor 2 (VEGFR2)-mediated endothelial differentiation of mouse ES cells (mESC)-derived Sca-1$^+$ progenitors [31], while these events can also signal through VEGR2-HDAC3 stabilisation in a ligand-independent manner through exposure to laminar shear flow [32]. These derived EC-like cells display increased angiogenic potential by significantly enhancing re-endothelialisation with the host vessels upon their transplantation into a mouse wire injury model and substantially attenuated the injury-induced neointimal hyperplasia [32]. In addition, HDAC3 is also essential for the survival of ECs under atherogenic disturbed flow, and knock-down of HDAC3 increases neointima formation in the atheroprone ApoE$^{-/-}$ mice [33]. Overall, these show HDAC3 plays a role in the angiogenic processes.

Angiogenic activation of ECs to migrate and to form sprouts is associated with characteristic changes in gene expression profiles [34], which can be modulated by the inhibition of HDAC. HDAC inhibitions by pan-HDAC inhibitors such as suberoylanilide hydroxamic acid (SAHA) and trichostatin A (TSA) can suppress VEGF-induced capillary-like structures formation in human umbilical vein endothelial cells (HUVEC) by suppressing angiogenic factors such as hypoxia-inducible factor 1 alpha (HIF-1α), VEGF, and eNOS while both HDACi also prevent the sprouting of capillaries from rat aorta [35]. Discrepant reports exist however, as another study has shown that treatment with SAHA or a more class I selective inhibitor valporic acid (VPA) in combination with VEGF indeed resulted in enhanced EC sprouting [36]. These discrepancies could be due to the contrasting roles that other HDACs within the same class and/or from the other classes might play in regulating angiogenesis.

In fact, it is common that completely opposite role has been reported for other HDACs in the regulation of angiogenesis. HDAC4, a class IIa HDAC, was reported to negatively regulate angiogenesis by reducing VEGF expression [37], while others have reported HDAC4 induces angiogenesis through an increase in stability of HIF-1γ [38]. In addition, Zhang et al. showed that HDAC4 inhibition facilitated c-kit+ cardiac stem cells (CSCs) into the differentiation of cardiac lineage commitments with EC potential in vitro [4].

Diverse role has also been reported in another class IIa HDAC HDAC5. On the one hand, HDAC5 has been shown to repress KLF2 an important regulator of EC homeostasis that is normally expressed in the laminar flow-exposed (therefore atheroprotective) segments of the vessels, which results in repressed eNOS expression in ECs [39]. This anti-angiogenic role of HDAC5 was validated by siRNA-mediated knock-down of HDAC5 that promoted migration and sprouting of ECs [40]. Conversely, phosphorylation-dependent nuclear exports of HDAC5 [40] and HDAC7 [41], thereby the de-repression of target genes, are crucial for the expression of VEGF or metalloproteinase-10 in ECs that lead to increased angiogenesis. Moreover, blockade of HDAC7 phosphorylation with a signal-resistant HDAC7 mutant represses EC proliferation and migration in response to VEGF, confirming the important role of both class IIa HDACs plays in VEGF-mediated angiogenesis [42]. In addition, HDAC7 has also been identified as a key modulator of EC migration at least in part by regulating PDGF-B/PDGF-beta gene expression [43].

Evidence from our laboratory demonstrated that mouse HDAC7 undergoes alternative translation during mouse ESCs differentiation, resulting in the production of a 7-amino acid peptide (*Data not publish yet*). This peptide was shown to enhance mouse vascular progenitor cell migration and VEGF-induced differentiation towards the EC lineage in vitro. Overall, HDAC7 appears to be pro-angiogenic, while the mediating role of HDAC5 in angiogenesis could be largely dependent on its translocation within the nucleus.

There is a limited research into the role of class IIb HDAC in angiogenesis, but nevertheless HDAC6 can be classified as a pro-angiogenic factor as it induces cell migration by the deacetylation of cytoskeletal proteins [44, 45]. Class III HDAC SIRT1 is also highly expressed in the vasculature during blood vessel growth where it controls the angiogenic activity of ECs. Loss of SIRT1 function leads to blockage of sprouting angiogenesis [46]. Furthermore, SIRT1 associates with and deacetylates transcription factor Foxo1 and hence restricts its anti-angiogenic activity [46].

6. The role of HDAC in therapeutic angiogenesis

Different strategies for therapeutic angiogenesis, including the direct delivery of angiogenic growth factors and the delivery of cells to ischemic tissues, have been developed. Moreover, there is a recent progress on therapeutic angiogenesis by utilising polymeric biomaterials, combined with stem cell and gene therapy as well as stimulation of endogenous stem cell homing (see Ref. [47] for a more comprehensive review).

Owing to the disadvantage of invasiveness, limited drug diffusion, and lack of selectivity towards targeted tissues, treatments with traditional drugs and surgery are becoming less commonly used [48]. An emerging technique, ultrasound-targeted microbubble destruction (UTMD), has been proposed as a non-invasive and specific targeting approach in angiogenic therapy of CVDs. UTMD might create a series of biological effects, including improving recovery of local tissue damages, improving transient membrane permeability, and extravasation to facilitate the entering of targeted genes or drugs into the tissues or cells of interest.

There are several approaches indicating that inhibition of HDAC protects the heart against injury in different cardiovascular-related diseases, including myocardial infarction, myocardial hypertrophy, and diabetic cardiomyopathy. In addition, HDACi also seem to play a therapeutic role in other CVDs with vascular remodelling as one of their main manifestations. Here, we review the role of HDACs in these diseases one by one in order to better understand the context-dependent effects of HDACs in angiogenesis regulation in these diseases.

6.1. Atherosclerosis

Atherosclerosis of the arteries is a main causative pathogenesis of various CVDs including coronary artery disease (CAD), peripheral vascular disease (PVD), and stroke. It is a chronic pathological condition of the arteries that is characterised by the accumulation of lipids, chronic inflammation, generation of a fibrous cap, proliferation of SMCs, calcification in vascular smooth muscle layer, with the resultant loss of elasticity of arteries. In addition, disturbed shear stress (the tangential force of the flowing blood on the endothelial surface of the blood vessel) contributes to several elements of atherosclerotic disease. As a result of the growth of atheroma, the lumen of the artery is gradually narrowed, which changes the local environment. Activated ECs within the injury lesions produce adhesion molecules [intercellular adhesion molecule (ICAM) and vascular cell adhesion molecule-1 (VCAM-1)], chemotactic proteins [monocyte chemotactic protein-1 (MCP-1)], E- and P-selectin, and growth factors [macrophage colony-stimulating factor (M-CSF)] that create a pro-inflammatory environment. The inflammatory molecules then recruit monocytes to the vessel wall and promote their transmigration across the endothelial monolayer into the intima, where they proliferate, differentiate into macrophages, and foam cells by taking up the lipoproteins, leading to neointimal formation. With time, the foam cells and macrophages die and release lipid-filled contents and tissue factors, contributing to the formation of the lipid-rich necrotic core, which is a key component of unstable plaques. Meanwhile, SMCs migrate from the medial layer and accumulate within the intima, where they synthesise and secrete interstitial collagen and elastin and form the fibrous cap over the lesion. Ultimately, the thin fibrous caps rupture, then expose, and release procoagulant materials into the blood, triggering the thrombosis that impedes blood flow and results in acute stenosis of the arteries, leading to clinical manifestations [49–51].

Because many patients are not candidates for the standard treatments such as angioplasty or bypass surgery, a great enthusiasm has emerged for the utilisation of angiogenesis as a therapeutic modality for atherosclerotic arterial disease. It must be taken into account that angiogenesis plays a vital part in the pathogenesis and treatment of CVDs and has become one of the hotspots that are being discussed in the past decades. Therapeutic angiogenesis provides a valuable tool for treating cardiovascular diseases by stimulating the growth of new blood vessels from pre-existing vessels.

This avenue needs to be explored with caution however, as the role of angiogenesis in athero-sclerosis remains a very contentious topic, and currently, there is no consensus as to whether angiogenesis is a way to treat coronary heart disease or in fact is a key causative factor in the pathogenesis of atherosclerotic plaque formation. The controversy surrounding the role of angiogenesis in ischemic heart disease reflects, in part, the complexity of the underlying disease process. There are lot of studies supporting the therapeutic role of angiogenesis in atherosclerosis since a key therapeutic objective has been to use the angiogenic cytokines such as VEGF or FGF to stimulate collateral blood vessel formation in the ischemic heart and limb [52]. But, on the other hand, the pathogenic role of angiogenesis has been suggested as VEGF, and other angiogenic growth factors can promote atherosclerosis in certain animal models and potentially destabilise coronary plaques by promoting intralesion angiogenesis [53].

Apolipoprotein E-deficient (ApoE$^{-/-}$) mice, created by homologous recombination in ES cells, was first described in 1992 [54, 55]. Since then, this model becomes the most commonly used mouse model of atherosclerosis that is able to develop severe hypercholesterolemia and lesions of ath-erosclerosis highly similar to those observed in humans. Endogenous SIRT1 has been shown to decrease macrophage foam cell formation and atherogenesis in ApoE$^{-/-}$mice [56], while endothe-lial-specific overexpression of human SIRT1 reduces atherogenesis in ApoE$^{-/-}$ mice and improves vascular function [57]. So, in the vasculature, *SIRT1* gain-of-function using *SIRT1* overexpression has been shown to improve endothelial function in mice. Subsequently, it was described that SIRT1 does not directly influence endothelium-dependent vascular function in ApoE−/− mice, but it improves vascular function by preventing superoxide production in ECs and reduces the expression of inflammatory adhesion molecules by suppressing NF-κB signalling [58].

HDACi TSA has been shown to exert contradictory role in the formation of atherosclerotic lesion. TSA successfully prevents neointima formation after injury [59, 60]. In contrast, how-ever, several reports have elucidated the proatherogenic effects of TSA [61]. Another example of the discrepancies in TSA roles is the reduction of angiogenesis through the decrease of NO level (a key second messenger in angiogenesis signalling) through downregulation of eNOS [62]. These contrasting findings reinforce the theory of the contesting role angiogen-esis plays in atherosclerosis. In addition, it was reported that TSA can reduce the cholesterol biosynthesis by repressing the genes involved in the cholesterol, fatty acids, and glycolysis pathways [63]. These evidences suggest that TSA could be used as a potential therapeutic agent for the control of cholesterol levels as high cholesterol level is one of the main triggers of atherosclerosis.

6.2. Myocardial infarction

Myocardial infarction (MI) occurs when blood flow stops to part of the heart causing damage to the cardiomyocytes. In physiological conditions, oxygen and nutrients are supplied to the ventricular myocytes by the coronary arteries. Under pathological condition, the coronary artery is often occluded by various pathological condition such as the growth of atheroma in the coronary artery, rupture of vulnerable plaque, thrombi from proximal lesions, emboli secondary to atrial fibrillation, or vegetation after endocarditis.

Several gene or protein therapies to deliver angiogenic factors such as VEGF, FGF2, or FGF4, as well as cell therapy using endothelial progenitor cells (EPCs), mesenchymal stem cells (MSCs), or induced pluripotent stem cells (iPSCs), have been developed as potential pro-angiogenic therapeutics for ischemic heart disease and peripheral vascular disease [64, 65]. HDAC4 inhibition has been demonstrated to promote cardiac stem cells mediated cardiac regeneration and improve the restoration of cardiac function in mice [4]. Granger et al. observed that ischemia induces HDAC activity in the heart resulting in increased deacetylation of histones H3/4 in vitro and in vivo that leads to injured cardiomyocytes [66]. Furthermore, HDACi exert direct antifibrotic activities that alter the response to ischemic cardiac injury and reduce infarct size, which are accompanied by improvement in cardiac functions in the mouse infarcted heart. However, it is unclear whether these therapeutic effects have any links with angiogenesis in these earlier studies.

TSA have exerted an increased angiogenic response in vivo in the mouse infarcted hearts. This indicates that TSA preserves cardiac performance and mitigates myocardial remodelling through stimulating cardiac endogenous regeneration that could be dependent on enhanced angiogenesis within the infarcted heart tissues [67]. The repression of ischemia-induced gene expression such as HIF-1α and VEGF has been suggested as possible mechanisms mediated by HDACi to stabilise vascular permeability [66]. Recruitment of stem cells has also been suggested as another main mechanism that TSA mediates through. After 8 weeks of TSA treatment in MI mice with or without c-kit deficiency, significantly improved neovascularisation and cardiac repair accompanied by cardiac functions and reduced cardiac remodelling can be observed in the wildtype infarcted heart compared to the c-kit-deficient mice [68]. It is also important to distinguish between the timing of the HDACi effects. Many reports show that long-term (8 weeks) administration of HDACi induces neovascularisation [67], while acute treatments (12 h) with HDACi inhibit angiogenesis [66].

6.3. Cardiac hypertrophy

Cardiac hypertrophy is a form of remodelling and is an adaptive response to the request for high workload from peripheral tissue or from intrinsic underlying disease conditions such as valvular dysfunction, hypertension, and MI. The heart responds to stresses by undergoing a remodelling process that is associated with myocyte hypertrophy, myocyte death, inflammation, and fibrosis, which often result in impaired cardiac function and heart failure. These are accompanied by activation of the myocyte enhancer factor-2 (MEF2) transcription factor and reprogramming of cardiac gene expression. Recent studies have revealed key roles for HDACs as both positive and negative regulators of pathological cardiac remodelling (**Figure 2**).

Members of MEF2 transcription factors family are some of the key regulators of myocardial hypertrophy. The first connection between HDACs and the regulation of pathological cardiac remodelling was provided by the discovery that class IIa HDACs interact with members of

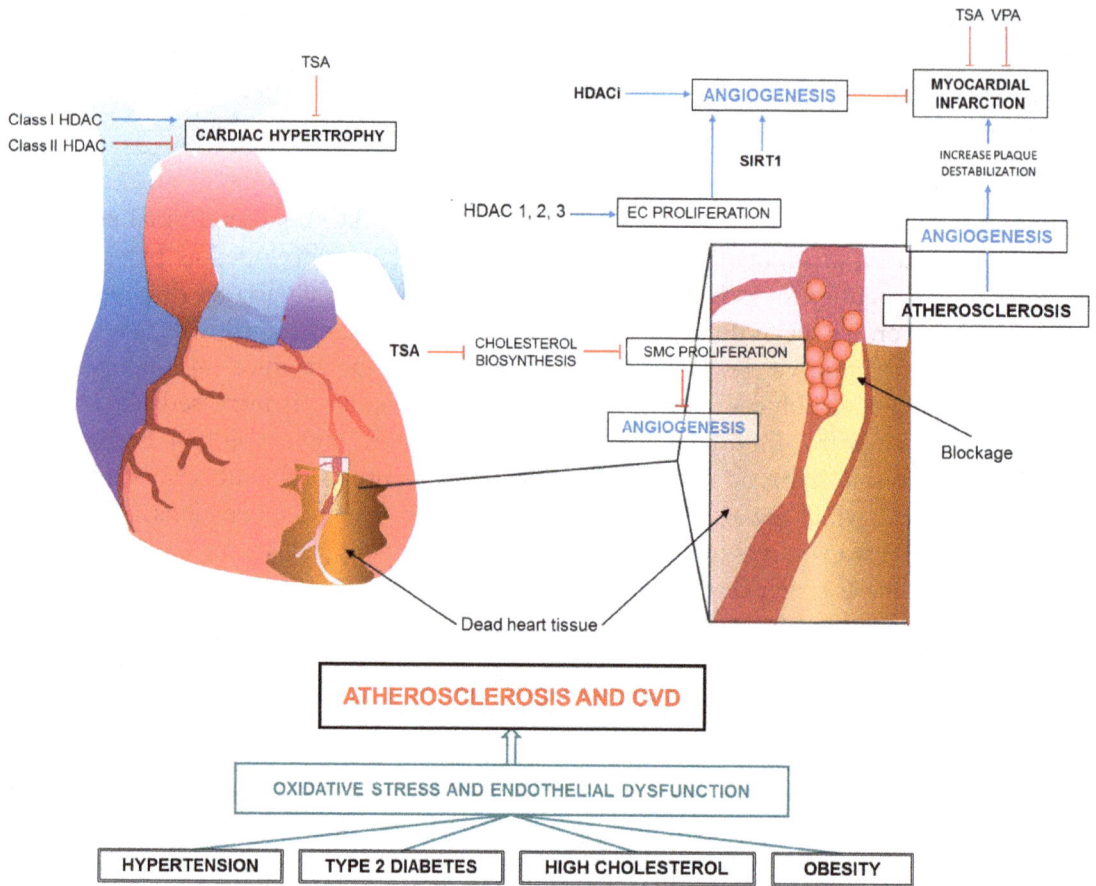

Figure 2. HDACs in cardiovascular disease. Different risk factors lead to the appearance of atheromatous plaques in the coronary arteries, and from these, other cardiovascular diseases such as myocardial infarction occur. The discovery that different HDAC enzymes are involved in processes such as angiogenesis has led to the development of inhibitors to modulate its effect as a therapeutic treatment (⟶ means induction; ⊣ means inhibition).

MEF2 transcription factor family [69]. The transcriptional activity of MEF2 factors is upregulated in response to pathological stress in the heart, and ectopic overexpression of constitutively active forms of MEF2 in mouse heart causes dilated cardiomyopathy. It was reported that class II HDACs are substrates for a stress-responsive kinase specific for conserved serines that regulate MEF2-HDAC interactions. Those kinases phosphorylate the signal-responsive sites in class II HDACs, and mutant proteins lacking these phosphorylation sites can act as signal-resistant repressors of cardiomyocyte hypertrophy and fetal cardiac gene expression in vitro [70]. These studies support a role for class IIa HDACs as endogenous repressors of cardiac hypertrophy. Conversely, the function of class IIb HDACs in the heart remains largely unknown in heart hypertrophy.

Nevertheless, administration of HDACi TSA 2 weeks after the induction of pressure overload can reverse cardiac hypertrophy in mice [71]. The class I selective HDACi MPT0E014 also improves cardiac contractibility and attenuates structural remodelling in isoproterenol-induced dilated cardiomyopathy [72]. As there is an intrinsic relationship between decreased capillary density and the transition of cardiac hypertrophy to cardiac failure [73], it remains to be investigated whether the cardioprotective effects exerted by HDACi are related to increased angiogenesis within the hypertrophic heart.

6.4. Peripheral artery disease

Peripheral artery disease (PAD) can be defined as the narrowing of the peripheral arteries that are not directly linked to the supply to the heart or the brain. PAD development is a multifactorial process with many different forms [74].

Different action mechanisms have been proposed for different HDACi in terms of regulating angiogenesis in the case of vascular diseases. It was reported in a mouse model of hindlimb ischaemia that the inhibition of class IIa HDACs is pro-angiogenic while class I HDAC inhibition is anti-angiogenic in mouse models of hindlimb ischemia [75].

6.5. Stroke

Stroke is a devastating illness and the second cause of death and disability worldwide after cardiac ischemia. A stroke occurs when a blood vessel that carries oxygen and nutrients to the brain is either blocked by a clot or bursts. As a consequence, part of the brain can die. Post-mortem studies have revealed that angiogenesis can be observed several days after cerebral ischemic stroke; it is noteworthy that higher microvessel density correlates with longer patient survival [76]. Enhanced angiogenesis facilities neurovascular remodelling processes and promotes brain functional recovery after stroke.

There are several studies testing the effects of HDACi in neurovascular remodelling processes and in brain functional recovery after stroke. Sun et al. showed that VPA treatment enhanced post-ischemic angiogenesis by increasing microvessel density, facilitating EC proliferation, and up-regulating rate of cerebral blood flow in the ipsilateral cortex. These events may be associated with up-regulation of HIF-1α and its downstream proangiogenic target VEGF as well as extracellular MMP2/9 [77]. Similar results were obtained by treating rats with VPA during permanent middle cerebral artery occlusion (pMCAO). They exhibit reduced infarct volume, promote functional recovery, enhance angiogenesis by upregulating VEGF [78], and reduce monocytes infiltration [79]. SIRT1 is proangiogenic and increases EC tube formation, especially in post-natal angiogenesis [46]. So loss of SIRT1 reduces angiogenesis and increases brain infarction, while SIRT1 was also demonstrated to play an important role in neuroprotection against brain ischemia by deacetylation and subsequent inhibition of p53-induced and nuclear factor κB-induced inflammatory and apoptotic pathways [80].

After pMCAO, sodium butyrate and TSA induce neurogenesis via HDACi in multiple ischemic brain regions in rats. Sodium butyrate also strongly upregulated VEGF, increasing angiogenesis and functional recovery after stroke. It was also described that sodium butyrate exhibits neuroprotective/neurogenic effects in rat model of neonatal hypoxia-ischemia [81]. All these results highlight that the inhibition of HDAC in brain after stroke enhances angiogenesis, and this may contribute to the long-term functional recovery after stroke.

6.6. HDACs role in angiogenesis in diabetes

Diabetes mellitus is a chronic disease where the lack of insulin leads to anomalies in the substrate metabolism, causing a range of acute and long-term complications. One of the main complication is the loss of small blood vessels. Another related secondary disease is diabetic glomerulomegaly or kidney disease. One of the predominant feature of diabetic glomerulomegaly is an increase in glomerular capillary volume [82], which can be controlled by anti-angiogenic therapies. As there is evidence of genetic association between diabetes and HDACs, treatment with HDACi exerts a reduction in glomerular endothelial markers expression, which demonstrates the anti-angiogenic benefit [83]. This effect seems to be opposite when it applies to the diabetic heart failure model, as another HDACi sodium butyrate exerts improved cardiac functions and increased microvessel density within the diabetic myocardium [84]. Moreover, HDACi also modulates cardiac peroxisome proliferator-activated receptors (PPARs) and fatty acid metabolism in diabetic cardiomyopathy [85].

7. Pathogenic role of angiogenesis

7.1. Cancer

There are more than 200 different kinds of cancers, and each type behaves and responds to treatments in different ways. Epigenetic enzymes are dysregulated in tumours through mutation or altered expression. More importantly, tumourigenesis is largely due to overexpression of oncogenes or the loss of function of tumour suppressor genes. The identification of these proteins has driven the rapid development of small-molecule inhibitors.

As we mention above, the function of HDACs is not solely on modifying histones, but they can also target many different cellular substrates and proteins, including those that are involved in tumour progression. Currently, many HDACi are in clinical trials for cancer therapeutics as HDACi result in hyperacetylation (and therefore repression) of genes related to tumour cell apoptosis, growth arrest, senescence, differentiation, cell invasion, and metastasis [86].

An exemplary role of HDACi play in modulating the tumour cells directly is its action on vasculogenic mimicry (VM). VM refers to the process by which highly aggressive tumour cells mimic ECs to form vessel-like structures that aid in supplying enough nutrients to rapidly growing tumours [87]. HDAC3 has demonstrated an important facilitative role on VM in gliomas, as HDAC3 expression is directly correlated with the number of VM in tumours with worsen tumour grade [88]. HDACi such as SAHA exert significant anti-VM effect in the progressive pancreatic cancer cells through its inhibition of AKT and ERK signalling pathways [89].

The role of HDACs play in tumour angiogenesis has also been studied. It is widely known that hypoxia induces tumour angiogenesis and cell survival through the up-regulation of VEGF expression in tumour cells [90]. Different studies have reported that inhibition of HDAC activity by TSA blocks hypoxia-induced tumour angiogenesis [91]. Other HDACi also exert similar effects, as exemplified by MPT0G157, a potent inhibitor of HDAC1, 2, 3, and 6, which was found to promote HIF-1α degradation followed by the downregulation of VEGF expression [92]. There are also reports of the anti-tumoural effects of other HDACi (TSA, sodium butyrate, and VPA) that are also partly mediated by the reduction of VEGFR-2 expression that might be related to repressing tumour angiogenesis [93].

SIRT1, a class III HDAC, also plays an important role in tumour initiation, progression, and development of drug resistance by hindering senescence, stress-induced apoptosis [94, 95], and activating cell growth and angiogenesis. MiR-34a, whose expression level was found to be reduced in various tumour cell lines [96, 97], was reported to exert its tumour suppression effect via direct binding onto SIRT1 mRNA and regulate cell apoptosis via SIRT1-p53 pathway [98]. miR-34a also exerts its anti-tumoural effect through inhibiting SIRT1 to induce the senescence of EPCs to suppress EPC-mediated tumour angiogenesis [99].

There are emerging HDACi for cancer therapy. HDACi-targeting class I, II, and IV HDACs to be used as anticancer agents are currently under development. One of them, vorinostat, has been approved by FDA for treating cutaneous T-cell lymphoma for patients with persistent or recurrent disease or following two systemic therapies. Other inhibitors, for example, FK228, PXD101, PCI-24781, ITF2357, MGCD0103, MS-275, valproic acid, and LBH589 have also demonstrated therapeutic potential as monotherapy or combination with other anti-tumour drugs [86, 100].

7.2. Age-related macular degeneration

Age-related macular degeneration (AMD) is the leading cause of blindness worldwide. AMD is characterised by the deposition of drusen aggregates under the retinal epithelium. Clusterin is one of the major proteins in drusens [101], and during aging, the expression of clusterin increases [102]. The impact of epigenetic modifications on the pathogenesis of AMD has been reported. It is known that aging affects histone acetylation status, so it is reasonable to presume that the epigenetic regulation might have a role in clusterin expression. It was reported that the treatment with HDACi induces prominent increases in the expression levels of clusterin mRNA and the secretion of clusterin protein. This result indicates that epigenetic factors regulate clusterin expression which could be affecting the pathogenesis of AMD via the inhibition of angiogenesis and inflammation [103].

7.3. Pulmonary arterial hypertension

Pulmonary arterial hypertension (PAH) is a condition characterised by increased pulmonary vascular resistance and pulmonary artery pressure leading to right heart failure and premature death [104]. During the process, there is a vascular remodelling caused by dysregulated cell proliferation, migration, and survival. The cause of PAH is complex, but the excessive proliferation of SMCs and ECs within the pulmonary artery is thought to play an essential role in its pathogenesis.

Elevated levels of HDAC1 and HDAC5 have been observed in the PAH lungs, and treatments with HDACi such as SAHA and VPA reduce disease worsening in rat models of pulmonary hypertension [105]. In addition, MEF2 might have a protective role in PAH progression as the expression of MEF2 and its transcriptional targets are significantly decreased in pulmonary artery ECs from patients with PAH. The impaired MEF2 activity in ECs from PAH was associated with increased nuclear accumulation of HDAC4 and HDAC5. So, increasing MEF2 activity by the selective inhibition of class IIa HDACs by MC1568 seems to suppress excessive EC migration and proliferation by PAH-ECs and can rescue experimental PAH model [106]. Although the increased migration and proliferation of pulmonary artery ECs in PAH are also hallmarks of angiogenesis, it is still contentious to link excessive angiogenesis with the pathogenesis of PAH [107], and any potential anti-angiogenic therapy for PAH should be proceeded with caution.

8. Concluding remarks and future perspectives

The past 15 years of research have significantly advanced our understanding of the functions and modes of regulation of HDACs in CVD. With all the studies discussed above, we can get an idea about how complex it is to translate HDACi as clinical therapeutics as they exert contradictory functions in many occasions. Extensive evidence for HDAC involvement in multiprotein complexes and cell-specific signalling indicates that a deeper understanding of these pathways will be crucial to effective pharmacological targeting in future.

Although angiogenesis seems to be a very promising therapeutic possibility for the majority of CVDs where patients are not responding to conventional treatments, there are also times that angiogenesis participates in the pathological processes. So in some diseases such as MI and diabetic cardiomyopathy, enhancement of angiogenesis is beneficial by improving recovery of injured myocardium. In the other circumstances where aberrant neoangiogensis is one of the main disease manifestations (such as cancer and AMD), potentiation of anti-angiogenic signalling could be beneficial. Thus, the crucial role that angiogenesis can play as a therapy can only be achieved by thoroughly understanding the underlying mechanisms.

In addition, the diverse and contrasting effects that the current available HDACi exert might be due to their low specificity to a particular HDAC. Class IIa HDACs are expressed in limited organs such as the muscles, brain, or bone, whereas class I HDACs exist ubiquitously. Thus, one may question the specificity and adverse effects of unspecific HDACi for therapeutic uses. Therefore in the future, creation of more specific HDACi, armed with better understanding of the underlying mechanisms of specific HDAC in angiogenesis within each pathological condition, could help the development of more targeted treatments to improve vascularisation and tissue repairs with higher efficiency and efficacy.

Alternative methods where HDAC modulation can be utilised in therapeutic angiogenesis are to modulate endothelial differentiation of stem or progenitor cells, which can be applied as cell therapy to enhance angiogenesis within the ischemic tissues. Next-generation gene-editing tool, such as CRISPR-Cas9, can also be extremely useful in accurately targeting specific gene responsible for suppressing or exacerbating angiogenesis depending on the diseases. Moreover, with diseases such as PAH that are characterised by both lack of angiogenesis (within the right ventricles) and excessive angiogenesis (within the pulmonary vasculature), the development of nanoparticles to deliver drugs to specific target tissues can be highly beneficial. This approach will also be extremely useful for patients that manifest both CVD and cancer.

We are currently in an exciting era for translational research with a lot of new inspiring technologies that can truly transform therapeutic approaches. With diligent efforts to devise the role of HDACs underlying angiogenesis robustly in various CVDs, in conjunction with the creation of more selective HDAC inhibitors, advanced engineering solutions, and gene-editing tools to correct genes responsible for repressing angiogenesis, and a commitment in rigorous placebo-controlled clinical trials, superior therapies for CVDs are on the horizon.

Author details

Ana Moraga, Ka Hou Lao and Lingfang Zeng*

*Address all correspondence to: lingfang.zeng@kcl.ac.uk

Cardiovascular Division, Faculty of Life Sciences and Medicine, King's College London, London, UK

References

[1] Goff DC, Lloyd-Jones DM, Bennett G, Coady S, D'Agostino RB, Gibbons R, et al. 2013 ACC/AHA guideline on the assessment of cardiovascular risk: a report of the American College of Cardiology/American Heart Association Task Force on Practice Guidelines. Circulation. 2014;129(25 Suppl 2):S49–73.

[2] O'Donnell CJ, Nabel EG. Genomics of cardiovascular disease. N Engl J Med. 2011;365(22):2098–109.

[3] Jones PA, Baylin SB. The fundamental role of epigenetic events in cancer. Nat Rev Genet. 2002;3(6):415–28.

[4] Zhang LX, DeNicola M, Qin X, Du J, Ma J, Tina Zhao Y, et al. Specific inhibition of HDAC4 in cardiac progenitor cells enhances myocardial repairs. Am J Physiol Cell Physiol. 2014;307(4):C358–72.

[5] Lehmann LH, Worst BC, Stanmore DA, Backs J. Histone deacetylase signaling in cardioprotection. Cell Mol Life Sci. 2014;71(9):1673–90.

[6] Aird WC. Phenotypic heterogeneity of the endothelium: I. Structure, function, and mechanisms. Circ Res. 2007;100(2):158–73.

[7] van Hinsbergh VW. Endothelium—role in regulation of coagulation and inflammation. Semin Immunopathol. 2012;34(1):93–106.

[8] Alderton WK, Cooper CE, Knowles RG. Nitric oxide synthases: structure, function and inhibition. Biochem J. 2001;357(Pt 3):593–615.

[9] Versari D, Daghini E, Virdis A, Ghiadoni L, Taddei S. Endothelial dysfunction as a target for prevention of cardiovascular disease. Diabetes Care. 2009;32 Suppl 2:S314–21.

[10] Risau W, Flamme I. Vasculogenesis. Annu Rev Cell Dev Biol. 1995;11:73–91.

[11] Carmeliet P. Mechanisms of angiogenesis and arteriogenesis. Nat Med. 2000;6(4):389–95.

[12] Al Sabti H. Therapeutic angiogenesis in cardiovascular disease. J Cardiothorac Surg. 2007;2:49.

[13] Sone H, Kawakami Y, Okuda Y, Kondo S, Hanatani M, Suzuki H, et al. Vascular endothelial growth factor is induced by long-term high glucose concentration and up-regulated by acute glucose deprivation in cultured bovine retinal pigmented epithelial cells. Biochem Biophys Res Commun. 1996;221(1):193–8.

[14] Sunderkötter C, Goebeler M, Schulze-Osthoff K, Bhardwaj R, Sorg C. Macrophage-derived angiogenesis factors. Pharmacol Ther. 1991;51(2):195–216.

[15] Tuder RM, Flook BE, Voelkel NF. Increased gene expression for VEGF and the VEGF receptors KDR/Flk and Flt in lungs exposed to acute or to chronic hypoxia. Modulation of gene expression by nitric oxide. J Clin Invest. 1995;95(4):1798–807.

[16] Carmeliet P, Jain RK. Molecular mechanisms and clinical applications of angiogenesis. Nature. 2011;473(7347):298–307.

[17] Fraineau S, Palii CG, Allan DS, Brand M. Epigenetic regulation of endothelial-cell-mediated vascular repair. FEBS J. 2015;282(9):1605–29.

[18] Schiano C, Vietri MT, Grimaldi V, Picascia A, Pascale MR, Napoli C. Epigenetic-related therapeutic challenges in cardiovascular disease. Trends Pharmacol Sci. 2015;36(4):226–35.

[19] Fish JE, Yan MS, Matouk CC, St Bernard R, Ho JJ, Gavryushova A, et al. Hypoxic repression of endothelial nitric-oxide synthase transcription is coupled with eviction of promoter histones. J Biol Chem. 2010;285(2):810–26.

[20] Miranda TB, Jones PA. DNA methylation: the nuts and bolts of repression. J Cell Physiol. 2007;213(2):384–90.

[21] Baccarelli A, Rienstra M, Benjamin EJ. Cardiovascular epigenetics: basic concepts and results from animal and human studies. Circ Cardiovasc Genet. 2010;3(6):567–73.

[22] Bassett SA, Barnett MP. The role of dietary histone deacetylases (HDACs) inhibitors in health and disease. Nutrients. 2014;6(10):4273–301.

[23] Zhou B, Margariti A, Zeng L, Xu Q. Role of histone deacetylases in vascular cell homeostasis and arteriosclerosis. Cardiovasc Res. 2011;90(3):413–20.

[24] Jin KL, Pak JH, Park JY, Choi WH, Lee JY, Kim JH, et al. Expression profile of histone deacetylases 1, 2 and 3 in ovarian cancer tissues. J Gynecol Oncol. 2008;19(3):185–90.

[25] Song Y, Shiota M, Tamiya S, Kuroiwa K, Naito S, Tsuneyoshi M. The significance of strong histone deacetylase 1 expression in the progression of prostate cancer. Histopathology. 2011;58(5):773–80.

[26] de Ruijter AJ, van Gennip AH, Caron HN, Kemp S, van Kuilenburg AB. Histone deacety-
      lases (HDACs): characterization of the classical HDAC family. Biochem J. 2003;370(Pt
      3):737–49.

[27] Bosch-Presegué L, Vaquero A. The dual role of sirtuins in cancer. Genes Cancer.
      2011;2(6):648–62.

[28] Tang J, Yan H, Zhuang S. Histone deacetylases as targets for treatment of multiple dis-
      eases. Clin Sci (Lond). 2013;124(11):651–62.

[29] Yang XJ, Seto E. HATs and HDACs: from structure, function and regulation to novel
      strategies for therapy and prevention. Oncogene. 2007;26(37):5310–8.

[30] Falkenberg KJ, Johnstone RW. Histone deacetylases and their inhibitors in cancer, neu-
      rological diseases and immune disorders. Nat Rev Drug Discov. 2014;13(9):673–91.

[31] Xiao Q, Zeng L, Zhang Z, Margariti A, Ali ZA, Channon KM, et al. Sca-1+ progenitors
      derived from embryonic stem cells differentiate into endothelial cells capable of vascular
      repair after arterial injury. Arterioscler Thromb Vasc Biol. 2006;26(10):2244–51.

[32] Zeng L, Xiao Q, Margariti A, Zhang Z, Zampetaki A, Patel S, et al. HDAC3 is crucial in
      shear- and VEGF-induced stem cell differentiation toward endothelial cells. J Cell Biol.
      2006;174(7):1059–69.

[33] Zampetaki A, Zeng L, Margariti A, Xiao Q, Li H, Zhang Z, et al. Histone deacetylase 3 is
      critical in endothelial survival and atherosclerosis development in response to disturbed
      flow. Circulation. 2010;121(1):132–42.

[34] Glesne DA, Zhang W, Mandava S, Ursos L, Buell ME, Makowski L, et al. Subtractive
      transcriptomics: establishing polarity drives in vitro human endothelial morphogenesis.
      Cancer Res. 2006;66(8):4030–40.

[35] Deroanne CF, Bonjean K, Servotte S, Devy L, Colige A, Clausse N, et al. Histone deacet-
      ylases inhibitors as anti-angiogenic agents altering vascular endothelial growth factor
      signaling. Oncogene. 2002;21(3):427–36.

[36] Jin G, Bausch D, Knightly T, Liu Z, Li Y, Liu B, et al. Histone deacetylase inhibitors
      enhance endothelial cell sprouting angiogenesis in vitro. Surgery. 2011;150(3):429–35.

[37] Sun X, Wei L, Chen Q, Terek RM. HDAC4 represses vascular endothelial growth fac-
      tor expression in chondrosarcoma by modulating RUNX2 activity. J Biol Chem.
      2009;284(33):21881–90.

[38] Geng H, Harvey CT, Pittsenbarger J, Liu Q, Beer TM, Xue C, et al. HDAC4 protein regu-
      lates HIF1α protein lysine acetylation and cancer cell response to hypoxia. J Biol Chem.
      2011;286(44):38095–102.

[39] Dekker RJ, van Soest S, Fontijn RD, Salamanca S, de Groot PG, VanBavel E, et al.
      Prolonged fluid shear stress induces a distinct set of endothelial cell genes, most specifi-
      cally lung Krüppel-like factor (KLF2). Blood. 2002;100(5):1689–98.

[40] Urbich C, Rössig L, Kaluza D, Potente M, Boeckel JN, Knau A, et al. HDAC5 is a repressor of angiogenesis and determines the angiogenic gene expression pattern of endothelial cells. Blood. 2009;113(22):5669–79.

[41] Margariti A, Zampetaki A, Xiao Q, Zhou B, Karamariti E, Martin D, et al. Histone deacetylase 7 controls endothelial cell growth through modulation of beta-catenin. Circ Res. 2010;106(7):1202–11.

[42] Wang S, Li X, Parra M, Verdin E, Bassel-Duby R, Olson EN. Control of endothelial cell proliferation and migration by VEGF signaling to histone deacetylase 7. Proc Natl Acad Sci USA. 2008;105(22):7738–43.

[43] Mottet D, Bellahcène A, Pirotte S, Waltregny D, Deroanne C, Lamour V, et al. Histone deacetylase 7 silencing alters endothelial cell migration, a key step in angiogenesis. Circ Res. 2007;101(12):1237–46.

[44] Kaluza D, Kroll J, Gesierich S, Yao TP, Boon RA, Hergenreider E, et al. Class IIb HDAC6 regulates endothelial cell migration and angiogenesis by deacetylation of cortactin. EMBO J. 2011;30(20):4142–56.

[45] Li D, Xie S, Ren Y, Huo L, Gao J, Cui D, et al. Microtubule-associated deacetylase HDAC6 promotes angiogenesis by regulating cell migration in an EB1-dependent manner. Protein Cell. 2011;2(2):150–60.

[46] Potente M, Ghaeni L, Baldessari D, Mostoslavsky R, Rossig L, Dequiedt F, et al. SIRT1 controls endothelial angiogenic functions during vascular growth. Genes Dev. 2007;21(20):2644–58.

[47] Deveza L, Choi J, Yang F. Therapeutic angiogenesis for treating cardiovascular diseases. Theranostics. 2012;2(8):801–14.

[48] Liao YY, Chen ZY, Wang YX, Lin Y, Yang F, Zhou QL. New progress in angiogenesis therapy of cardiovascular disease by ultrasound targeted microbubble destruction. Biomed Res Int. 2014;2014:872984.

[49] Libby P, Ridker PM, Hansson GK. Progress and challenges in translating the biology of atherosclerosis. Nature. 2011;473(7347):317–25.

[50] Lusis AJ. Atherosclerosis. Nature. 2000;407(6801):233–41.

[51] Glass CK, Witztum JL. Atherosclerosis. the road ahead. Cell. 2001;104(4):503–16.

[52] Simons M, Ware JA. Therapeutic angiogenesis in cardiovascular disease. Nat Rev Drug Discov. 2003;2(11):863–71.

[53] Celletti FL, Waugh JM, Amabile PG, Brendolan A, Hilfiker PR, Dake MD. Vascular endothelial growth factor enhances atherosclerotic plaque progression. Nat Med. 2001;7(4):425–9.

[54] Plump AS, Smith JD, Hayek T, Aalto-Setälä K, Walsh A, Verstuyft JG, et al. Severe hypercholesterolemia and atherosclerosis in apolipoprotein E-deficient mice created by homologous recombination in ES cells. Cell. 1992;71(2):343–53.

[55] Zhang SH, Reddick RL, Piedrahita JA, Maeda N. Spontaneous hypercholesterolemia and arterial lesions in mice lacking apolipoprotein E. Science. 1992;258(5081):468–71.

[56] Stein S, Lohmann C, Schäfer N, Hofmann J, Rohrer L, Besler C, et al. SIRT1 decreases Lox-1-mediated foam cell formation in atherogenesis. Eur Heart J. 2010;31(18):2301–9.

[57] Zhang QJ, Wang Z, Chen HZ, Zhou S, Zheng W, Liu G, et al. Endothelium-specific over-expression of class III deacetylase SIRT1 decreases atherosclerosis in apolipoprotein E-deficient mice. Cardiovasc Res. 2008;80(2):191–9.

[58] Stein S, Schäfer N, Breitenstein A, Besler C, Winnik S, Lohmann C, et al. SIRT1 reduces endothelial activation without affecting vascular function in ApoE−/− mice. Aging (Albany, NY). 2010;2(6):353–60.

[59] Okamoto H, Fujioka Y, Takahashi A, Takahashi T, Taniguchi T, Ishikawa Y, et al. Trichostatin A, an inhibitor of histone deacetylase, inhibits smooth muscle cell prolifera-tion via induction of p21(WAF1). J Atheroscler Thromb. 2006;13(4):183–91.

[60] Findeisen HM, Gizard F, Zhao Y, Qing H, Heywood EB, Jones KL, et al. Epigenetic regu-lation of vascular smooth muscle cell proliferation and neointima formation by histone deacetylase inhibition. Arterioscler Thromb Vasc Biol. 2011;31(4):851–60.

[61] Song S, Kang SW, Choi C. Trichostatin A enhances proliferation and migration of vascular smooth muscle cells by downregulating thioredoxin 1. Cardiovasc Res. 2010;85(1):241–9.

[62] Rössig L, Li H, Fisslthaler B, Urbich C, Fleming I, Förstermann U, et al. Inhibitors of histone deacetylation downregulate the expression of endothelial nitric oxide synthase and compromise endothelial cell function in vasorelaxation and angiogenesis. Circ Res. 2002;91(9):837–44.

[63] Chittur SV, Sangster-Guity N, McCormick PJ. Histone deacetylase inhibitors: a new mode for inhibition of cholesterol metabolism. BMC Genomics. 2008;9:507.

[64] Aranguren XL, McCue JD, Hendrickx B, Zhu XH, Du F, Chen E, et al. Multipotent adult progenitor cells sustain function of ischemic limbs in mice. J Clin Invest. 2008;118(2):505–14.

[65] Suzuki H, Shibata R, Kito T, Yamamoto T, Ishii M, Nishio N, et al. Comparative angio-genic activities of induced pluripotent stem cells derived from young and old mice. PLoS One. 2012;7(6):e39562.

[66] Granger A, Abdullah I, Huebner F, Stout A, Wang T, Huebner T, et al. Histone deacet-ylase inhibition reduces myocardial ischemia-reperfusion injury in mice. FASEB J. 2008;22(10):3549–60.

[67] Zhang L, Qin X, Zhao Y, Fast L, Zhuang S, Liu P, et al. Inhibition of histone deacetylases preserves myocardial performance and prevents cardiac remodeling through stimula-tion of endogenous angiomyogenesis. J Pharmacol Exp Ther. 2012;341(1):285–93.

[68] Zhang L, Chen B, Zhao Y, Dubielecka PM, Wei L, Qin GJ, et al. Inhibition of histone deacetylase-induced myocardial repair is mediated by c-kit in infarcted hearts. J Biol Chem. 2012;287(47):39338–48.

[69] McKinsey TA, Zhang CL, Olson EN. MEF2: a calcium-dependent regulator of cell division, differentiation and death. Trends Biochem Sci. 2002;27(1):40–7.

[70] Zhang CL, McKinsey TA, Chang S, Antos CL, Hill JA, Olson EN. Class II histone deacetylases act as signal-responsive repressors of cardiac hypertrophy. Cell. 2002;110(4):479–88.

[71] Kee HJ, Sohn IS, Nam KI, Park JE, Qian YR, Yin Z, et al. Inhibition of histone deacetylation blocks cardiac hypertrophy induced by angiotensin II infusion and aortic banding. Circulation. 2006;113(1):51–9.

[72] Kao YH, Liou JP, Chung CC, Lien GS, Kuo CC, Chen SA, et al. Histone deacetylase inhibition improved cardiac functions with direct antifibrotic activity in heart failure. Int J Cardiol. 2013;168(4):4178–83.

[73] Oka T, Akazawa H, Naito AT, Komuro I. Angiogenesis and cardiac hypertrophy: maintenance of cardiac function and causative roles in heart failure. Circ Res. 2014;114(3):565–71.

[74] Lin JB, Phillips EH, Riggins TE, Sangha GS, Chakraborty S, Lee JY, et al. Imaging of small animal peripheral artery disease models: recent advancements and translational potential. Int J Mol Sci. 2015;16(5):11131–77.

[75] Spallotta F, Tardivo S, Nanni S, Rosati JD, Straino S, Mai A, et al. Detrimental effect of class-selective histone deacetylase inhibitors during tissue regeneration following hindlimb ischemia. J Biol Chem. 2013;288(32):22915–29.

[76] Krupinski J, Kaluza J, Kumar P, Kumar S, Wang JM. Role of angiogenesis in patients with cerebral ischemic stroke. Stroke. 1994;25(9):1794–8.

[77] Sun Y, Jin K, Xie L, Childs J, Mao XO, Logvinova A, et al. VEGF-induced neuroprotection, neurogenesis, and angiogenesis after focal cerebral ischemia. J Clin Invest. 2003;111(12):1843–51.

[78] Wang Z, Tsai LK, Munasinghe J, Leng Y, Fessler EB, Chibane F, et al. Chronic valproate treatment enhances postischemic angiogenesis and promotes functional recovery in a rat model of ischemic stroke. Stroke. 2012;43(9):2430–6.

[79] Kim HJ, Rowe M, Ren M, Hong JS, Chen PS, Chuang DM. Histone deacetylase inhibitors exhibit anti-inflammatory and neuroprotective effects in a rat permanent ischemic model of stroke: multiple mechanisms of action. J Pharmacol Exp Ther. 2007;321(3):892–901.

[80] Hernández-Jiménez M, Hurtado O, Cuartero MI, Ballesteros I, Moraga A, Pradillo JM, et al. Silent information regulator 1 protects the brain against cerebral ischemic damage. Stroke. 2013;44(8):2333–7.

[81] Ziemka-Nalecz M, Jaworska J, Sypecka J, Polowy R, Filipkowski RK, Zalewska T. Sodium butyrate, a histone deacetylase inhibitor, exhibits neuroprotective/neurogenic effects in a rat model of neonatal hypoxia-ischemia. Mol Neurobiol. 2016.

[82] Nyengaard JR, Rasch R. The impact of experimental diabetes mellitus in rats on glomerular capillary number and sizes. Diabetologia. 1993;36(3):189–94.

[83] Gilbert RE, Huang Q, Thai K, Advani SL, Lee K, Yuen DA, et al. Histone deacetylase inhibition attenuates diabetes-associated kidney growth: potential role for epigenetic modification of the epidermal growth factor receptor. Kidney Int. 2011;79(12):1312–21.

[84] Chen Y, Du J, Zhao YT, Zhang L, Lv G, Zhuang S, et al. Histone deacetylase (HDAC) inhibition improves myocardial function and prevents cardiac remodeling in diabetic mice. Cardiovasc Diabetol. 2015;14:99.

[85] Lee TI, Kao YH, Tsai WC, Chung CC, Chen YC, Chen YJ. HDAC inhibition modulates cardiac PPARs and fatty acid metabolism in diabetic cardiomyopathy. PPAR Res. 2016;2016:5938740.

[86] West AC, Johnstone RW. New and emerging HDAC inhibitors for cancer treatment. J Clin Invest. 2014;124(1):30–9.

[87] Maniotis AJ, Folberg R, Hess A, Seftor EA, Gardner LM, Pe'er J, et al. Vascular channel formation by human melanoma cells in vivo and in vitro: vasculogenic mimicry. Am J Pathol. 1999;155(3):739–52.

[88] Liu X, Wang JH, Li S, Li LL, Huang M, Zhang YH, et al. Histone deacetylase 3 expression correlates with vasculogenic mimicry through the phosphoinositide3-kinase/ERK-MMP-laminin5γ2 signaling pathway. Cancer Sci. 2015;106(7):857–66.

[89] Xu XD, Yang L, Zheng LY, Pan YY, Cao ZF, Zhang ZQ, et al. Suberoylanilide hydroxamic acid, an inhibitor of histone deacetylase, suppresses vasculogenic mimicry and proliferation of highly aggressive pancreatic cancer PaTu8988 cells. BMC Cancer. 2014;14:373.

[90] Harris AL. Hypoxia—a key regulatory factor in tumour growth. Nat Rev Cancer. 2002;2(1):38–47.

[91] Sawa H, Murakami H, Ohshima Y, Murakami M, Yamazaki I, Tamura Y, et al. Histone deacetylase inhibitors such as sodium butyrate and trichostatin A inhibit vascular endothelial growth factor (VEGF) secretion from human glioblastoma cells. Brain Tumor Pathol. 2002;19(2):77–81.

[92] Huang YC, Huang FI, Mehndiratta S, Lai SC, Liou JP, Yang CR. Anticancer activity of MPT0G157, a derivative of indolylbenzenesulfonamide, inhibits tumor growth and angiogenesis. Oncotarget. 2015;6(21):18590–601.

[93] Hrgovic I, Doll M, Pinter A, Kaufmann R, Kippenberger S, Meissner M. Histone deacet-ylase inhibitors interfere with angiogenesis by decreasing endothelial VEGFR-2 protein half-life in part via a VE-cadherin dependent mechanism. Exp Dermatol. 2016.

[94] Luo J, Nikolaev AY, Imai S, Chen D, Su F, Shiloh A, et al. Negative control of p53 by Sir2alpha promotes cell survival under stress. Cell. 2001;107(2):137–48.

[95] Huffman DM, Grizzle WE, Bamman MM, Kim JS, Eltoum IA, Elgavish A, et al. SIRT1 is significantly elevated in mouse and human prostate cancer. Cancer Res. 2007;67(14):6612–8.

[96] Li N, Fu H, Tie Y, Hu Z, Kong W, Wu Y, et al. miR-34a inhibits migration and inva-sion by down-regulation of c-Met expression in human hepatocellular carcinoma cells. Cancer Lett. 2009;275(1):44–53.

[97] Tazawa H, Tsuchiya N, Izumiya M, Nakagama H. Tumor-suppressive miR-34a induces senescence-like growth arrest through modulation of the E2F pathway in human colon cancer cells. Proc Natl Acad Sci USA. 2007;104(39):15472–7.

[98] Yamakuchi M, Lowenstein CJ. MiR-34, SIRT1 and p53: the feedback loop. Cell Cycle. 2009;8(5):712–5.

[99] Zhao T, Li J, Chen AF. MicroRNA-34a induces endothelial progenitor cell senescence and impedes its angiogenesis via suppressing silent information regulator 1. Am J Physiol Endocrinol Metab. 2010;299(1):E110–6.

[100] Tan J, Cang S, Ma Y, Petrillo RL, Liu D. Novel histone deacetylase inhibitors in clinical trials as anti-cancer agents. J Hematol Oncol. 2010;3:5.

[101] Crabb JW, Miyagi M, Gu X, Shadrach K, West KA, Sakaguchi H, et al. Drusen proteome analysis: an approach to the etiology of age-related macular degeneration. Proc Natl Acad Sci USA. 2002;99(23):14682–7.

[102] Trougakos IP, Gonos ES. Regulation of clusterin/apolipoprotein J, a functional homo-logue to the small heat shock proteins, by oxidative stress in ageing and age-related diseases. Free Radic Res. 2006;40(12):1324–34.

[103] Suuronen T, Nuutinen T, Ryhänen T, Kaarniranta K, Salminen A. Epigenetic regula-tion of clusterin/apolipoprotein J expression in retinal pigment epithelial cells. Biochem Biophys Res Commun. 2007;357(2):397–401.

[104] Voelkel NF, Gomez-Arroyo J, Abbate A, Bogaard HJ, Nicolls MR. Pathobiology of pulmonary arterial hypertension and right ventricular failure. Eur Respir J. 2012;40(6):1555–65.

[105] Zhao L, Chen CN, Hajji N, Oliver E, Cotroneo E, Wharton J, et al. Histone deacetylation inhibition in pulmonary hypertension: therapeutic potential of valproic acid and sube-roylanilide hydroxamic acid. Circulation. 2012;126(4):455–67.

[106] Kim J, Hwangbo +C, Hu X, Kang Y, Papangeli I, Mehrotra D, et al. Restoration of impaired endothelial myocyte enhancer factor 2 function rescues pulmonary arterial hypertension. Circulation. 2015;131(2):190–9.

[107] Voelkel NF, Gomez-Arroyo J. The role of vascular endothelial growth factor in pulmonary arterial hypertension. The angiogenesis paradox. Am J Respir Cell Mol Biol. 2014;51(4):474–84.

4

Antiangiogenic Therapy for Hepatocellular Carcinoma

Kosuke Kaji and Hitoshi Yoshiji

Additional information is available at the end of the chapter

Abstract

Angiogenesis plays a pivotal role in many pathological processes, including hepatocellular carcinoma (HCC). This indicates that antiangiogenic agents could be promising candidates for chemoprevention against HCC. Several inhibitors targeting receptor tyrosine kinases (RTKs) for the regulation of tumoral vascularization have been developed and employed in clinical practice, including sorafenib. However, there seem to be several issues for the long-term use of this agent as some patients have experienced adverse effects while taking sorafenib. Therefore, it is desirable for patients with chronic liver diseases to be administered sorafenib as little as possible by combining other safe-to-use antiangiogenic compounds. Various factors, such as renin-angiotensin-aldosterone system (RAAS) and insulin resistance (IR), reciprocally contribute to the promotion of angiogenesis. A blockade of RAAS with an angiotensin-converting enzyme inhibitor (ACE-I) or angiotensin-II (AT-II) receptor blocker (ARB) markedly attenuates HCC in conjunction with the suppression of angiogenesis. Moreover, the IR status has demonstrated direct acceleration in the progression of HCC via the augmentation of tumoral neovascularization. These findings suggest that a combination therapy involving a lower dose of sorafenib with other clinically used agents [e.g., RAAS blockers, insulin sensitizer agents, and branched-chain amino acids (BCAA)] may reduce the adverse effects of sorafenib without attenuating the inhibitory effect against HCC in comparison to a high-dose administration.

Keywords: hepatocellular carcinoma, fibrosis, renin-angiotensin system

1. Introduction

Angiogenesis is the development of new vasculature from preexisting blood vessels or circulating endothelial cell (EC) stem cells. Emerging evidence indicates that angiogenesis develops in many organs and under multiple pathologic situations, as well as during conditions of tissue growth and regeneration. Abnormal pathological angiogenesis is observed in patients with rheumatoid arthritis, psoriasis, diabetic retinopathy, fibrogenesis, and tumor growth [1]. Although early studies were conducted to determine the molecular processes associated with carcinogenesis and angiogenesis that were performed independently, more recent studies have revealed that both biological phenomena emerge synergistically [2].

Hepatocellular carcinoma (HCC) is the sixth most common cancer and the second leading cause of cancer-related mortality worldwide, accounting for more than 600,000 new cases annually. The greatest risk factors for developing HCC include liver cirrhosis induced by hepatitis B virus (HBV) or hepatitis C virus (HCV) infections, excessive alcohol intake, and metabolic syndrome. Regardless of the etiology, since HCC commonly develops in patients with a chronic liver disease (e.g., liver cirrhosis) only approximately one-third of the patients diagnosed with HCC are eligible for curative treatments (e.g., surgical resection) [3]. Consequently, several alternative therapies have been employed, including percutaneous radiofrequency ablation (RFA) and transarterial chemoembolization (TACE). However, no satisfactory improvement of HCC prognosis has been achieved to date. The notable characteristic of HCC that accounts for its poor prognosis is the risk of high frequency in recurrence attributed to intrahepatic metastasis or the multicentric development. The key feature of HCC progression is also hypervascularity formed by intratumoral angiogenesis as well as the frequent recurrence. Several studies have demonstrated that angiogenesis is implicated in the survival and growth of HCC. It has also been reported that angiogenesis can be induced during the early stages of tumor formation and the various carcinogenic mechanisms have been demonstrated in several different experimental models [4–7]. Therefore, several antiangiogenic agents (i.e., sorafenib) have been developed as novel treatment options for HCC.

In this chapter, mechanistic insights into angiogenesis and its contribution to hepatocarcinogenesis will initially be reviewed. In addition, newly developed antiangiogenic agents will be described in detail.

2. Angiogenesis in HCC

In HCC, tumor angiogenesis leads to a pathologic vascularization pattern, of which intratumoral vascularization is critical for the diagnosis and treatment of HCC, as well as for pathogenesis and patient prognosis [1, 8, 9]. In general, HCC is supplied with blood flow primarily via the hepatic arteries, while noncancerous lesions and the normal liver parenchyma are supplied predominantly by the portal vein. This distinct vascularization is clinically utilized to diagnose HCC radiographically by emphasizing the tumor lesions. Any tumor mass more than 1–2 mm^3 depends entirely on the formation of a vascular network that provides the growing tumor with oxygen and essential nutrients [10].

Of the various proangiogenic factors, vascular endothelial growth factor (VEGF) is one of the most potent and required for both physiological and pathological angiogenesis [11]. VEGF induces EC proliferation, promotes migration and differentiation as well as stimulates permeabilization of blood vessels and vasculogenesis. The several forms of VEGF bind to two tyrosine kinase receptors, *fms*-like tyrosine kinase (flt-1: VEGFR-1) and the kinase insert domain-containing receptor/murine homolog, fetal liver kinase-1 (KDR/Flk-1: VEGFR-2) [11, 12]. Recent reports have demonstrated that upregulated VEGF expression is more frequently observed in the tumor lesions of HCC than noncancerous lesions [13–15]. Moreover, the marked increase of VEGF expression is shown during both hepatocarcino-genesis and HCC growth in accordance with the augmented neovascularization. Our basic studies elucidated that monoclonal antibodies (mAb) against both VEGFR-1 and VEGFR-2 ameliorated the HCC development with antiangiogenic activity in rodents [16]. These findings indicate that a blockade of the VEGF-VEGFR axis contributes to the suppressive effect on HCC development.

In tumor neovascularization, VEGF often coordinates with other angiogenic pathways. The angiopoietins (Ang) bind with receptor tyrosine kinases (RTKs) with immunoglobulin-like and EGF-like domains (Tie1 and Tie2). Increased levels of Ang2 promote tumor angiogenesis, metastasis, and inflammation with augmentation of VEGF activity. VEGF-A is also upregu-lated by interaction with multiple growth factors, including fibroblast growth factor (FGF), insulin-like growth factor-1 (IGF-1), platelet-derived growth factor (PDGF), and the trans-forming growth factors (TGF) [17]. Tissue hypoxia also stimulates VEGF-A upregulation via the hypoxia-inducible factors (HIF)-1α and HIF-2α [17].

3. Molecular targeted therapy

Several small-molecule, orally available RTK inhibitors exhibit an antiangiogenic effect of inhibiting VEGF and other kinases. They are expected to have high clinical utility and are currently being tested in clinical trials of varying stages for the treatment of advanced HCC (**Table 1**).

Agent	Target
Sorafenib	A-RAF, B-RAF, C-RAF/Raf-1VEGFR-2, VEGFR-3, PDGFR-β, Flt-3, c-Kit
Sunitinib	VEGFR-1, 2, and 3, PDGFR-α, β, c-Kit, Flt3
Brivanib	VEGFR-1, 2, and 3, FGFR-1, 2, and 3
Lenvatinib	VEGFR-1, 2, and 3, FGFR-1, 2, 3, and 4,PDGFR-α, c-Kit, RET
Cabozantinib	VEGFR-2, MET, RET

Table 1. Molecularly targeted antiangiogenic agents for advanced HCC.

3.1. Sorafenib

Sorafenib (Nexavar®) was developed in 1995 and is the only chemotherapeutic drug that has demonstrated to improve the survival rate in patients with HCC [18, 19]. Sorafenib acts by inhibiting the RAF serine/threonine kinases that play a key role in the transduction of mito-genic and oncogenic pathways through the Raf/mitogen-activated protein kinase (MEK)/

extracellular signal-regulated kinase (ERK)/mitogen-activated protein kinase (MAPK) signaling pathway [20]. Such signaling results in a lower cyclin D1 expression as well as cell cycle arrest. Sorafenib also potently inhibits VEGFR-2, VEGFR-3, PDGFR-β, Flt-3, and c-Kit, which promote angiogenesis [19, 20]. The repression blocks a broad spectrum of different processes involved in proliferation, angiogenesis, or apoptosis, causing a reduction in the blood vessel regions of the tumor and the starving of cancerous cells. Furthermore, sorafenib enhances tumor necrosis factor (TNF)-related apoptosis-inducing ligand (TRAIL)-induced cell death through an SH2 domain, which causes a tyrosine phosphatase (SHP-1)-dependent reduction of signal transducers and activators of transcription type 3 (STAT3) phosphorylation and the related protein myeloid cell leukemia 1 (Mcl-1) (i.e., survivin and cyclin D1) in HCC cells [21]. Sorafenib is also able to repress Mcl-1 activity through an MAPK-independent mechanism, which increases the intrinsic apoptosis pathway in tumor cells. Moreover, recent studies have claimed that the eukaryotic translation initiation factor 4E (eIF4E) might be implicated in sorafenib-dependent Mcl-1 inhibition [22]. Clinically, sorafenib can extend the mean patient survival from 7.9 to 10.7 months [19]. Representative adverse events caused by the treatment of sorafenib consist of diarrhea, weight loss, hand-foot skin reaction, and hypophosphatemia. Currently, sorafenib is the first and only agent to demonstrate a beneficial overall survival (OS) and be approved by regulators globally in patients with advanced HCC [19].

3.2. Sunitinib

Sunitinib (Sutent®) is an oral multi-RTK inhibitor targeting VEGFR-1, 2, and 3, PDGFRs, c-Kit, and other RTKs associated with angiogenesis [23]. Several phase II clinical trials have shown favorable results regarding the antitumor activity of this drug against advanced HCC. In one phase III trial, the median OS was 7.9 and 10.2 in the sunitinib and sorafenib groups, respectively [24]. This indicates that sunitinib had no benefit over sorafenib as a first-line therapy for advanced HCC.

3.3. Brivanib

Brivanib, a dual tyrosine kinase inhibitor, shows potent and selective inhibition of VEGFR and FGFR [25]. Brivanib has exerted an anticancerous effect in xenograft human HCC models expressing FGF receptors [26]. Two phase III trials have been performed: (1) the BRISK-FL study, in which brivanib vs. sorafenib as first-line therapy was evaluated in patients with advanced HCC and (2) the BRISK-PS study, in which brivanib was administered to patients with advanced HCC who were resistant to sorafenib [27, 28]. However, both trials failed to meet the primary endpoint of statistically improving the OS rate.

3.4. Lenvatinib

Lenvatinib (Lenvima®) is an oral multityrosine kinase inhibitor with potent antiangiogenic effects that has recently been approved for use in differentiated thyroid cancer [29]. The drug was established in patient-derived xenograft models that reliably recapitulated the genetic and phenotypic features of HCC [30]. Moreover, in models expressing high levels of FGF receptor

1, lenvatinib exhibited a greater efficacy than sorafenib. Lenvatinib has also shown highly promising data in phase I/II clinical trials involving patients with advanced HCC [31].

3.5. Cabozantinib

Cabozantinib (Cometriq®) was approved in 2012 by the FDA and is a small-molecule RTK inhibitor with potent activity toward VEGFR-2, MET, and RET (rearranged during transfection), leading to the inhibition of tumor angiogenesis [32]. In a phase II study, the observed disease control rate following 12 weeks of treatment with cabozantinib was found to be 68 or 78% of the patients with or without prior sorafenib treatment exhibited tumor regression. A phase III randomized double-blind, controlled trial is ongoing to compare the efficacy of cabozantinib with a placebo as the second-line treatment modality for advanced HCC patients who have previously received sorafenib.

4. Alternative therapy

Sorafenib is the standard therapeutic agent administered for the treatment of advanced stages of HCC and it is likely that other RTK inhibitors will also become commonly utilized drugs. However, chronic liver damage usually lowers the capacity of drug metabolism in patients, and the long-term administration of sorafenib may induce excessive adverse effects. Therefore, to reduce dosage of sorafenib, an alternative approach may be required to identify a clinically available compound targeting tumor angiogenesis. Among the various factors to affect angiogenic activities, many researchers have focused their attention on the mechanisms of angiotensin-II (AT-II) and insulin resistance (IR). These factors have been shown to affect angiogenesis in the liver via close interactions [33]. Moreover, since these factors could also be involved in the HCC, the regulation of these factors might contribute to suppressing the progression of the chronic liver disease.

4.1. RAAS blockers

The renin-angiotensin-aldosterone system (RAAS) is a hormone system that is involved in the regulation of the plasma sodium concentration and arterial blood pressure to maintain body fluid homeostasis [34]. Recent reports have demonstrated that RAAS is locally expressed in a number of tissues, including the kidneys, adrenal glands, heart, vasculature and nervous system, and liver. Actually, RAAS is frequently activated in patients with chronic liver diseases, such as liver cirrhosis [35, 36]. AT-II is an octapeptide derived from its precursor, AT-I, after AT-I converting enzyme (ACE) acts AT-I, proteolytically cleaving the C-terminal dipeptide. During the progression of chronic liver diseases, AT-II is considered to be a potential mediator of portal hypertension. It has been reported that AT-II plasma levels are clinically increased in patients with cirrhosis, and an animal study has shown the elevation of the portal pressure by AT-II administration [37, 38].

AT-II plays a crucial role in the development of several cancers, including HCC. Lever et al. has previously shown the outcome of a retrospective cohort study consisting of 5207 patients with treatment of either an ACE inhibitor (ACE-I) or other antihypertensive agents such as calcium channel blockers, diuretics, and β-blockers with a 10-year follow-up (Glasgow study). Interestingly, in their study, the incidence of cancer and fetal cancer was decreased in the patients with ACE-I treatment as compared with those with other drugs [39]. A recent cohort study has also demonstrated a lower incidence of cancer in patients using ACE-I or an AT-II receptor blocker (ARB) than nonusers [40]. Furthermore, it has been reported that the addition of ACE-I or ARB provided the prolonged survival for the patients with advanced non–small cell lung cancer undergoing platinum-based chemotherapy [41]. Additionally, inhibition of RAAS possibly exerted the beneficial effects on the prognosis of patients with advanced hormone-refractory prostate cancer and pancreatic cancer receiving gemcitabine [42, 43]. In regard to liver cancer, ACE-I showed the suppressive effect on the tumor growth in a murine HCC experimental model [44].

The RAAS, especially AT-II, is potently involved in the regulation of both rarefaction and expansion of the vascular network. Circulating AT-II leads to drive a variety of signaling cascades leading to VEGF, FGF, IGF, and TGF-β expression through mainly binding to the AT1R on ECs [45–47]. AT-II/AT1-R axis plays a key role in the regulation of angiogenic activity in various pathological events, including tumor neovascularization. Actually, inhibition of AT-II by ACE-I and ARB reportedly attenuates **intratumoral neovascularization with down-regulation of** VEGF expression in several cancers [48–50]. These findings indicate that ACE-I and ARB can be candidates for novel antiangiogenic agents against HCC. However, previous report has suggested that monotherapy with only antiangiogenic agent does not exert the sufficient effect on the prognosis in patients with advanced cancer [51]. Therefore, the combination treatment of antiangiogenic agents has been approached to show a synergistic inhibitory effect on cancer progression [51, 52]. For example, the combination of ACE-I and interferon (IFN) suppressed HCC growth more potently than monotherapy with ACE-I [53]. Our report demonstrated that the antitumoral effect of 5-fluorouracil (5-FU) is also enhanced by combination with ACE-I [54].

As well as tumor growth and metastasis, the early stages of carcinogenesis are also regulated by RAAS-mediated angiogenesis [5, 55]. Our animal study has shown that ACE-I significantly suppressed hepatocarcinogenesis at a clinically comparable low dose together with an attenuated neovascularization [56]. Additionally, a combination of ACE-I with supplementation of vitamin K (VK), which is often administered to the patients with osteoporosis, showed a more potent inhibitory effect on rat hepatocarcinogenesis than ACE-I monotherapy [57]. This combination regimen consisting of ACE-I and VK also exhibited the beneficial effect on ameliorating hepatocarcinogenesis in our clinical study [58]. A 48-month follow-up study revealed that a combined ACE-I with VK significantly suppressed the cumulative recurrence of HCC with reduced serum VEGF levels. The serum level of lectin-reactive α-fetoprotein (AFP-L3), known as one of the HCC tumor markers, was also decreased in parallel with VEGF. Accordingly, this combination regimen may represent a new strategy for chemoprevention against HCC.

Aldosterone (Ald), a downstream component of AT-II in RAAS, also affects in the regulation of angiogenesis. **Endocrinologically**, Ald is a mineralocorticoid hormone regulating the plasma sodium (Na$^+$), the extracellular potassium (K$^+$) and arterial blood pressure, blood pressure, and electrolyte balance via mineralocorticoid receptors (MR) [59]. Recent data have suggested that Ald plays a key role in endothelial dysfunction, as well as a suggested involvement in the pathogenesis of hypertension [60]. Moreover, the possible involvement of Ald and the MR systems in pathological ocular neovascularization has been reported [61]. Ald was shown to stimulate the proliferation and tubulogenesis of EC, and exacerbated angiogenesis in oxygen-induced retinopathy. In addition, these events could be attenuated by spironolactone. Eplerenone, a selective Ald blocker (SAB), is clinically used as a novel option for the treatment of hypertension. SAB is a selective MR antagonist with higher affinity than spironolactone, contributing to lower side effect by binding the progesterone and androgen receptors. The animal study revealed that murine hepatocarcinogenesis was markedly suppressed by the treatment of SAB with attenuation of VEGF-mediated angiogenesis [62]. These results indicate that SAB is also a viable option for treatment of HCC.

4.2. Regulation of insulin resistance

Recent studies have revealed a close relationship between IR and the progression of liver disease, including HCC [63, 64]. In general, chronic liver diseases impair the metabolic homeostasis of glucose as a result of IR, glucose intolerance, and DM [65]. Several clinical studies have also identified the hyperinsulinemia in patients with chronic hepatitis C (CHC) [66–68]. Experimental evidence with the HCV-transgenic mouse model confirms the contribution of HCV in the development of IR and DM [69]. In this model, the overproduced TNF-α appears to play a pivotal role in the induction of IR and DM. TNF-α is a proinflammatory cytokine, dramatically elevated during inflammation-induced disease pathology. HCV itself induces the phosphorylation of the serine residues associated with the insulin receptor substrate (IRS)-1 and -2 and stimulates the overproduction of suppressor of cytokine-3 (SOC-3), inhibiting the phosphorylation of Akt/PI3K, leading to the blockade of transactivation of GLUT-4, which contributes to inhibit intracellular glucose uptake. Additionally, nonalcoholic fatty liver disease (NAFLD) is a common liver disorder associated with IR and DM [70]. Various factors participate in the progression of NAFLD, such as oxidative stress, endotoxemia, obesity, genetic factors, and IR. Several reports have suggested the association of IR and mitochondrial abnormalities [71].

Recently, a reciprocal relationship between diabetes and HCC has been noticed. A two to threefold increase in the risk of HCC has been observed in the patients with DM, regardless of the etiology of chronic liver diseases [72–74]. A large longitudinal study in the United States demonstrated the twofold higher incidence of HCC in the diabetic patients [74]. Moreover, a recent study has elucidated that the IR status directly facilitated hepatocarcinogenesis [64]. Hyperinsulinemia can generally induce the synthesis and activation of IGF-1, which has a potential to progress a variety of cancer [75]. The altered expression pattern of IGF-1 signaling has been found in human HCC as well as hepatocarcinogenesis in rodent models [76]. Furthermore, IR status may progress hepatocarcinogenesis through the augmentation of hepatic neovascularization and VEGF expression in a rat carcinogenesis model [64].

The diabetic patients with compensated liver diseases initially are treated by a lifestyle change. However, restrictive diets may be liable to aggravate malnutrition in some patients. Thus, the oral antidiabetic drugs are administered to treat the diabetic patients with advanced liver diseases such as cirrhosis [77, 78]. To avoid hyperinsulinemia affecting adversely HCC growth, the drugs exerting insulin-sensitizing effects are preferable such as metformin, pioglitazone, dipeptidyl peptidase 4 inhibitor, or sodium glucose cotransporter inhibitor. Another report has demonstrated that the use of statins, a class of lipid-lowering medications by inhibiting HMG-CoA reductase that plays a central role in the production of cholesterol, significantly lowered the risk of HCC in the patients with DM [79].

The branched-chain amino acid (BCAA), an amino acid having aliphatic side chains with a branch (a central carbon atom bound to three or more carbon atoms), comprises three essential amino acids: leucine, isoleucine, and valine. Several clinical studies have suggested the beneficial effect of the long-term supplementation with BCAA granules on hypoalbuminemia and event-free survival in the patients with cirrhosis [80, 81]. BCAAs have also been shown to induce glucose uptake and improve glucose metabolism in a rat cirrhotic model. Intriguingly, the animal study using obese diabetic rat showed a chemopreventive effect of BCAAs against HCC with the downregulation of VEGF and antiangiogenic activity [82, 83]. Multicenter study in Japan also revealed that BCAAs decreased the incidence of HCC in patients with HCV-related cirrhosis as well as the type 2 DM and obesity [84]. However, a monotherapy with BCAA did not inhibit the recurrence of HCC after curative treatment. Therefore, to utilize BCAAs with sufficient effect against HCC, it is strongly recommended to combine them with other drugs. From previous research, AT-II also plays a key role in the development of IR. Actually, mice genetically lacking ACE exhibited the improvement of glucose tolerance through the reduced fat mass [85]. Moreover, additional administration of ACE-I or ARB to BCAAs is also shown to improve the IR status [33, 86]. Our randomized control trial study demonstrated that the combined BCAAs with ACE-I suppresses the cumulative recurrence of HCC in the patients with IR [87].

Taken together, these findings indicate that the combination of BCAAs supplementation and RAAS blockade may represent a potentially novel therapeutic strategy against HCC in the patients with IR.

5. Conclusions and future perspectives

Angiogenesis plays a crucial role in hepatocarcinogenesis and HCC progression, indicating the requirement of an antiangiogenic therapy as a tool for suppressing HCC. Sorafenib has become a breakthrough drug in the field of HCC, with an improvement in the median survival of almost 3 months. This represents a reduction of greater than 30% for the probability of death during the follow-up period.

However, when using RTK inhibitors, including sorafenib for patients with chronic liver diseases, many patients exhibit adverse effects, and several symptoms are very severe. Since the adverse effects induced by RTK inhibitors emerge in a dose-dependent manner, it is desirable for patients with chronic liver diseases to avoid these drugs as much as possible. Therefore, to lower the dose of such treatments, a clinically available compound to use in combination with RTK inhibitors may be required.

ACE-I, ARB, and SAB are extensively employed as antihypertensive agents in clinical practice without serious adverse effects. Thus, these RAAS blocking agents may provide a novel strategy targeting HCC. However, several reports also suggest that there is a close relationship between AT-II polymorphisms and the progression of chronic liver diseases and cancers. In certain types of cancers, the elevated ACE genetic polymorphisms are significantly involved in their poor prognosis [88, 89]. Additionally, AT-II type I receptor polymorphism reportedly contributes to the occurrence of nonalcoholic steatohepatitis (NASH) [90]. These evidences suggest that the efficacy of RAAS inhibition may vary in each case. Since combination treatment of ACE-I and VK exerted substantially more potent inhibitory effects, a combination treatment involving these agents may be preferable for future clinical applications. Furthermore, under IR conditions, the combination treatment of BCAA and ACE-I would be a promising approach against HCC via the suppression of VEGF-mediated angiogenesis. Since these agents are widely used in clinical practice, the combination of these agents with RTK inhibitors such as sorafenib represents a potential alternative approach against HCC.

Author details

Kosuke Kaji* and Hitoshi Yoshiji

*Address all correspondence to: kajik@naramed-u.ac.jp

Third Department of Internal Medicine, Nara Medical University, Shijo-cho, Kashihara, Nara, Japan

References

[1] Carmeliet P. Angiogenesis in life, disease and medicine. Nature. 2005;438(7070):932–6.

[2] Kalluri R, Sukhatme VP. Fibrosis and angiogenesis. Current Opinion in Nephrology and Hypertension. 2000;9(4):413–8.

[3] Llovet JM, Schwartz M, Mazzaferro V. Resection and liver transplantation for hepato-cellular carcinoma. Seminars in Liver Disease. 2005;25(2):181–200.

[4] Li CY, Shan S, Huang Q, Braun RD, Lanzen J, Hu K, et al. Initial stages of tumor cell-induced angiogenesis: evaluation via skin window chambers in rodent models. Journal of the National Cancer Institute. 2000;92(2):143–7.

[5]   Bergers G, Benjamin LE. Tumorigenesis and the angiogenic switch. Nature Reviews Cancer. 2003;3(6):401–10.

[6]   Bergers G, Javaherian K, Lo KM, Folkman J, Hanahan D. Effects of angiogenesis inhibitors on multistage carcinogenesis in mice. Science. 1999;284(5415):808–12.

[7]   Brandvold KA, Neiman P, Ruddell A. Angiogenesis is an early event in the generation of myc-induced lymphomas. Oncogene. 2000;19(23):2780–5.

[8]   Carr BI. Hepatocellular carcinoma: current management and future trends. Gastroen-terology. 2004;127(5 Suppl 1):S218–24.

[9]   Kerbel RS. Tumor angiogenesis. The New England Journal of Medicine. 2008;358(19): 2039–49.

[10] Carmeliet P. VEGF as a key mediator of angiogenesis in cancer. Oncology. 2005;69(Suppl 3):4–10.

[11] Shibuya M. Structure and function of VEGF/VEGF-receptor system involved in angiogenesis. Cell Structure and Function. 2001;26(1):25–35.

[12] Karkkainen MJ, Petrova TV. Vascular endothelial growth factor receptors in the regulation of angiogenesis and lymphangiogenesis. Oncogene. 2000;19(49):5598–605.

[13] Miura H, Miyazaki T, Kuroda M, Oka T, Machinami R, Kodama T, et al. Increased expression of vascular endothelial growth factor in human hepatocellular carcinoma. Journal of Hepatology. 1997;27(5):854–61.

[14] Yamaguchi R, Yano H, Iemura A, Ogasawara S, Haramaki M, Kojiro M. Expression of vascular endothelial growth factor in human hepatocellular carcinoma. Hepatology. 1998;28(1):68–77.

[15] Yamaguchi R, Yano H, Nakashima Y, Ogasawara S, Higaki K, Akiba J, et al. Expression and localization of vascular endothelial growth factor receptors in human hepatocel-lular carcinoma and non-HCC tissues. Oncology Reports. 2000;7(4):725–9.

[16] Yoshiji H, Kuriyama S, Yoshii J, Ikenaka Y, Noguchi R, Hicklin DJ, et al. Halting the interaction between vascular endothelial growth factor and its receptors attenuates liver carcinogenesis in mice. Hepatology. 2004;39(6):1517–24.

[17] Cook KM, Figg WD. Angiogenesis inhibitors: current strategies and future prospects. CA: Cancer Journal for Clinicians. 2010;60(4):222–43.

[18] Forner A, Llovet JM, Bruix J. Hepatocellular carcinoma. Lancet. 2012;379(9822):1245–55.

[19] Llovet JM, Ricci S, Mazzaferro V, Hilgard P, Gane E, Blanc JF, et al. Sorafenib in advanced hepatocellular carcinoma. The New England Journal of Medicine. 2008;359(4):378–90.

[20] Wilhelm S, Carter C, Lynch M, Lowinger T, Dumas J, Smith RA, et al. Discovery and development of sorafenib: a multikinase inhibitor for treating cancer. Nature Reviews Drug Discovery. 2006;5(10):835–44.

[21] Chen KF, Tai WT, Liu TH, Huang HP, Lin YC, Shiau CW, et al. Sorafenib overcomes TRAIL resistance of hepatocellular carcinoma cells through the inhibition of STAT- Clinical Cancer Research: An Official Journal of the American Association for Cancer Research. 2010;16(21):5189–99.

[22] Rosato RR, Almenara JA, Coe S, Grant S. The multikinase inhibitor sorafenib potenti- ates TRAIL lethality in human leukemia cells in association with Mcl-1 and cFLIPL down-regulation. Cancer Research. 2007;67(19):9490–500.

[23] Zhu AX, Raymond E. Early development of sunitinib in hepatocellular carcinoma. Expert Review of Anticancer Therapy. 2009;9(1):143–50.

[24] Cheng AL, Kang YK, Lin DY, Park JW, Kudo M, Qin S, et al. Sunitinib versus sorafenib in advanced hepatocellular cancer: results of a randomized phase III trial. Journal of Clinical Oncology: Official Journal of the American Society of Clinical Oncology. 2013;31(32):4067–75.

[25] Bhide RS, Cai ZW, Zhang YZ, Qian L, Wei D, Barbosa S, et al. Discovery and preclinical studies of (R)-1-(4-(4-fluoro-2-methyl-1H-indol-5-yloxy)-5- methylpyrrolo[2,1-f] [1,2,4]triazin-6-yloxy)propan-2-ol (BMS-540215), an in vivo active potent VEGFR-2 inhibitor. Journal of Medicinal Chemistry. 2006;49(7):2143–6.

[26] Huynh H, Ngo VC, Fargnoli J, Ayers M, Soo KC, Koong HN, et al. Brivanib alaninate, a dual inhibitor of vascular endothelial growth factor receptor and fibroblast growth factor receptor tyrosine kinases, induces growth inhibition in mouse models of human hepatocellular carcinoma. Clinical Cancer Research: An Official Journal of the Ameri- can Association for Cancer Research. 2008;14(19):6146–53.

[27] Johnson PJ, Qin S, Park JW, Poon RT, Raoul JL, Philip PA, et al. Brivanib versus sorafenib as first-line therapy in patients with unresectable, advanced hepatocellular carcinoma: results from the randomized phase III BRISK-FL study. Journal of Clinical Oncology: Official Journal of the American Society of Clinical Oncology. 2013;31(28):3517–24.

[28] Llovet JM, Decaens T, Raoul JL, Boucher E, Kudo M, Chang C, et al. Brivanib in patients with advanced hepatocellular carcinoma who were intolerant to sorafenib or for whom sorafenib failed: results from the randomized phase III BRISK-PS study. Journal of Clinical Oncology: Official Journal of the American Society of Clinical Oncology. 2013;31(28):3509–16.

[29] Yeung KT, Cohen EE. Lenvatinib in advanced, radioactive iodine-refractory, differen- tiated thyroid carcinoma. Clinical Cancer Research: An Official Journal of the American Association for Cancer Research. 2015;21(24):5420–6.

[30] Gu Q, Zhang B, Sun H, Xu Q, Tan Y, Wang G, et al. Genomic characterization of a large panel of patient-derived hepatocellular carcinoma xenograft tumor models for pre- clinical development. Oncotarget. 2015;6(24):20160–76.

[31] Oikonomopoulos G, Aravind P, Sarker D. Lenvatinib: a potential breakthrough in advanced hepatocellular carcinoma? Future Oncology. 2016;12(4):465–76.

[32] Xiang Q, Chen W, Ren M, Wang J, Zhang H, Deng DY, et al. Cabozantinib suppresses tumor growth and metastasis in hepatocellular carcinoma by a dual blockade of VEGFR2 and MET. Clinical Cancer Research: An Official Journal of the American Association for Cancer Research. 2014;20(11):2959–70.

[33] de Kloet AD, Krause EG, Woods SC. The renin angiotensin system and the metabolic syndrome. Physiology & Behavior. 2010;100(5):525–34.

[34] Ardaillou R. Angiotensin II receptors. Journal of the American Society of Nephrology: JASN. 1999;10(Suppl 11):S30–9.

[35] Helmy A, Jalan R, Newby DE, Hayes PC, Webb DJ. Role of angiotensin II in regulation of basal and sympathetically stimulated vascular tone in early and advanced cirrhosis. Gastroenterology. 2000;118(3):565–72.

[36] Munshi MK, Uddin MN, Glaser SS. The role of the renin-angiotensin system in liver fibrosis. Experimental Biology and Medicine. 2011;236(5):557–66.

[37] Beyazit Y, Ibis M, Purnak T, Turhan T, Kekilli M, Kurt M, et al. Elevated levels of circulating angiotensin converting enzyme in patients with hepatoportal sclerosis. Digestive Diseases and Sciences. 2011;56(7):2160–5.

[38] Lugo-Baruqui A, Munoz-Valle JF, Arevalo-Gallegos S, Armendariz-Borunda J. Role of angiotensin II in liver fibrosis-induced portal hypertension and therapeutic implications. Hepatology Research: the Official Journal of the Japan Society of Hepatology. 2010;40(1):95–104.

[39] Lever AF, Hole DJ, Gillis CR, McCallum IR, McInnes GT, MacKinnon PL, et al. Do inhibitors of angiotensin-I-converting enzyme protect against risk of cancer? Lancet. 1998;352(9123):179–84.

[40] Christian JB, Lapane KL, Hume AL, Eaton CB, Weinstock MA, Trial V. Association of ACE inhibitors and angiotensin receptor blockers with keratinocyte cancer prevention in the randomized VATTC trial. Journal of the National Cancer Institute. 2008;100(17): 1223–32.

[41] Wilop S, von Hobe S, Crysandt M, Esser A, Osieka R, Jost E. Impact of angiotensin I converting enzyme inhibitors and angiotensin II type 1 receptor blockers on survival in patients with advanced non-small-cell lung cancer undergoing first-line platinum-based chemotherapy. Journal of Cancer Research and Clinical Oncology. 2009;135(10): 1429–35.

[42] Uemura H, Hasumi H, Kawahara T, Sugiura S, Miyoshi Y, Nakaigawa N, et al. Pilot study of angiotensin II receptor blocker in advanced hormone-refractory prostate cancer. International Journal of Clinical Oncology. 2005;10(6):405–10.

[43] Nakai Y, Isayama H, Ijichi H, Sasaki T, Sasahira N, Hirano K, et al. Inhibition of renin-angiotensin system affects prognosis of advanced pancreatic cancer receiving gemcitabine. British Journal of Cancer. 2010;103(11):1644–8.

[44] Yoshiji H, Kuriyama S, Kawata M, Yoshii J, Ikenaka Y, Noguchi R, et al. The angiotensin-I-converting enzyme inhibitor perindopril suppresses tumor growth and angiogenesis: possible role of the vascular endothelial growth factor. Clinical cancer Research: An Official Journal of the American Association for Cancer Research. 2001;7(4):1073–8.

[45] Miura S, Saku K. Regulation of angiogenesis and angiogenic factors by cardiovascular medications. Current Pharmaceutical Design. 2007;13(20):2113–7.

[46] Heffelfinger SC. The renin angiotensin system in the regulation of angiogenesis. Current Pharmaceutical Design. 2007;13(12):1215–29.

[47] Greene AS, Amaral SL. Microvascular angiogenesis and the renin-angiotensin system. Current Hypertension Reports. 2002;4(1):56–62.

[48] Huang W, Wu YL, Zhong J, Jiang FX, Tian XL, Yu LF. Angiotensin II type 1 receptor antagonist suppress angiogenesis and growth of gastric cancer xenografts. Digestive Diseases and Sciences. 2008;53(5):1206–10.

[49] Kosaka T, Miyajima A, Takayama E, Kikuchi E, Nakashima J, Ohigashi T, et al. Angiotensin II type 1 receptor antagonist as an angiogenic inhibitor in prostate cancer. The Prostate. 2007;67(1):41–9.

[50] Noguchi R, Yoshiji H, Ikenaka Y, Namisaki T, Kitade M, Kaji K, et al. Synergistic inhibitory effect of gemcitabine and angiotensin type-1 receptor blocker, losartan, on murine pancreatic tumor growth via antiangiogenic activities. Oncology Reports. 2009;22(2):355–60.

[51] Kerbel RS. Clinical trials of antiangiogenic drugs: opportunities, problems, and assessment of initial results. Journal of Clinical Oncology: Official Journal of the American Society of Clinical Oncology. 2001;19(18 Suppl):45S–51S.

[52] Scappaticci FA. Mechanisms and future directions for angiogenesis-based cancer therapies. Journal of Clinical Oncology: Official Journal of the American Society of Clinical Oncology. 2002;20(18):3906–27.

[53] Noguchi R, Yoshiji H, Kuriyama S, Yoshii J, Ikenaka Y, Yanase K, et al. Combination of interferon-beta and the angiotensin-converting enzyme inhibitor, perindopril, attenuates murine hepatocellular carcinoma development and angiogenesis. Clinical Cancer Research: An Official Journal of the American Association for Cancer Research. 2003;9(16 Pt 1):6038–45.

[54] Yanase K, Yoshiji H, Ikenaka Y, Noguchi R, Kitade M, Kaji K, et al. Synergistic inhibition of hepatocellular carcinoma growth and hepatocarcinogenesis by combination of 5-fluorouracil and angiotensin-converting enzyme inhibitor via anti-angiogenic activities. Oncology Reports. 2007;17(2):441–6.

[55] Staton CA, Chetwood AS, Cameron IC, Cross SS, Brown NJ, Reed MW. The angiogenic switch occurs at the adenoma stage of the adenoma carcinoma sequence in colorectal cancer. Gut. 2007;56(10):1426–32.

[56] Yoshiji H, Yoshii J, Ikenaka Y, Noguchi R, Yanase K, Tsujinoue H, et al. Suppression of the renin-angiotensin system attenuates vascular endothelial growth factor-mediated tumor development and angiogenesis in murine hepatocellular carcinoma cells. International Journal of Oncology. 2002;20(6):1227–31.

[57] Yoshiji H, Kuriyama S, Noguchi R, Yoshii J, Ikenaka Y, Yanase K, et al. Combination of vitamin K2 and the angiotensin-converting enzyme inhibitor, perindopril, attenuates the liver enzyme-altered preneoplastic lesions in rats via angiogenesis suppression. Journal of Hepatology. 2005;42(5):687–93.

[58] Yoshiji H, Noguchi R, Toyohara M, Ikenaka Y, Kitade M, Kaji K, et al. Combination of vitamin K2 and angiotensin-converting enzyme inhibitor ameliorates cumulative recurrence of hepatocellular carcinoma. Journal of Hepatology. 2009;51(2):315–21.

[59] Williams GH. Aldosterone biosynthesis, regulation, and classical mechanism of action. Heart Failure Reviews. 2005;10(1):7–13.

[60] Funder JW. Minireview: Aldosterone and mineralocorticoid receptors: past, present, and future. Endocrinology. 2010;151(11):5098–102.

[61] Wilkinson-Berka JL, Tan G, Jaworski K, Miller AG. Identification of a retinal aldosterone system and the protective effects of mineralocorticoid receptor antagonism on retinal vascular pathology. Circulation Research. 2009;104(1):124–33.

[62] Kaji K, Yoshiji H, Kitade M, Ikenaka Y, Noguchi R, Shirai Y, et al. Selective aldosterone blocker, eplerenone, attenuates hepatocellular carcinoma growth and angiogenesis in mice. Hepatology Research: The Official Journal of the Japan Society of Hepatology. 2010;40(5):540–9.

[63] Llovet JM, Bruix J. Novel advancements in the management of hepatocellular carcinoma in Journal of Hepatology. 2008;48 Suppl 1:S20–37.

[64] Kaji K, Yoshiji H, Kitade M, Ikenaka Y, Noguchi R, Yoshii J, et al. Impact of insulin resistance on the progression of chronic liver diseases. International Journal of Molecular Medicine. 2008;22(6):801–8.

[65] Nielsen MF, Caumo A, Aagaard NK, Chandramouli V, Schumann WC, Landau BR, et al. Contribution of defects in glucose uptake to carbohydrate intolerance in liver cirrhosis: assessment during physiological glucose and insulin concentrations. American journal of physiology Gastrointestinal and Liver Physiology. 2005;288(6):G1135–43.

[66] Kawaguchi T, Yoshida T, Harada M, Hisamoto T, Nagao Y, Ide T, et al. Hepatitis C virus down-regulates insulin receptor substrates 1 and 2 through up-regulation of suppressor of cytokine signaling The American Journal of Pathology. 2004;165(5):1499–508.

[67] Hui JM, Sud A, Farrell GC, Bandara P, Byth K, Kench JG, et al. Insulin resistance is associated with chronic hepatitis C virus infection and fibrosis progression [corrected]. Gastroenterology. 2003;125(6):1695–704.

[68] Petit JM, Bour JB, Galland-Jos C, Minello A, Verges B, Guiguet M, et al. Risk factors for diabetes mellitus and early insulin resistance in chronic hepatitis C. Journal of Hepatology. 2001;35(2):279–83.

[69] Shintani Y, Fujie H, Miyoshi H, Tsutsumi T, Tsukamoto K, Kimura S, et al. Hepatitis C virus infection and diabetes: direct involvement of the virus in the development of insulin resistance. Gastroenterology. 2004;126(3):840–8.

[70] Bugianesi E, McCullough AJ, Marchesini G. Insulin resistance: a metabolic pathway to chronic liver disease. Hepatology. 2005;42(5):987–1000.

[71] Sanyal AJ, Campbell-Sargent C, Mirshahi F, Rizzo WB, Contos MJ, Sterling RK, et al. Nonalcoholic steatohepatitis: association of insulin resistance and mitochondrial abnormalities. Gastroenterology. 2001;120(5):1183–92.

[72] Davila JA, Morgan RO, Shaib Y, McGlynn KA, El-Serag HB. Diabetes increases the risk of hepatocellular carcinoma in the United States: a population based case control study. Gut. 2005;54(4):533–9.

[73] El-Serag HB, Tran T, Everhart JE. Diabetes increases the risk of chronic liver disease and hepatocellular carcinoma. Gastroenterology. 2004;126(2):460–8.

[74] El-Serag HB, Richardson PA, Everhart JE. The role of diabetes in hepatocellular carcinoma: a case-control study among United States Veterans. The American Journal of Gastroenterology. 2001;96(8):2462–7.

[75] Siddique A, Kowdley KV. Insulin resistance and other metabolic risk factors in the pathogenesis of hepatocellular carcinoma. Clinics in Liver Disease. 2011;15(2):281–96, vii-x.

[76] Alexia C, Fallot G, Lasfer M, Schweizer-Groyer G, Groyer A. An evaluation of the role of insulin-like growth factors (IGF) and of type-I IGF receptor signalling in hepatocarcinogenesis and in the resistance of hepatocarcinoma cells against drug-induced apoptosis. Biochemical Pharmacology. 2004;68(6):1003–15.

[77] Donadon V, Balbi M, Mas MD, Casarin P, Zanette G. Metformin and reduced risk of hepatocellular carcinoma in diabetic patients with chronic liver disease. Liver International: Official Journal of the International Association for the Study of the Liver. 2010;30(5):750–8.

[78] Khattab M, Emad M, Abdelaleem A, Eslam M, Atef R, Shaker Y, et al. Pioglitazone improves virological response to peginterferon alpha-2b/ribavirin combination therapy in hepatitis C genotype 4 patients with insulin resistance. Liver International: Official Journal of the International Association for the Study of the Liver. 2010;30(3): 447–54.

[79] El-Serag HB, Johnson ML, Hachem C, Morgana RO. Statins are associated with a reduced risk of hepatocellular carcinoma in a large cohort of patients with diabetes. Gastroenterology. 2009;136(5):1601–8.

[80] Marchesini G, Bianchi G, Merli M, Amodio P, Panella C, Loguercio C, et al. Nutritional supplementation with branched-chain amino acids in advanced cirrhosis: a double-blind, randomized trial. Gastroenterology. 2003;124(7):1792–801.

[81] Muto Y, Sato S, Watanabe A, Moriwaki H, Suzuki K, Kato A, et al. Effects of oral branched-chain amino acid granules on event-free survival in patients with liver cirrhosis. Clinical Gastroenterology and Hepatology: The Official Clinical Practice Journal of the American Gastroenterological Association. 2005;3(7):705–13.

[82] Yoshiji H, Noguchi R, Kaji K, Ikenaka Y, Shirai Y, Namisaki T, et al. Attenuation of insulin-resistance-based hepatocarcinogenesis and angiogenesis by combined treatment with branched-chain amino acids and angiotensin-converting enzyme inhibitor in obese diabetic rats. Journal of Gastroenterology. 2010;45(4):443–50.

[83] Yoshiji H, Noguchi R, Kitade M, Kaji K, Ikenaka Y, Namisaki T, et al. Branched-chain amino acids suppress insulin-resistance-based hepatocarcinogenesis in obese diabetic rats. Journal of Gastroenterology. 2009;44(5):483–91.

[84] Muto Y, Sato S, Watanabe A, Moriwaki H, Suzuki K, Kato A, et al. Overweight and obesity increase the risk for liver cancer in patients with liver cirrhosis and long-term oral supplementation with branched-chain amino acid granules inhibits liver carcinogenesis in heavier patients with liver cirrhosis. Hepatology Research: The Official Journal of the Japan Society of Hepatology. 2006;35(3):204–14.

[85] Jayasooriya AP, Mathai ML, Walker LL, Begg DP, Denton DA, Cameron-Smith D, et al. Mice lacking angiotensin-converting enzyme have increased energy expenditure, with reduced fat mass and improved glucose clearance. Proceedings of the National Academy of Sciences of the United States of America. 2008;105(18):6531–6.

[86] Manrique C, Lastra G, Gardner M, Sowers JR. The renin angiotensin aldosterone system in hypertension: roles of insulin resistance and oxidative stress. The Medical Clinics of North America. 2009;93(3):569–82.

[87] Yoshiji H, Noguchi R, Ikenaka Y, Kaji K, Aihara Y, Yamazaki M, et al. Combination of branched-chain amino acids and angiotensin-converting enzyme inhibitor suppresses the cumulative recurrence of hepatocellular carcinoma: a randomized control trial. Oncology Reports. 2011;26(6):1547–53.

[88] Fabris C, Smirne C, Fangazio S, Toniutto P, Burlone M, Minisini R, et al. Influence of angiotensin-converting enzyme I/D gene polymorphism on clinical and histological correlates of chronic hepatitis C. Hepatology Research: The Official Journal of the Japan Society of Hepatology. 2009;39(8):795–804.

[89] Medeiros R, Vasconcelos A, Costa S, Pinto D, Lobo F, Morais A, et al. Linkage of angiotensin I-converting enzyme gene insertion/deletion polymorphism to the progression of human prostate cancer. The Journal of Pathology. 2004;202(3):330–5.

[90] Yoneda M, Hotta K, Nozaki Y, Endo H, Uchiyama T, Mawatari H, et al. Association between angiotensin II type 1 receptor polymorphisms and the occurrence of nonalcoholic fatty liver disease. Liver International: Official Journal of the International Association for the Study of the Liver. 2009;29(7):1078–85.

5

Therapeutic Angiogenesis: Foundations and Practical Application

Pavel Igorevich Makarevich and
Yelena Viktorovna Parfyonova

Abstract

Angiogenesis as therapeutic target has emerged since early works by Judah Folkman, yet his "holy grail" was inhibiting vascular growth to block tumor nutrition. However, in modern biomedicine, "therapeutic angiogenesis" became a large field focusing on stimulation of blood vessel growth for ischemia relief to reduce its detrimental effects in the tissues. In this review, we introduce basic principles of tissue vascularization in response to ischemia exploited in this field. An overview of recent status in therapeutic angiogenesis is given with introduction to emerging technologies, including gene therapy, genetic modification of cells ex vivo and tissue engineering.

Keywords: therapeutic angiogenesis, growth factors, cytokines, gene therapy, cell therapy, plasmid, viral vector

1. Introduction

Blood vessel growth is a natural process driven by multiple stimuli of which hypoxia is one of the strongest inducing potent response until O_2 pressure is normalized by the blood coming through de novo formed vasculature. However, a large group of diseases is caused by hypoxic or ischemic state of tissue. These include peripheral artery disease (PAD) and intermittent claudication (IC), coronary heart disease (CHD), myocardial infarction (MI) and ischemic stroke. Accompanied by endothelial dysfunction and age-related reduction of angiogenic response, they result in disabilities and mortality rate of 25–25% annually. Existing strategies for surgical bypass or endovascular interventions have limited efficacy as far as a cohort of non-option patients expands reaching 25–50% after certain extent of disease progression. Moreover, long-term prognosis after most interventions is negative as grafts undergo restenosis and vascular biocompatible prosthetics are yet to come for wide application. This drew attention of physicians and researchers to the concept of angiogenic therapy to stimulate body's own resource and form new blood vessels to relieve ischemia. During recent decade the field of biomedicine known as *therapeutic angiogenesis* evolved rapidly using protein delivery, gene therapy, cell therapy and tissue engineering for induction of vessel growth and overview of its basic concepts and recent achievements will be presented to the reader in chapters below.

2. Biological foundations of therapeutic angiogenesis

Postnatal growth of blood vessels is mediated by three mechanisms: vasculogenesis, angiogenesis and arteriogenesis [1]. Vasculogenesis is de novo formation of vasculature from specific progenitor or stem cells; however, it is attributed to prenatal period and after birth its role is unclear [2] and major extent of blood vessel formation involves two other mechanisms focusing our attention on them. Molecular and cellular basics underlying these processes became the cornerstones of therapeutic angiogenesis and become the source of novel objects for applied researchers and translational medicine.

2.1. Angiogenesis: hypoxia-driven growth of blood vessels

Angiogenesis is the formation of a blood vessel de novo, yet in contrast to vasculogenesis, it relies on migration, proliferation and sprouting of existing endothelial cells (EC) comprising capillaries. The latter are small (8–15 μm) vessels lacking tunica media responsible for majority of tissue blood supply and O_2/CO_2 exchange [3]. Reduction of tissue O_2 induces angiogenesis response in health (intense exercise, tissue growth, etc.) and in disease: in the case of interrupted or declining supply due to atherosclerotic lesions or anemia [4]. Under normal condition, capillaries are stabilized by autocrine and paracrine stimuli (Notch1 axis, angiopoietins, thrombospondin, angiostatin, transforming growth factor (TGF)-β, etc.) that balance influence of pro-angiogenic cytokines within blood vessels' vicinity (vascular endothelial growth factors (VEGFs), fibroblast growth factors (FGFs), hepatocyte growth factor (HGF), platelet-derived growth factor (PDGF)). Hypoxia dislodges this balance toward angiogenic events and this is mediated by O_2-sensitive system existing in a variety of cells including EC themselves, smooth muscle cells (SMC), pericytes and fibroblasts. Cells respond to hypoxia via a system of hypoxia-induced factors (HIFs) [5]—a group of heterodimeric transcription regulators controlled by O_2-sensitive prolyl hydroxylases. Briefly, stability of HIFs is increased drastically in hypoxic environment resulting in their binding to hypoxia-responsive elements within promoter regions of genes increasing their expression [6]. HIF-dependent genes include a vast array of cytokines stimulating EC proliferation, blood vessel sprouting and, thus, labeled "angiogenic growth factors" [7, 8]. The latter include soluble growth factors associated with EC proliferation and differentiation (acidic FGF (aFGF), basic FGF (bFGF), HGF, VEGFs) [9, 10] and cytokines bound to extracellular matrix (ECM) and released during its cleavage [11]. These changes induce EC proliferation and migration forming a vascular sprout guided by a "tip cell." This cell follows a gradient of concentration and produces matrix metalloproteinases (MMPs) and urokinase (uPA) to cleave the ECM [12], releasing growth factors and basically tunneling ECM followed by "stalk cells" that form a new capillary [13]. After lumen formation occurs normalized blood supply switches off hypoxic stimuli, "tip cells" lose their phenotype and proteolytic potential [14] commencing microenvironment stabilization. Expression of tissue metalloproteinase inhibitors and Dll4-Notch1 axis [15] induction in EC is followed by reestablishment of a balanced state between pro- and antiangiogenic molecules in the tissue leaving a new capillary-sized blood vessel [16]. However, it should be mentioned that this sequence of events never occurs as a perfectly tuned mechanism. "Stub" branches are formed and must be removed, certain "tip cells" fail to form a sprout and maturation of vascular network includes dissociation of certain anastomoses [16], which overall describes angiogenesis as a dynamic process modulated by multiple stimuli [17]. Finally, under influence of stabilizing signals from surrounding EC, pericytes and stromal cells, the vascular bed returns to normal steady state.

2.2. Arteriogenesis: shear stress-induced vascular remodeling

Arteriogenesis is triggered by rise of shear stress after an occlusion and induces collateral vessel remodeling forming a bypass 20–100 μm in diameter with developed tunica media. Arteriogenesis may occur gradually (e.g., in increasing stenosis of a large-caliber artery) or can be triggered by a rapidly developed occlusion with both situations are to result in effective blood flow delivery "around an obstacle" to distal portions of the limb or organ [18]. Certain studies show that collateral remodeling can be reversible till certain point of this process in case shear stress drops to normal after thrombolysis or surgical thrombectomy [19]. Effective arteriogenesis may bypass up to 30–40% of basal blood flow in critical stenosis and thrombosis, which is sufficient for tissue survival. However, its efficacy is drastically reduced in disease and with aging [20]. Smoking-related hypercoagulation, hypertension and diabetes also limit arteriogenic response resulting in critical level of ischemia and tissue loss [21].

After pressure rise in collaterals above the site of thrombosis, shear stress induces EC membrane deformation and flow-sensitive ion channels activate downstream MAP-kinase (ERK1/2, Rho, etc.) phosphorylation and expression of, growth factors, adhesion molecules and chemokines (interleukin-8, macrophage chemoattractant proteins, etc.) [20]. Eventually leukocytes begin to "roll" on EC surface resembling inflammatory changes of vascular function and infiltrate the collateral's wall [22]. Pivotal role in wall thickening is played by monocytes and their differentiated forms—macrophages and dendritic cells. Their function is not limited to ECM and basal lamina cleavage by MMP and uPA production to destabilize the collateral and make it "flexible" [23], but they seem to profoundly change the properties of the blood vessel by induction of SMC proliferation and hypertrophy [24]. Under these influences, media thickness may increase 3- to 4-fold and collateral vessel's volume can enlarge up to 20-fold [25]. Moreover, monocytes produce a wide spectrum of angiogenic and mitogenic cytokines, some of which have antiapoptotic properties required for tissue protection [26]. The role of monocytes and macrophages has been especially emphasized in cardiac arteriogenesis where immunosuppressive steroid hormones [27], anti-inflammatory therapies and even aspirin [28] have been shown to negatively impact the outcomes and collateral remodeling. Toxic depletion of monocytes by clodronate reduced arteriogenesis in cryo-injured myocardium and led to decreased ventricular function and higher mortality [29]. As collaterals increase shear stress stimulus is relieved and EC reduce production of chemokines and lose their "adhesive" phenotype. Macrophages limit production of proteolytic enzymes and start

ECM reconstruction producing collagens, laminin and elastin and forming adventitial and medial portions of a new arterial vessel.

Typically, we mention "therapeutic angiogenesis" referring gene or cell therapy to relieve ischemia. Nevertheless, one may see that angiogenesis and arteriogenesis share common mediators—namely growth factors and enzymes, ECM components, EC activation, etc. Eventually, for adequate function therapeutic angiogenesis has to rebuild both—medium/large-caliber arteries providing influx of blood and capillary-sized vessels that deliver it to the cells.

3. Therapeutic angiogenesis: methods and approaches

3.1. Protein-based therapeutics

After the discovery of proteins with angiogenic effects, the concept of their therapeutic application was introduced by the 1990s and a vast array of animal studies was published to demonstrate angiogenic efficacy of recombinant protein delivery. Going beyond the VEGF family, experimental works showed induction of angiogenesis by FGFs, HGF, PDGF and placental growth factor (PlGF) in small rodents and rabbits [30, 31]. Injection of these cytokines to ischemic tissue or blood vessels increased perfusion and vascular density. However, promise of this method was questioned as far as achievement of local pharmacological concentration by injection was extremely expensive (especially for human body mass) and half-life of most cytokines was too low to render potent effects [32]. Furthermore, little was known on pharmacokinetics of recombinant proteins delivered intravascularly and their potential involvement in tumor growth and chance of "washout" to systemic blood flow raised safety concerns.

In 2000, the first clinical trials of recombinant human bFGF were initiated in PAD/IC patients after a pilot study showing safety and tolerance of intra-arterial delivery of bFGF solution. Unfortunately, it was halted prior to completion of protocol due to urinalysis data revealing proteinuria in bFGF-treated subjects and no positive changes of endpoints at the moment when the trial was put to a premature end [33]. The final attempt to achieve success in the field was the Therapeutic angiogenesis with recombinant fibroblast growth Factor-2 for intermittent claudication (TRAFFIC) randomized placebo-controlled trial in patients with PAD showing significant improvement in walking time and ankle-brachial index (ABI) in bFGF group. However, safety profile was compromised and yet no cardiac adverse effects or evidence for tumor formation was found in recurrent cases of proteinuria and signs of nephrotoxicity were an issue [34].

These results were as disappointing as valuable for the field and suggested that gene therapy with its local sustained expression of desired protein is the best alternative possible [32]. Recently, no further attempts to implicate protein delivery for therapeutic angiogenesis were made in clinics and advantages of other methods are exploited to patients' benefit.

3.2. Gene therapy for angiogenesis

Gene therapy relies on delivery of genetic information by introduction of nucleic acids to target cells/tissues using vector systems. This results in local expression and production of desired protein over a certain period depending on vector used and properties of tissue. First experiments indicating possibility of in vivo gene delivery using simple injection of a recombinant plasmid DNA (pDNA) opened the gate for hundreds of studies published within the last two decades [35].

As far as the "cornerstone" of gene therapy is the vector system, a brief overview of existing options is required. General concept in the field is that all vectors can be divided into "viral" and "nonviral" subgroups covering nearly any possible way of genetic material delivery. Among nonviral vectors, pDNA is the most widely used due to its long-studied safety profile, ease of production and low immunogenicity allowing repetitive administration [31, 36]. Moreover, plasmids are feasible for combined delivery of several growth factors by mixing them in a formulation or generating a multicistronic vector. However, low transfection efficacy (0.5–2.0% in various tissues) in large mammals including human is an efficacy-limiting issue for pDNA [37]. Viral delivery systems comprise a broad spectrum of recombinant or chimeric viruses of different capacity having a great potential. The latter is due to high transduction efficacy and long expression period accompanied by tissue tropism in certain viruses. However, disadvantages are safety issues: immune reactions and risk of carcinogenesis due to integration to host genome. The most widely spread vectors include adeno- [38], adeno-associated [39] and retroviruses, yet in therapeutic angiogenesis, the latter have limited application due to high risk of insertional mutagenesis [40]. Recent progress of molecular engineering allowed development of optimized viral systems exploiting their advantages as well as novel more effective pDNA systems [41, 42].

Period of growth factor-based gene delivery dates back to the seminal study by Dr. J. Isner [43] who used injection of pDNA encoding VEGF-A 165 (VEGF165) isoform to succeed in treatment of a non-option patient with critical limb ischemia. "First in-human" data were supported by Baumgartner et al. who found increased collateral formation after intramuscular delivery of VEGF165 and EC proliferation in amputation material providing proof of mechanism [44]. Later a number of vectors using VEGF-A and its isoforms were evaluated in experimental and clinical trials making it the most intensively studied object in therapeutic angiogenesis.

Among numerous clinical examples, one may highlight the first "head-to-head" comparison of adenovirus with VEGF165 (Ad-VEGF165) and liposome-packed pDNA-VEGF165 in PAD patients undergoing angioplasty. The trial showed low clinical efficacy of both approaches — Rutherford severity class stayed comparable to control group yet vascular density was increased after treatment [45]. This and other studies using catheter delivery hinted that this method lacks site specificity and intramuscular injection technique was generally adopted. However, initial Groningen double-blind placebo-controlled trial intramuscular injection of pDNA-VEGF165 in PAD patients with diabetes mellitus failed the primary endpoint (amputation rate), yet improvements in ulcer healing, TcO_2 and ABI were observed [46].

Later, Regional angiogenesis with VEGF (RAVE) trial was the first double-blind placebo-controlled trial of VEGF-A 121 isoform (VEGF121). This cytokine is considered to have better solubility than VEGF165 isoform as it lacks a heparin-binding domain [47]. Key feature of this study was an attempt to perform dose optimization of Ad-VEGF121 dividing 105 patients with PAD/IC into three subgroups that received a single session of 20 intramuscular injections of AdVEGF165 delivering low dose (4×10^9 particles), high dose (4×10^{10} particles), or placebo. Final assessment after 12 weeks revealed no significant differences in endpoints between control and treatment subgroups, yet dose-dependent increase of edema adverse effect was observed. Indeed, since first studies delivery of VEGF-A isoforms was haunted by evidence of edema formation due to its influence on endothelial permeability [48] with certain authors claiming this was a putative reason for low efficacy of therapy [49].

Trials in MI patients were initiated as early as in 1998 using a pDNA-VEGF165 showing good safety profile and no positive changes [50]. It was followed by Kuopio Angiogenesis Trial [51] using a comparative design with Ad-VEGF165 or pDNA-VEGF165 delivery by intramyocardial injection during transcutaneous angioplasty. In this trial, no differences between control and treatment groups were found, yet at 6 months after injection of Ad-VEGF165, myocardium perfusion was higher than pDNA-VEGF165, which was attributed to its high transduction efficacy. EuroInject One trial gave similar results showing no significant improvement of myocardial perfusion after injection of pDNA-VEGF165, yet local contractility was higher than control [52].

Trials using delivery of HGF were initiated and conducted by Dr. Morishita's group aiming to treat PAD by intramuscular injection of pDNA-HGF. Encouraging results in animal models [31, 53] promoted clinical translation and after safety assessment a Phase II trial was initiated comparing single and repeated dose of pDNA-HGF in favor of multiple injections: only this dosing regimen showed improvement of TcO_2 compared to control [54]. Further results in a placebo-controlled I/IIa phase trial showed good safety with no traces of secreted HGF in peripheral blood and repeated injection of 8 mg pDNA-HGF showed significant improvements of secondary endpoints (ulcer size, ABI and pain reduction) [55]. Similar results were obtained in a placebo-controlled trial in PAD patients where by the end of week 12, 70% decrease of ulcer size was observed [56]. Further attempts to increase efficacy included the use of a bicistronic plasmid encoding two forms of HGF named dHGF and cHGF. They were evaluated in animal models showing better perfusion after expression of dHGF + cHGF than each one alone [57]. Clinical trial of this approach in PAD patients showed that multifocal intramuscular injections of 4–16 mg of pDNA-dHGF/cHGF resulted in improvement within 3 months independently of dose: rest and walking pains reduced and a trend toward ulcer healing and increase of TcO_2 was observed [58].

Overall, we may expect HGF-based drugs to become the first widely marketed for PAD—in Japan it has been registered under "Collategene" name and now undergoes stage III clinical trial in PAD cohort. Furthermore, despite HGF has never been tested for MI treatment in clinical settings, preclinical assessments indicate that it may be effective as it has antifibrotic and angiogenic mode of action that can be a good option for this disease or subsequent ventricular failure due to tissue scarring [53, 59].

Fibroblast growth factor has been the first used in protein delivery and gene therapy studies were to follow as soon as it gained attention. Therapeutic angiogenesis leg ischemia study for the management of arteriopathy and non-healing ulcer (TALISMAN-201) have evaluated pDNA-FGF-1 in no-option PAD patients [60] and showed improvements as decreased amputation rate within 1 year after treatment [61] and its prospective part showed reduced general mortality in treated subjects [62]. However, phase III placebo-controlled "TAMARIS" (n = 525) trial drew disappointing results and all primary endpoints including amputation events failed to improve after treatment by pDNA-FGF-1 [62, 63]. Similar results obtained in OPTIMIST and

EuroOPTIMIST trials indicated safety and lack of efficacy after treatment and lead to wrapping up of this prospective drug testing. Nevertheless, in a follow-up stage, important safety data showing no increased cancer, stroke, or MI in FGF-treated patients was obtained and positively impacted new proceedings in the field [64].

In MI patients, FGF-4 was delivered using an intracoronary injection of an adenovirus with this gene (Ad-FGF-4) in an Angiogenic gene therapy (AGENT) trial. Result evaluation showed that the only subgroup with reduced size of ischemic myocardium after treatment was female patients when compared to male subgroup. The authors speculated that it may be attributed to higher extent of microcirculatory disorders in females [65, 66] accompanied by fewer critical stenosis typical in men [67]. As far as FGF-4 is known to positively influence endothelial function, this might have been the mechanism for observed changes in the trial. Among other therapeutic factors used for stimulation of angiogenesis, HIF-1α and development endothelial locus-1 (DEL) are both worth a mention as far as they made it to the bedside in recent years using adenovirus or pDNA vectors. However, trials showed minimal improvement in PAD patients and further evaluations were ceased up to date [68, 69].

Overall despite failure to show expected efficacy in clinic, gene therapy is safe and well tolerated by patients showing little evidence although long-term evaluations are yet to be completed. Key obstacle in pDNA-mediated gene therapy relates to transfection efficacy and thus protein production levels after administration [70]. Viral vectors show some promise in solving the problem, yet optimization of dosage regimen, delivery routes and administration protocols also provide a field for further development.

From the point of translational potential, pDNA-based gene therapy has the best safety profile and the best results are definitely yet to come in the following years yet points for improvement are obvious. Efficacy improvement in gene therapy can be achieved by combined approaches basing on the point that angiogenesis is a dynamic process controlled by numerous cytokines, each playing its party in initiation/cessation of different stages. This puts the basis for combined gene therapy to treat ischemia with higher efficacy and it has been supported by experimental findings using VEGF165 combined with another pro-angiogenic growth factor: bFGF [71], PDGF [72], angiopoietin-1 [73], or Stromal cell-derived factor-1α (SDF-1α) [74]. Our previous experience in mouse hind limb ischemia model showed that combination of VEGF165 and uPA [75] or HGF [76] induced angiogenic response more effectively than each factor alone or allowed to reduce pDNA dose for combined delivery [75]. A crucial transcription factor in angiogenesis, HIF-1α, was also used for combined gene therapy with VEGF165 showing good results in animal model [77] as well as bFGF + heme oxygenase-1 (HO-1) [78]. Regarding the latter, it is known that HO-1 is an important regulator of endothelial function with protective function. Its expression is known to induce angiogenesis in ischemic tissues and blockade or knockout reduces EC proliferation and motility and thus capillary growth [79].

Triple combined gene therapy has not been evaluated for angiogenesis, yet a study was published where controlled release scaffolds containing a mix of VEGF165, HGF and angiopoietin-1 or their double combinations were evaluated for enhancing efficacy of endothelial progenitor cell (EPC) therapy. Triple combinations resulted in significantly higher

SMC counts indicating more efficient vessel stabilization due to angiopoietin-1 effects on perivascular cell chemotaxis [80].

Authors claimed that the use of VEGF165 + another cytokine typically leads to decreased edema and vascular permeability: this has been shown for a well-known stabilizing cytokines—angiopoietin-1 [73] and HGF [81]. Thus, another rationale for combined therapy is decrease of certain "side effects" observed in "monotherapy" by VEGF as a key player in gene therapy. The latter point is not limited to reduction of adverse reactions, but also arises from a large spectrum of pleiotropic effects of cytokines. For example, VEGF may act as a pro-inflammatory cytokine by induction of nuclear factor κ-B, while HGF [82] or angiopoietin-1 shows antagonistic effects leading to reduction of VEGF-driven cell adhesion and inflammation [83]. Indeed, this has been confirmed in a number of in vitro tests and skin inflammation model indicating that these properties may be utilized for development of next-generation gene therapy drugs for angiogenesis exploiting pleiotropy of cytokines besides their main angiogenic effect. Another approach is delivery of growth factors in two sessions apart in time: for example, pre-treatment by angiopoietin-1 pDNA resulted in better angiogenic response after subsequent pDNA-VEGF165 injection in mouse hind limb ischemia model hinting time of administration as an important factor for efficacy [84].

3.3. Cell therapy and *ex vivo* modified cells

Cell therapy is a promising tool for regenerative medicine and therapeutic angiogenesis using progenitor or stem cells' ability to self-renew and mediate tissue repair. For potential use of cell therapy for vascular repair, one of the most intriguing findings was the discovery of endothelial progenitor cells (EPC) in circulating blood which hinted involvement of postnatal vasculogenesis in perfusion restoration [85]. However, further works sparkled controversy about EPC phenotype, origin [86], role in recovery from disease and even existence. Report by Prokopi et al. [87] claimed that EPC can be false-detected as endothelium-like (CD31/vWF+) monocytes in cultures due to phagocytosis of residual platelets rich with these protein markers.

Clinical trials up to date focus on delivery of bone marrow (BM) cells for induction of angiogenesis. These studies evaluated effects of BM mesenchymal stem cells (BM-MSC) or mononuclear cells (BM-MNC) delivered by intramuscular or intravascular injection in PAD patients. Most studies supported efficacy and indicated improvement in evaluated endpoints: ABI, pain-free walking distance, TcO_2, ulcer healing, or amputation-free period. However, some pivotal trials are to be mentioned in detail for better understanding of the field's status.

First set of crucial data was obtained during "head-to-head" comparison of different cell types to identify the optimal cell source. In a double-blind randomized study, administration of BM-MSC to diabetic PAD patients with foot ulcerations showed efficacy superior to BM-MNC [88]. Subjects that received BM-MSC showed complete ulcer healing 4 weeks earlier than BM-MNC; perfusion assessment, pain-free walking time, ABI and angiography data also spoke in favor of BM-MSC as a more effective cellular angiogenic agent [88].

However, limitation of BM-based treatment is invasive procedure to obtain material and alternative approach was proposed using peripheral blood mononuclear cells (PB-MNC) mobilized by granulocyte colony-stimulating factor (G-CSF) pre-administration. Feasibility of this approach was obvious and a trial was initiated to confirm its efficacy compared to BM-MNC enrolling a total of 150 patients split in two groups. After 12 weeks of observation, PB-MNC patients showed significantly higher limb temperature, ABI and reduced rest pains than BM-MNC. Yet no difference was found in TcO_2, ulcer healing rate and amputation frequency hinting that two methods showed comparable efficacy profile with a trend to PB-MNC application due to feasibility and endpoint improvements [89]. Interestingly, a trial of conventional therapy + G-CSF monotherapy was compared to BM cells and in these groups, improvements in ABI and TcO_2 were comparable and significantly better than in conventional drug therapy control. This was an intriguing finding which showed that mobilization of endogenous mononuclear cells (MNC) was sufficient to replace BM grafting and injection [90].

Another source of cells for therapeutic angiogenesis is adipose-derived mesenchymal stromal cells (AD-MSC). Despite sources of mesenchymal stem cells (MSC) are not limited to adipose tissue, these adult stromal cells can be isolated from samples obtained during lipoaspiration or surgery. Taken together with ease of expansion, well-established phenotype and abundance in healthy individuals, it makes AD-MSC an excellent object for autologous and allogeneic use for angiogenesis stimulation [91]. Published experimental studies show that AD-MSC use their paracrine potential for induction of angiogenesis and support of collateral remodeling [92]. This is referred as "bystander effect" to emphasize that AD-MSC render their effects by paracrine mechanism in contrast to previously existing opinion about their significant ability to differentiate into specific vascular cells and EC in particular [93].

These cells have not been evaluated in PAD or MI clinical trials yet and considered to be a very attractive option to complement existing strategies. Certain factors limiting potency of AD-MSC exist including donors' age [94], comorbidities and effects of *ex vivo* culture [95]. However, improvement can be achieved by manipulation of cells' paracrine activity, e.g., by viral transduction to increase expression of cytokines forming an "alliance of gene and cell therapy" for higher efficacy [96]. This approach has become possible after development of effective viral gene delivery systems as far as pDNA transfection in primary human cultures was extremely low or at the level of toxicity exerted by transfection reagents [97]. Modification of cells intended for therapy use in performed *ex vivo* after sufficient amount of material is obtained in appropriate culture condition. Selection of a viral vector depends on safety precautions and vector capacity for genetic material; however, cDNA of most angiogenic cytokines "fit" into commonly used adenoviruses or adeno-associated virus (AAV).

This method has been tested in animal models of ischemia using exogenous delivery of VEGF165 [98], insulin-like growth factor-1 [99], HO-1 [100], or other genes to different types of cells: AD-MSC, EC, BM-MSC, etc. In majority of reports, modification resulted in improvement of response after delivery to ischemic tissue. In our experience, administration of human VEGF165-expressing AD-MSC to ischemic limb of immunodeficient mice resulted in enhanced perfusion and vascular density superior to control cells. Furthermore, muscle necrosis was minimal in this group indicating enhanced blood supply and antiapoptotic effects of VEGF165 as mode of action [98].

Application of modified stem cells for induction of angiogenesis may be limited in coming years unless safety of modification and full extent of its influence on biological properties of cells is understood. *Ex vivo* modified cells are widely used for treatment of oncology and hereditary disease where benefit for patient overwhelms existing risks [101]; however, for treatment of PAD and MI, additional measures of precaution will be required prior to active clinical trials. Nevertheless, recently a group led by Dr. J. Laird began a phase I trial to evaluate the use of VEGF-expressing MSC in patients with critical limb ischemia. The trial is now ongoing with expected completion in 2017 and preclinical data indicated good safety profile with long-term expression of VEGF in MSC after viral modification [102]. Recent progress in virus biology and gene engineering allowed development of safer vector systems with controlled expression, integration, or directed insertion to genomic "safe harbors" where they induce minimal to none disturbances [103]. Preclinical evaluation of these systems is expected to give more data on long-term impact of modification and facilitate translation.

4. Cell sheets: minimal tissue-engineered constructs

Cell sheets (CS) were first introduced by Dr. Okano's group and occupied a niche between 3D tissue engineering and 2D cell cultures used to obtain therapeutic cellular materials [104]. Briefly, CS is an attached mono- or multilayered xeno-free construct that consists of viable cells with ECM produced by these cells. Application of this method allowed to circumvent a crucial setback observed in a number of experimental works—poor survival of cells used for therapeutic interventions. One of main reasons for this is procedure of detachment by proteolytic enzymes leading to disruption of ECM (along with deposited cytokines) and loss of intercellular contacts resulting in anoikis and high prevalence of cell death aggravated by passage of cells through a catheter or needle causing mechanical damage. Loss of cells implanted to the tissue by injection in suspended form is estimated as 40–75% within the first 3 days [105], while CS limits this damage to minimum keeping the cells viable after delivery and enhancing their engraftment [106]. Furthermore, ECM proteins delivered as a part of the construct are known to have a beneficial impact on regeneration and do not have toxic or immunogenic features of chemical or xenogeneic scaffolds. Generation of CS is possible from MSC, fibroblasts, EC, skeletal myoblasts, induced pluripotent stem cells and cardiomyocytes derived from them, BM cells and cardiac progenitor cells [107]—literally, any adherent cell culture after it produces enough ECM to stand mechanical manipulation [108]. CS can be used to cover a significant surface making it a good technique for superficial lesions, cardiomyoplasty and ophthalmologic and microsurgical manipulations. Numerous clinical trials are being run in Japan these years to reveal their full potential in a wide array of disorders [109].

In relation to angiogenesis, this technique was evaluated in MI models using CS from skeletal myoblasts, AD-MSC, or cardiac progenitor cells showing their ability to generate vascularized additional layer of tissue and facilitate vascular growth in underlying tissue [110, 111]. This resulted in improved ventricular function, limited MI size and fibrosis and favorable outcomes in experimental animals. Comparative study of CS vs. injection of suspended cells showed CS to be superior in terms of most functional and histological endpoints analyzed and using a bioluminescent method, the authors reported higher survival of transplanted rat neonatal cardiomyocytes after CS delivery compared to injection [112]. Recently, clinical application of CS from autologous skeletal myoblasts has begun to treat severe heart failure patients with left ventricular assist devices. Delivery of multilayered constructs resulted in ejection fraction increase sufficient to remove the device and postpone heart transplant as well showing good potential of this approach [113].

In limb ischemia and diabetes, CS are generally considered to be a tool for ulcer treatment and indeed numerous clinical trials have been initiated within last years. However, our group has been extensively investigating application of CS as an angiogenic therapy in PAD. We have found that subcutaneous delivery of CS from AD-MSC to mice with limb ischemia resulted in robust angiogenic response and CS were superior to dispersed cells in terms of tissue perfusion and vessel density [114]. This piece of evidence provided basis for CS application in PAD indicating that their potential is not limited to cutaneous healing but that paracrine factors are capable to induce angiogenic response in ischemic muscle. Our data were supported almost at the same time in a study by Bak et al. who used mixed CS from SMC and EC for successful treatment of experimental limb ischemia in mice by subcutaneous delivery [115].

Further improvement of CS potential is possible by application of *ex vivo* modification to express growth factors and discussed above. Our group's experience with viral vectors expressing VEGF165 suggested robust increase of angiogenesis in MI and limb ischemia after delivery of sheets from AD-MSC expressing VEGF165 after viral transduction [114, 116]. Effect of these constructs was superior to control CS and we observed no changes in immune response to genetically modified sheets or cell proliferation/viability within them [114].

Overall, application of CS for therapeutic angiogenesis is a new field and its expansion is expected within next years. These constructs are feasible from a translational point of view as far as they do not contain xenogeneic, artificial, or cadaveric materials circumventing many ethical and safety problems in translation.

5. Concluding remarks

Overall, therapeutic angiogenesis has accumulated a "critical mass" of evidence and approaches that would allow its application in practice within the next 10–15 years expanding the capabilities of treatment. However, possibility to shift from initially used non-option or critical patients may lead to better results in clinical trials, especially in gene therapy, where numerous failures put the whole concept under question several years ago. Development of cell therapy was accompanied by a large framework of regulatory, legal, ethical and industrial work to ensure safety and patients' benefit. Number of clinical trials is growing every year and fortunately no serious evidence for adverse events or other risks for subjects' health and well-being was found up-to-date.

Therapeutic angiogenesis has become one of the pioneer methods in translational medicine and its full potential is yet to be unleashed especially in the field of *ex vivo* modification and tissue-engineered approaches to increase efficacy and ensure safety.

Funding

Study and publication was supported by a grant from Russian Scientific Foundation (RSF) №16-45-03007.

Abbreviations

AAV	adeno-associated virus
(a/b)FGF	(acidic/basic) fibroblast growth factor
ABI	ankle-brachial (pressure) index
AD-MSC	adipose-derived mesenchymal stem cells
BM-MNC	bone marrow mononuclear cell(s)
BM-MSC	bone marrow mesenchymal stem cell(s)
CHD	coronary heart disease
CS	cell sheet
EC	endothelial cell(s)
ECM	extracellular matrix
G-CSD	granulocyte colony-stimulating factor
HGF	hepatocyte growth factor
HIFs	hypoxia-induced factors
HO-1	heme oxygenase-1
IC	intermittent claudication
MI	myocardial infarction
MMP	matrix metalloproteinase
MSC	mesenchymal stem cell(s)
PAD	peripheral artery disease
PB-MNC	peripheral blood mononuclear cell(s)
pDNA	plasmid DNA
PlGF	placental growth factor
SDF-1α	Stromal cell-derived factor-1α
SMC	smooth muscle cell(s)
TcO$_2$	transcutaneous O$_2$ pressure
TGF	transforming growth factor
uPA	urokinase plasminogen activator
VEGF	vascular endothelial growth factor
vWF	von Willebrand factor
PDGF	platelet-derived growth factor

Author details

Pavel Igorevich Makarevich[1-3*] and Yelena Viktorovna Parfyonova[1, 3]

*Address all correspondence to: pmakarevich@mc.msu.ru

1 Institute of Regenerative Medicine, Lomonosov Moscow State University, Moscow, Russia

2 Faculty of Medicine, Lomonosov Moscow State University, Moscow, Russia

3 Institute of Experimental Cardiology, Russian Cardiology Research and Production Complex, Russia

References

[1] Carmeliet P, Jain RK. Molecular mechanisms and clinical applications of angiogenesis. Nature. 2011;473(7347):298–307.

[2] Beck H, Voswinckel R, Wagner S, Ziegelhoeffer T, Heil M, Helisch A, et al. Participation of bone marrow-derived cells in long-term repair processes after experimental stroke. Journal of cerebral blood flow and metabolism: official journal of the International Society of Cerebral Blood Flow and Metabolism. 2003;23(6):709–17.

[3] Folkman J. Angiogenesis in cancer, vascular, rheumatoid and other disease. Nature medicine. 1995;1(1):27–31.

[4] Fong GH. Regulation of angiogenesis by oxygen sensing mechanisms. Journal of molecular medicine (Berlin). 2009;87(6):549–60.

[5] Deveza L, Choi J, Yang F. Therapeutic angiogenesis for treating cardiovascular diseases. Theranostics. 2012;2(8):801–14.

[6] Semenza GL. Oxygen sensing, hypoxia-inducible factors and disease pathophysiology. Annual review of pathology. 2014;9:47–71.

[7] Murakami M, Simons M. Fibroblast growth factor regulation of neovascularization. Current opinion in hematology. 2008;15(3):215–20.

[8] Taimeh Z, Loughran J, Birks EJ, Bolli R. Vascular endothelial growth factor in heart failure. Nature reviews cardiology. 2013;10(9):519–30.

[9] Ferrara N, Gerber HP, LeCouter J. The biology of VEGF and its receptors. Nature medicine. 2003;9(6):669–76.

[10] Xin X, Yang S, Ingle G, Zlot C, Rangell L, Kowalski J, et al. Hepatocyte growth factor enhances vascular endothelial growth factor-induced angiogenesis in vitro and in vivo. The American journal of pathology. 2001;158(3):1111–20.

[11] Menshikov M, Torosyan N, Elizarova E, Plakida K, Vorotnikov A, Parfyonova Y, et al. Urokinase induces matrix metalloproteinase-9/gelatinase B expression in THP-1

monocytes via ERK1/2 and cytosolic phospholipase A2 activation and eicosanoid production. Journal of vascular research. 2006;43(5):482–90.

[12] Adams RH, Alitalo K. Molecular regulation of angiogenesis and lymphangiogenesis. Nature reviews molecular cell biology. 2007;8(6):464–78.

[13] Gerhardt H, Golding M, Fruttiger M, Ruhrberg C, Lundkvist A, Abramsson A, et al. VEGF guides angiogenic sprouting utilizing endothelial tip cell filopodia. The journal of cell biology. 2003;161(6):1163–77.

[14] Fischer C, Schneider M, Carmeliet P. Principles and Therapeutic Implications of Angiogenesis, Vasculogenesis and Arteriogenesis. In: Moncada S, Higgs A, editors. The Vascular Endothelium II. Berlin, Heidelberg: Springer Berlin Heidelberg; 2006. p. 157–212.

[15] Hellstrom M, Phng LK, Hofmann JJ, Wallgard E, Coultas L, Lindblom P, et al. Dll4 signalling through Notch1 regulates formation of tip cells during angiogenesis. Nature. 2007;445(7129):776–80.

[16] Chung AS, Lee J, Ferrara N. Targeting the tumour vasculature: insights from physiological angiogenesis. Nature reviews cancer. 2010;10(7):505–14.

[17] Jain RK. Molecular regulation of vessel maturation. Nature medicine. 2003;9(6):685–93.

[18] Persson AB, Buschmann IR. Vascular growth in health and disease. Frontiers in molecular neuroscience. 2011;4:14.

[19] Heil M, Eitenmuller I, Schmitz-Rixen T, Schaper W. Arteriogenesis versus angiogenesis: similarities and differences. Journal of cellular and molecular medicine. 2006;10(1):45–55.

[20] Schaper W. Collateral circulation: past and present. Basic research in cardiology. 2009;104(1):5–21.

[21] de Groot D, Pasterkamp G, Hoefer IE. Cardiovascular risk factors and collateral artery formation. European journal of clinical investigation. 2009;39(12):1036–47.

[22] Hillmeister P, Lehmann KE, Bondke A, Witt H, Duelsner A, Gruber C, et al. Induction of cerebral arteriogenesis leads to early-phase expression of protease inhibitors in growing collaterals of the brain. Journal of cerebral blood flow and metabolism: official journal of the International Society of Cerebral Blood Flow and Metabolism. 2008;28(11):1811–23.

[23] Tkachuk V, Stepanova V, Little PJ, Bobik A. Regulation and role of urokinase plasminogen activator in vascular remodelling. Clinical and experimental pharmacology & physiology. 1996;23(9):759–65.

[24] Parfyonova YV, Plekhanova OS, Tkachuk VA. Plasminogen activators in vascular remodeling and angiogenesis. Biochemistry Biokhimiia. 2002;67(1):119–34.

[25] Scholz D, Ito W, Fleming I, Deindl E, Sauer A, Wiesnet M, et al. Ultrastructure and molecular histology of rabbit hind-limb collateral artery growth (arteriogenesis). Virchows Archiv: an international journal of pathology. 2000;436(3):257–70.

[26] Jaipersad AS, Lip GY, Silverman S, Shantsila E. The role of monocytes in angiogenesis and atherosclerosis. Journal of the American College of Cardiology. 2014;63(1):1–11.

[27] Roberts R, DeMello V, Sobel BE. Deleterious effects of methylprednisolone in patients with myocardial infarction. Circulation. 1976;53(3 Suppl):I204–6.

[28] Duelsner A, Gatzke N, Glaser J, Hillmeister P, Li M, Lee EJ, et al. Acetylsalicylic acid, but not clopidogrel, inhibits therapeutically induced cerebral arteriogenesis in the hypo-perfused rat brain. Journal of cerebral blood flow and metabolism: official journal of the International Society of Cerebral Blood Flow and Metabolism. 2012;32(1):105–14.

[29] van Amerongen MJ, Harmsen MC, van Rooijen N, Petersen AH, van Luyn MJ. Macrophage depletion impairs wound healing and increases left ventricular remodeling after myocardial injury in mice. The American journal of pathology. 2007;170(3):818–29.

[30] Baffour R, Berman J, Garb JL, Rhee SW, Kaufman J, Friedmann P. Enhanced angiogen-esis and growth of collaterals by in vivo administration of recombinant basic fibroblast growth factor in a rabbit model of acute lower limb ischemia: dose–response effect of basic fibroblast growth factor. Journal of vascular surgery: official publication, the Society for Vascular Surgery [and] International Society for Cardiovascular Surgery, North American Chapter. 1992;16(2):181–91.

[31] Morishita R, Nakamura S, Hayashi S, Taniyama Y, Moriguchi A, Nagano T, et al. Therapeutic angiogenesis induced by human recombinant hepatocyte growth factor in rabbit hind limb ischemia model as cytokine supplement therapy. Hypertension. 1999;33(6):1379–84.

[32] Grochot-Przeczek A, Dulak J, Jozkowicz A. Therapeutic angiogenesis for revasculariza-tion in peripheral artery disease. Gene. 2013;525(2):220–8.

[33] Lazarous DF, Unger EF, Epstein SE, Stine A, Arevalo JL, Chew EY, et al. Basic fibroblast growth factor in patients with intermittent claudication: results of a phase I trial. Journal of the American College of Cardiology. 2000;36(4):1239–44.

[34] Lederman RJ, Mendelsohn FO, Anderson RD, Saucedo JF, Tenaglia AN, Hermiller JB, et al. Therapeutic angiogenesis with recombinant fibroblast growth factor-2 for intermittent claudication (the TRAFFIC study): a randomised trial. Lancet. 2002;359(9323):2053–8.

[35] Wolff JA, Malone RW, Williams P, Chong W, Acsadi G, Jani A, et al. Direct gene transfer into mouse muscle in vivo. Science. 1990;247(4949 Pt 1):1465–8.

[36] Morishita R, Aoki M, Hashiya N, Makino H, Yamasaki K, Azuma J, et al. Safety evalua-tion of clinical gene therapy using hepatocyte growth factor to treat peripheral arterial disease. Hypertension. 2004;44(2):203–9.

[37] van Gaal EV, Hennink WE, Crommelin DJ, Mastrobattista E. Plasmid engineering for controlled and sustained gene expression for nonviral gene therapy. Pharmaceutical research. 2006;23(6):1053–74.

[38] Khare R, Chen CY, Weaver EA, Barry MA. Advances and future challenges in adenoviral vector pharmacology and targeting. Current gene therapy. 2011;11(4):241–58.

[39] Dismuke DJ, Tenenbaum L, Samulski RJ. Biosafety of recombinant adeno-associated virus vectors. Current gene therapy. 2013;13(6):434–52.

[40] Verma IM, Weitzman MD. Gene therapy: twenty-first century medicine. Annual review of biochemistry. 2005;74:711–38.

[41] MacColl GS, Novo FJ, Marshall NJ, Waters M, Goldspink G, Bouloux PM. Optimisation of growth hormone production by muscle cells using plasmid DNA. Journal of endocrinology. 2000;165(2):329–36.

[42] Makarevich PI, Rubina KA, Diykanov DT, Tkachuk VA, Parfyonova YV. Therapeutic angiogenesis using growth factors: current state and prospects for development. Kardiologiia. 2015;55(9):59–71.

[43] Takeshita S, Zheng LP, Brogi E, Kearney M, Pu LQ, Bunting S, et al. Therapeutic angiogenesis. A single intraarterial bolus of vascular endothelial growth factor augments revascularization in a rabbit ischemic hind limb model. The journal of clinical investigation. 1994;93(2):662–70.

[44] Baumgartner I, Pieczek A, Manor O, Blair R, Kearney M, Walsh K, et al. Constitutive expression of phVEGF165 after intramuscular gene transfer promotes collateral vessel development in patients with critical limb ischemia. Circulation. 1998;97(12):1114–23.

[45] Makinen K, Manninen H, Hedman M, Matsi P, Mussalo H, Alhava E, et al. Increased vascularity detected by digital subtraction angiography after VEGF gene transfer to human lower limb artery: a randomized, placebo-controlled, double-blinded phase II study. Molecular therapy: the journal of the American Society of Gene Therapy. 2002;6(1):127–33.

[46] Kusumanto YH, van Weel V, Mulder NH, Smit AJ, van den Dungen JJ, Hooymans JM, et al. Treatment with intramuscular vascular endothelial growth factor gene compared with placebo for patients with diabetes mellitus and critical limb ischemia: a double-blind randomized trial. Human gene therapy. 2006;17(6):683–91.

[47] Rajagopalan S, Mohler ER, 3rd, Lederman RJ, Mendelsohn FO, Saucedo JF, Goldman CK, et al. Regional angiogenesis with vascular endothelial growth factor in peripheral arterial disease: a phase II randomized, double-blind, controlled study of adenoviral delivery of vascular endothelial growth factor 121 in patients with disabling intermittent claudication. Circulation. 2003;108(16):1933–8.

[48] Vajanto I, Rissanen TT, Rutanen J, Hiltunen MO, Tuomisto TT, Arve K, et al. Evaluation of angiogenesis and side effects in ischemic rabbit hindlimbs after intramuscular injection of adenoviral vectors encoding VEGF and LacZ. The journal of gene medicine. 2002;4(4):371–80.

[49] Shimamura M, Nakagami H, Koriyama H, Morishita R. Gene therapy and cell-based therapies for therapeutic angiogenesis in peripheral artery disease. BioMed research international. 2013;2013:186215.

[50] Losordo DW, Vale PR, Symes JF, Dunnington CH, Esakof DD, Maysky M, et al. Gene therapy for myocardial angiogenesis: initial clinical results with direct myocardial injection of phVEGF165 as sole therapy for myocardial ischemia. Circulation. 1998;98(25):2800–4.

[51] Hedman M, Hartikainen J, Syvanne M, Stjernvall J, Hedman A, Kivela A, et al. Safety and feasibility of catheter-based local intracoronary vascular endothelial growth factor gene transfer in the prevention of postangioplasty and in-stent restenosis and in the treatment of chronic myocardial ischemia: phase II results of the Kuopio Angiogenesis Trial (KAT). Circulation. 2003;107(21):2677–83.

[52] Gyongyosi M, Khorsand A, Zamini S, Sperker W, Strehblow C, Kastrup J, et al. NOGA-guided analysis of regional myocardial perfusion abnormalities treated with intramyocardial injections of plasmid encoding vascular endothelial growth factor A-165 in patients with chronic myocardial ischemia: subanalysis of the EUROINJECT-ONE multicenter double-blind randomized study. Circulation. 2005;112(9 Suppl):I157–65.

[53] Aoki M, Morishita R, Taniyama Y, Kida I, Moriguchi A, Matsumoto K, et al. Angiogenesis induced by hepatocyte growth factor in non-infarcted myocardium and infarcted myocardium: up-regulation of essential transcription factor for angiogenesis, ets. Gene therapy. 2000;7(5):417–27.

[54] Morishita R, Aoki M, Hashiya N, Yamasaki K, Kurinami H, Shimizu S, et al. Therapeutic angiogenesis using hepatocyte growth factor (HGF). Current gene therapy. 2004;4(2):199–206.

[55] Morishita R, Makino H, Aoki M, Hashiya N, Yamasaki K, Azuma J, et al. Phase I/IIa clinical trial of therapeutic angiogenesis using hepatocyte growth factor gene transfer to treat critical limb ischemia. Arteriosclerosis, thrombosis and vascular biology. 2011;31(3):713–20.

[56] Shigematsu H, Yasuda K, Iwai T, Sasajima T, Ishimaru S, Ohashi Y, et al. Randomized, double-blind, placebo-controlled clinical trial of hepatocyte growth factor plasmid for critical limb ischemia. Gene therapy. 2010;17(9):1152–61.

[57] Pyun WB, Hahn W, Kim DS, Yoo WS, Lee SD, Won JH, et al. Naked DNA expressing two isoforms of hepatocyte growth factor induces collateral artery augmentation in a rabbit model of limb ischemia. Gene therapy. 2010;17(12):1442–52.

[58] Gu Y, Zhang J, Guo L, Cui S, Li X, Ding D, et al. A phase I clinical study of naked DNA expressing two isoforms of hepatocyte growth factor to treat patients with critical limb ischemia. The journal of gene medicine. 2011;13(11):602–10.

[59] Taniyama Y, Morishita R, Nakagami H, Moriguchi A, Sakonjo H, Shokei K, et al. Potential contribution of a novel antifibrotic factor, hepatocyte growth factor, to prevention of myocardial fibrosis by angiotensin II blockade in cardiomyopathic hamsters. Circulation. 2000;102(2):246–52.

[60] Nikol S, Baumgartner I, Van Belle E, Diehm C, Visona A, Capogrossi MC, et al. Therapeutic angiogenesis with intramuscular NV1FGF improves amputation-free

survival in patients with critical limb ischemia. Molecular therapy: the journal of the American Society of Gene Therapy. 2008;16(5):972–8.

[61] Comerota AJ, Throm RC, Miller KA, Henry T, Chronos N, Laird J, et al. Naked plasmid DNA encoding fibroblast growth factor type 1 for the treatment of end-stage unreconstructible lower extremity ischemia: preliminary results of a phase I trial. Journal of vascular surgery: official publication, the Society for Vascular Surgery [and] International Society for Cardiovascular Surgery, North American Chapter. 2002;35(5):930–6.

[62] Fowkes FG, Price JF. Gene therapy for critical limb ischaemia: the TAMARIS trial. Lancet. 2011;377(9781):1894–6.

[63] Belch J, Hiatt WR, Baumgartner I, Driver IV, Nikol S, Norgren L, et al. Effect of fibroblast growth factor NV1FGF on amputation and death: a randomised placebo-controlled trial of gene therapy in critical limb ischaemia. Lancet. 2011;377(9781):1929–37.

[64] Niebuhr A, Henry T, Goldman J, Baumgartner I, van Belle E, Gerss J, et al. Long-term safety of intramuscular gene transfer of non-viral FGF1 for peripheral artery disease. Gene therapy. 2012;19(3):264–70.

[65] Reis SE, Holubkov R, Conrad Smith AJ, Kelsey SF, Sharaf BL, Reichek N, et al. Coronary microvascular dysfunction is highly prevalent in women with chest pain in the absence of coronary artery disease: results from the NHLBI WISE study. American heart journal. 2001;141(5):735–41.

[66] Handberg E, Johnson BD, Arant CB, Wessel TR, Kerensky RA, von Mering G, et al. Impaired coronary vascular reactivity and functional capacity in women: results from the NHLBI Women's Ischemia Syndrome Evaluation (WISE) Study. Journal of the American College of Cardiology. 2006;47(3 Suppl):S44–9.

[67] Hochman JS, Tamis JE, Thompson TD, Weaver WD, White HD, Van de Werf F, et al. Sex, clinical presentation and outcome in patients with acute coronary syndromes. Global Use of Strategies to Open Occluded Coronary Arteries in Acute Coronary Syndromes IIb Investigators. The New England journal of medicine. 1999;341(4):226–32.

[68] Yonemitsu Y, Matsumoto T, Itoh H, Okazaki J, Uchiyama M, Yoshida K, et al. DVC1-0101 to treat peripheral arterial disease: a Phase I/IIa open-label dose-escalation clinical trial. Molecular therapy: the journal of the American Society of Gene Therapy. 2013;21(3):707–14.

[69] Creager MA, Olin JW, Belch JJ, Moneta GL, Henry TD, Rajagopalan S, et al. Effect of hypoxia-inducible factor-1 alpha gene therapy on walking performance in patients with intermittent claudication. Circulation. 2011;124(16):1765–73.

[70] Yla-Herttuala S, Markkanen JE, Rissanen TT. Gene therapy for ischemic cardiovascular diseases: some lessons learned from the first clinical trials. Trends in cardiovascular medicine. 2004;14(8):295–300.

[71] Spanholtz TA, Theodorou P, Holzbach T, Wutzler S, Giunta RE, Machens HG. Vascular endothelial growth factor (VEGF165) plus basic fibroblast growth factor (bFGF) producing cells induce a mature and stable vascular network--a future therapy for ischemically challenged tissue. The journal of surgical research. 2011;171(1):329–38.

[72] Kupatt C, Hinkel R, Pfosser A, El-Aouni C, Wuchrer A, Fritz A, et al. Cotransfection of vascular endothelial growth factor-A and platelet-derived growth factor-B via recombinant adeno-associated virus resolves chronic ischemic malperfusion role of vessel maturation. Journal of the American College of Cardiology. 2010;56(5):414–22.

[73] Arsic N, Zentilin L, Zacchigna S, Santoro D, Stanta G, Salvi A, et al. Induction of functional neovascularization by combined VEGF and angiopoietin-1 gene transfer using AAV vectors. Molecular therapy: the journal of the American Society of Gene Therapy. 2003;7(4):450–9.

[74] Yu JX, Huang XF, Lv WM, Ye CS, Peng XZ, Zhang H, et al. Combination of stromal-derived factor-1 alpha and vascular endothelial growth factor gene-modified endothelial progenitor cells is more effective for ischemic neovascularization. Journal of vascular surgery: official publication, the Society for Vascular Surgery [and] International Society for Cardiovascular Surgery, North American Chapter. 2009;50(3):608–16.

[75] Traktuev DO, Tsokolaeva ZI, Shevelev AA, Talitskiy KA, Stepanova VV, Johnstone BH, et al. Urokinase gene transfer augments angiogenesis in ischemic skeletal and myocardial muscle. Molecular therapy: the journal of the American Society of Gene Therapy. 2007;15(11):1939–46.

[76] Makarevich P, Tsokolaeva Z, Shevelev A, Rybalkin I, Shevchenko E, Beloglazova I, et al. Combined transfer of human VEGF165 and HGF genes renders potent angiogenic effect in ischemic skeletal muscle. PLoS one. 2012;7(6):e38776.

[77] Lee S, Kim K, Kim HA, Kim SW, Lee M. Augmentation of erythropoietin enhancer-mediated hypoxia-inducible gene expression by co-transfection of a plasmid encoding hypoxia-inducible factor 1 alpha for ischemic tissue targeting gene therapy. Journal of drug targeting. 2008;16(1):43–50.

[78] Bhang SH, Kim JH, Yang HS, La WG, Lee TJ, Sun AY, et al. Combined delivery of heme oxygenase-1 gene and fibroblast growth factor-2 protein for therapeutic angiogenesis. Biomaterials. 2009;30(31):6247–56.

[79] Dulak J, Jozkowicz A, Foresti R, Kasza A, Frick M, Huk I, et al. Heme oxygenase activity modulates vascular endothelial growth factor synthesis in vascular smooth muscle cells. Antioxidants & redox signaling. 2002;4(2):229–40.

[80] Saif J, Schwarz TM, Chau DY, Henstock J, Sami P, Leicht SF, et al. Combination of injectable multiple growth factor-releasing scaffolds and cell therapy as an advanced modality to enhance tissue neovascularization. Arteriosclerosis, thrombosis and vascular biology. 2010;30(10):1897–904.

[81] Yang Y, Chen QH, Liu AR, Xu XP, Han JB, Qiu HB. Synergism of MSC-secreted HGF and VEGF in stabilising endothelial barrier function upon lipopolysaccharide stimulation via the Rac1 pathway. Stem cell research & therapy. 2015;6:250.

[82] Min JK, Lee YM, Kim JH, Kim YM, Kim SW, Lee SY, et al. Hepatocyte growth factor suppresses vascular endothelial growth factor-induced expression of endothelial ICAM-1 and VCAM-1 by inhibiting the nuclear factor-kappaB pathway. Circulation research. 2005;96(3):300-7.

[83] Kim I, Moon SO, Park SK, Chae SW, Koh GY. Angiopoietin-1 reduces VEGF-stimulated leukocyte adhesion to endothelial cells by reducing ICAM-1, VCAM-1 and E-selectin expression. Circulation research. 2001;89(6):477-9.

[84] Yamauchi A, Ito Y, Morikawa M, Kobune M, Huang J, Sasaki K, et al. Pre-administration of angiopoietin-1 followed by VEGF induces functional and mature vascular formation in a rabbit ischemic model. The journal of gene medicine. 2003;5(11):994-1004.

[85] Asahara T, Murohara T, Sullivan A, Silver M, van der Zee R, Li T, et al. Isolation of putative progenitor endothelial cells for angiogenesis. Science. 1997;275(5302):964-7.

[86] Rohde E, Malischnik C, Thaler D, Maierhofer T, Linkesch W, Lanzer G, et al. Blood monocytes mimic endothelial progenitor cells. Stem cells. 2006;24(2):357-67.

[87] Prokopi M, Pula G, Mayr U, Devue C, Gallagher J, Xiao Q, et al. Proteomic analysis reveals presence of platelet microparticles in endothelial progenitor cell cultures. Blood. 2009;114(3):723-32.

[88] Lu D, Chen B, Liang Z, Deng W, Jiang Y, Li S, et al. Comparison of bone marrow mesenchymal stem cells with bone marrow-derived mononuclear cells for treatment of diabetic critical limb ischemia and foot ulcer: a double-blind, randomized, controlled trial. Diabetes research and clinical practice. 2011;92(1):26-36.

[89] Huang PP, Yang XF, Li SZ, Wen JC, Zhang Y, Han ZC. Randomised comparison of G-CSF-mobilized peripheral blood mononuclear cells versus bone marrow-mononuclear cells for the treatment of patients with lower limb arteriosclerosis obliterans. Thrombosis and haemostasis. 2007;98(6):1335-42.

[90] Arai M, Misao Y, Nagai H, Kawasaki M, Nagashima K, Suzuki K, et al. Granulocyte colony-stimulating factor: a noninvasive regeneration therapy for treating atherosclerotic peripheral artery disease. Circulation journal: official journal of the Japanese Circulation Society. 2006;70(9):1093-8.

[91] Bourin P, Bunnell BA, Casteilla L, Dominici M, Katz AJ, March KL, et al. Stromal cells from the adipose tissue-derived stromal vascular fraction and culture expanded adipose tissue-derived stromal/stem cells: a joint statement of the International Federation for Adipose Therapeutics and Science (IFATS) and the International Society for Cellular Therapy (ISCT). Cytotherapy. 2013;15(6):641-8.

[92] Rubina K, Kalinina N, Efimenko A, Lopatina T, Melikhova V, Tsokolaeva Z, et al. Adipose stromal cells stimulate angiogenesis via promoting progenitor cell differentia-

tion, secretion of angiogenic factors and enhancing vessel maturation. Tissue engineering Part A. 2009;15(8):2039–50.

[93] Yang D, Wang W, Li L, Peng Y, Chen P, Huang H, et al. The relative contribution of paracrine effect versus direct differentiation on adipose-derived stem cell transplantation mediated cardiac repair. PLoS one. 2013;8(3):e59020.

[94] Efimenko A, Starostina E, Kalinina N, Stolzing A. Angiogenic properties of aged adipose derived mesenchymal stem cells after hypoxic conditioning. Journal of translational medicine. 2011;9:10.

[95] Efimenko A, Dzhoyashvili N, Kalinina N, Kochegura T, Akchurin R, Tkachuk V, et al. Adipose-derived mesenchymal stromal cells from aged patients with coronary artery disease keep mesenchymal stromal cell properties but exhibit characteristics of aging and have impaired angiogenic potential. Stem cells translational medicine. 2014;3(1):32–41.

[96] Makarevich PI, Dergilev KV, Tsokolaeva ZI, Efimenko AY, Gluhanuk EV, Gallinger JO, et al. Delivery of genetically engineered adipose-derived cell sheets for treatment of ischemic disorders-development of application in animal models. Molecular therapy; Nature Publishing Group: New York, NY, USA; 2015. p. S262-S.

[97] Merdan T, Kopecek J, Kissel T. Prospects for cationic polymers in gene and oligonucleotide therapy against cancer. Advanced drug delivery reviews. 2002;54(5):715–58.

[98] Shevchenko EK, Makarevich PI, Tsokolaeva ZI, Boldyreva MA, Sysoeva VY, Tkachuk VA, et al. Transplantation of modified human adipose derived stromal cells expressing VEGF165 results in more efficient angiogenic response in ischemic skeletal muscle. Journal of translational medicine. 2013;11:138.

[99] Sen S, Merchan J, Dean J, Ii M, Gavin M, Silver M, et al. Autologous transplantation of endothelial progenitor cells genetically modified by adeno-associated viral vector delivering insulin-like growth factor-1 gene after myocardial infarction. Human gene therapy. 2010;21(10):1327–34.

[100] Suzuki M, Iso-o N, Takeshita S, Tsukamoto K, Mori I, Sato T, et al. Facilitated angiogenesis induced by heme oxygenase-1 gene transfer in a rat model of hindlimb ischemia. Biochemical and biophysical research communications. 2003;302(1):138–43.

[101] Holzinger A, Barden M, Abken H. The growing world of CAR T cell trials: a systematic review. Cancer Immunol Immunother. 2016;65(12):1433–50.

[102] Phase I study of IM injection of VEGF-producing MSC for the treatment of critical limb ischemia [Available from: https://www.cirm.ca.gov/our-progress/awards/phase-i-study-im-injection-vegf-producing-msc-treatment-critical-limb-ischemia-0.

[103] Papapetrou EP, Lee G, Malani N, Setty M, Riviere I, Tirunagari LM, et al. Genomic safe harbors permit high beta-globin transgene expression in thalassemia induced pluripotent stem cells. Nature biotechnology. 2011;29(1):73–8.

[104] Kumashiro Y, Fukumori K, Takahashi H, Nakayama M, Akiyama Y, Yamato M, et al. Modulation of cell adhesion and detachment on thermo-responsive polymeric surfaces through the observation of surface dynamics. Colloids and surfaces B: biointerfaces. 2013;106:198–207.

[105] Aguado BA, Mulyasasmita W, Su J, Lampe KJ, Heilshorn SC. Improving viability of stem cells during syringe needle flow through the design of hydrogel cell carriers. Tissue engineering Part A. 2012;18(7–8):806–15.

[106] Lin CY, Lin KJ, Li KC, Sung LY, Hsueh S, Lu CH, et al. Immune responses during healing of massive segmental femoral bone defects mediated by hybrid baculovirus-engineered ASCs. Biomaterials. 2012;33(30):7422–34.

[107] Dergilev K, Tsokolaeva Z, Rubina K, Sysoeva V, Makarevich P, Boldyreva M, et al. Isolation and characterization of cardiac progenitor cells from myocardial right atrial appendage tissue. Cell and tissue biology. 2016;10(5):349–56.

[108] Elloumi-Hannachi I, Yamato M, Okano T. Cell sheet engineering: a unique nanotechnology for scaffold-free tissue reconstruction with clinical applications in regenerative medicine. Journal of internal medicine. 2010;267(1):54–70.

[109] Matsuura K, Utoh R, Nagase K, Okano T. Cell sheet approach for tissue engineering and regenerative medicine. Journal of controlled release: official journal of the Controlled Release Society. 2014;190:228–39.

[110] Yang J, Yamato M, Shimizu T, Sekine H, Ohashi K, Kanzaki M, et al. Reconstruction of functional tissues with cell sheet engineering. Biomaterials. 2007;28(34):5033–43.

[111] Yang J, Yamato M, Kohno C, Nishimoto A, Sekine H, Fukai F, et al. Cell sheet engineering: recreating tissues without biodegradable scaffolds. Biomaterials. 2005;26(33):6415–22.

[112] Sekine H, Shimizu T, Dobashi I, Matsuura K, Hagiwara N, Takahashi M, et al. Cardiac cell sheet transplantation improves damaged heart function via superior cell survival in comparison with dissociated cell injection. Tissue engineering Part A. 2011;17(23–24):2973–80.

[113] Mitamura Y. Current status of left ventricular assist devices and cell sheet engineering for treatment of severe heart disease in Japan. Artificial organs. 2015;39(7):543–9.

[114] Makarevich P, Boldyreva M, Dergilev K, Gluhanyuk E, Gallinger J, Efimenko A, et al. Transplantation of cell sheets from adipose-derived mesenchymal stromal cells effectively induces angiogenesis in ischemic skeletal muscle. Genes and cells. 2015;10(3):68–77.

[115] Bak S, Ahmad T, Lee YB, Lee JY, Kim EM, Shin H. Delivery of a cell patch of cocultured endothelial cells and smooth muscle cells using thermoresponsive hydrogels for enhanced angiogenesis. Tissue engineering Part A. 2016;22(1–2):182–93.

[116] Yeh TS, Fang YH, Lu CH, Chiu SC, Yeh CL, Yen TC, et al. Baculovirus-transduced, VEGF-expressing adipose-derived stem cell sheet for the treatment of myocardium infarction. Biomaterials. 2014;35(1):174–84.

6

Noncoding RNAs in Lung Cancer Angiogenesis

Ioana Berindan-Neagoe, Cornelia Braicu,
Diana Gulei, Ciprian Tomuleasa and
George Adrian Calin

Abstract

Lung cancer is the major death-related cancer in both men and women, due to late diagnostic and limited treatment efficacy. The angiogenic process that is responsible for the support of tumor progression and metastasis represents one of the main hallmarks of cancer. The role of VEGF signaling in angiogenesis is well-established, and we summarize the role of semaphorins and their related receptors or hypoxia-related factors role as prone of tumor microenvironment in angiogenic mechanisms. Newly, noncoding RNA transcripts (ncRNA) were identified to have vital functions in miscellaneous biological processes, including lung cancer angiogenesis. Therefore, due to their capacity to regulate almost all molecular pathways related with altered key genes, including those involved in angiogenesis and its microenvironment, ncRNAs can serve as diagnosis and prognosis markers or therapeutic targets. We intend to summarize the latest progress in the field of ncRNAs in lung cancer and their relation with hypoxia-related factors and angiogenic genes, with a particular focus on ncRNAs relation to semaphorins.

Keywords: noncoding RNAs, angiogenesis, lung cancer, semaphorins, therapy

1. Introduction

1.1. Noncoding RNAs (ncRNAs)—definition, biogenesis and classification

The noncoding RNAs evolved in the last few years as important regulators of numerous physiological and pathological processes with increased attention regarding cancer diagnosis, prognosis, and therapeutics [1]. The concept known as "dark matter" defined by the lack of function and lack of genetic information is now long gone, being replaced by the regulatory ncRNAs involved in cancer development and progression [1]. The transcription of the noncoding regions produces RNA sequences that can vary in size, short, mid-size, and long noncoding RNAs, and are able to influence the expression of tumor suppressor or tumor promoting coding genes, activity that further classifies this class of RNAs into oncogenic or tumor suppressor sequences [2].

The noncoding niche is rapidly expanding as new sequences are discovered and characterized. The ncRNAs, as their name underline, are RNAs that do not codify for proteins but new molecular concepts are revealed regarding the interplay between these types of RNA sequences and protein coding genes [3]. ncRNAs are also known as regulatory RNAs.

One of the most studied ncRNAs class is represented by microRNAs (miRNAs) that are small single-stranded nucleotide sequences (18–22 nucleotide length) capable of gene regulation through sequence complementarity [2], being involved in all hallmarks of cancer [4]. The biogenesis mechanism is presented in **Figure 1**. The discovery of miRNAs has enabled new

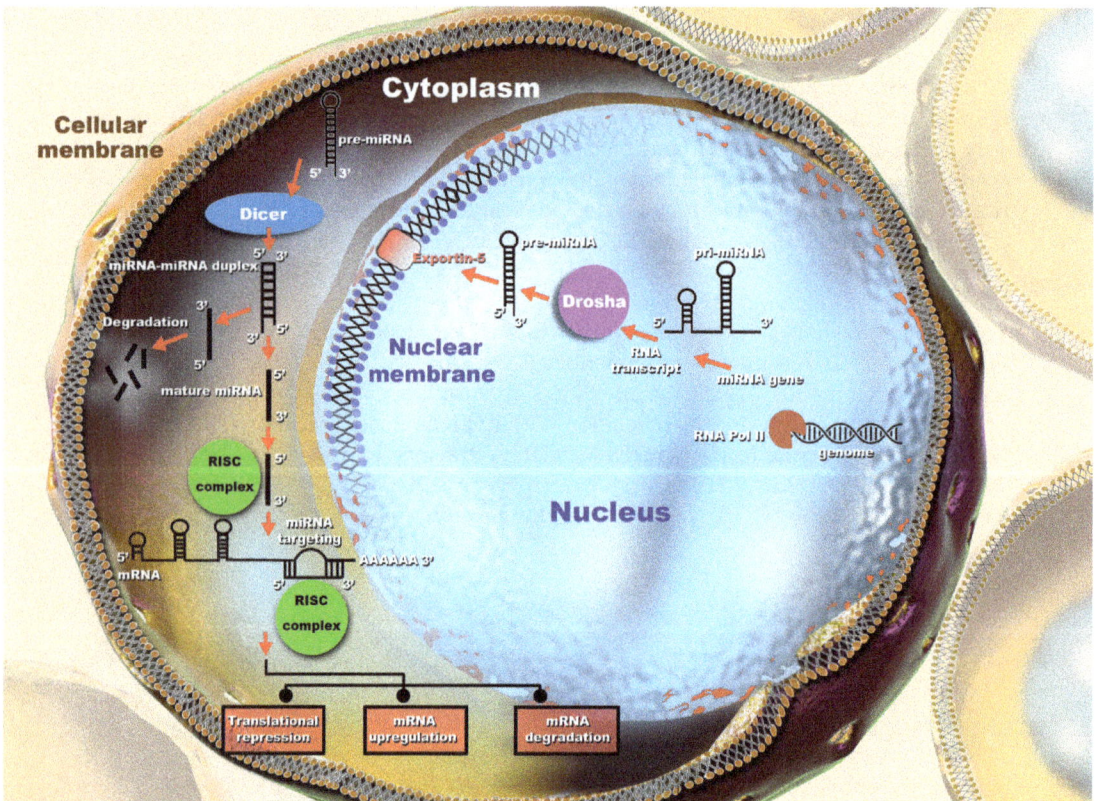

Figure 1. miRNA biogenesis mechanism. microRNAs are situated in the genome of the host as individual transcriptional units but also as clusters of a number of distinct microRNAs. For the first step, RNA polymerase II transcribes the target sequence resulting in a primary transcript named pri-miRNAs. This unprocessed sequence is then subjected to the activity of RNase III-type enzyme Drosha that transforms the pri-miRNA sequence into a transcript of approximatively 70 nt, pre-miRNA. This precursor is then transferred in the cytoplasm via Exportin-5, followed by another miRNA manipulation step governed by the RNase III protein Dicer, resulting in a double stranded RNA called miRNA-miRNA duplex. The less stable strand is further captured by the RISC complex, association that facilitates specific gene regulation through complementary interactions.

noninvasive diagnosis methods and also has conducted towards the development of more targeted therapeutics alternatives in a large number of cancers and other pathological states [4, 5]. Despite numerous discoveries in the ncRNA field, the two main noncoding fronts in cancer are still represented by microRNAs and the more recent characterized long noncoding RNAs (lncRNAs) [6]. As the technology advances, these last sequences are increasingly mentioned in pathological contexts, where differential expression levels are associated with malignant states and other diseases [6]. Despite the associations between lncRNAs expression patterns and different types of cancers, there are still many unknowns regarding the complex mechanism of action.

MiRNAs revolution has stimulated the investigation of other types of small ncRNAs such as small interfering RNAs (siRNAs), and Piwi-interacting RNAs (piRNAs) [3, 7, 8]. These last two types of molecules are similar to miRNAs in length and function, where siRNAs mediate posttranscriptional inhibitory processes and piRNAs act particularly on transposable elements and are capable of forming complexes with Piwi proteins [7, 8]. piRNAs transcribed from kiwi clusters together with Piwi proteins are capable of transposon modulation through interruption of the specific transcript that will be no longer able to exercise their specific activity. Other types of ncRNAs, circularRNA (ciRNA) are formed through base pairing of intronic repeats that ends up with a complete circular fragment that is able to act as a miRNA sponge through complementary interactions [3, 9].

Supplementing the complex regulatory networks of miRNAs, ciRNAs have recently emerged as new cancer modeling tools through miRNA targeting, escaping from the initial characterization as transcriptional "noise" [9, 10]. These types of transcripts are ubiquitous present in eukaryotic cells and competitively bind microRNAs sequences, functioning like an inhibitory sponge; process that could attribute a significant therapeutic potential to these circular fragments [9, 10, 11, 12]. In this sense, specific microRNAs are eliminated from the regulatory networks, influencing the expression scheme of target genes. Competitive endogenous RNA (ceRNA) describes a new mechanism of gene regulation, being involved in physiological and pathological processes [13].

The traditional concept that RNA molecules are just intermediary sequences between DNA and proteins is now replaced with more advanced molecular data, where short- and long-noncoding sequences play a key role in normal development and disease progression [14]. SiRNAs and miRNAs are similar in length, approximatively 22 nucleotides, and are both processed by Dicer through cleavage. SiRNAs are derived from complementary dsRNA duplexes, where miRNAs originate from imperfect RNA hairpins from short introns or long transcripts [15–18]. Both small noncoding types of sequences associate with Argonaute proteins in order to manipulate gene expression (generally through 3'UTRs) [19], although siRNAs are also involved in viral defense and transposon regulation. piRNAs are the longest fragments from the small RNAs group, having approximatively 26–30 in length. This class associates with PIWI-clade Argonaute proteins in order to guide transposon activity and chromatin status [15, 17]. Long noncoding RNA group consist in all RNA sequences that are not responsible for protein generation and their length exceed

200 nucleotides, being further grouped in concordance with their genomic localization: intronic, intergenic, sense, and antisense ncRNAs to host gene locus [6, 20]. Biogenesis of lncRNAs is very similar with the processing activity of mRNAs molecule, being transcribed by RNA Pol II and also being subjected to the same epigenetic modifications and splicing signals. The functional roles of lncRNAs are more extended than in the case of small ncRNAs, a significant part being still incompletely understood. Briefly, this type of sequences is not so well conserved as miRNAs and also can control gene activity at different levels in a more complex scheme [2, 6, 16].

2. Lung cancer—molecular classification and survival rates

Lung cancer occupies the first place regarding the mortality rates from the oncological field, being characterized by an aggressive profile that ends with numerous deadly metastatic sites. One of the main reasons for the high mortality rates consists in the late diagnosis [21]. According to the characteristics of the cancer cells, this malignancy presents itself in two major forms, one being *small-cell lung cancer* (SCLC), and the other being named *non-small-cell lung cancer* (NSCLC) according to the histological classification and another rare subtype, *lung carcinoid tumor* (*LCT*) [22, 23]. NSCLC ranks as the number one diagnosed type of lung cancer in the oncological field, being further divided into three histologic types: *squamous cell carcinoma, large-cell carcinoma, and adenocarcinoma. Adenocarcinomas* represent the most common subtype of NSCLC, with an incidence of 35–40% from all lung cancer cases, being the most lethal type of cancer in male population, and the second in women. This type of pulmonary malignancy frequently presents distant metastases and pleural effusions. Between a quarter and 30% of all lung cancer cases belong to the squamous cell carcinoma category. These particular tumors are mostly located in the central areas of the lungs, and were shown to be connected to tobacco smoking [24]. Lung carcinoid tumors are very rare and represent about 5% of the lung cancers which grows very slowly and are rarely associated with metastasis [25]. Despite the frequency drop, pulmonary tumors remain the major cause of death and morbidity around the world, being very aggressive and refractory to standard oncologic therapy [26], due to the late diagnostic [27].

Environmental and occupational exposure to different agents and an individual's susceptibility for these agents were associated with a risk of lung cancer in approximately 9–15% of cases. The cigarette smoke is the primary risk factor for the development of lung cancer and is estimated to be responsible for approximately 90% of all lung cancers [24], followed by asbestos [28], and radon [27]. More than 300 harmful substances with 40 known potent carcinogens were discovered in tobacco smoke.

The classical therapeutic strategies like surgery and chemotherapy or radiation fail to accomplish their purpose in advanced pathological states. In the case of patients diagnosed early in the disease, the chances of survival are more promising, being observed a partial response to drugs based on platinum. However, even in this case, the final outcome is not necessary a positive one due to acquisition of treatment resistance. According to National Cancer Institute, survival rates for early stages of NSCLC are extremely low compared to other types of cancer, where the rate for the late stages of the same malignancy can reach even 1%: the 5 years survival rate for stage IA is approximately 49%, 45% for stage IB, 30% for stage IIA and 31% for IIB. The next stages, IIIA and IIIB, are associated with even more dramatically numbers, 14% and 5% respectively (**Figure 2**). For the case of metastatic lung cancer, where the tumor has spread within different body sites, the survival rates are extremely low (1%) [29, 30]. Therefore, a critical part of lung cancer management is represented by the discovery of specific molecular carcinogenic pathways in order to precisely target key molecules that are responsible for tumor development and avoid treatment resistance. ncRNAs study represents an important research direction for achieving these goals.

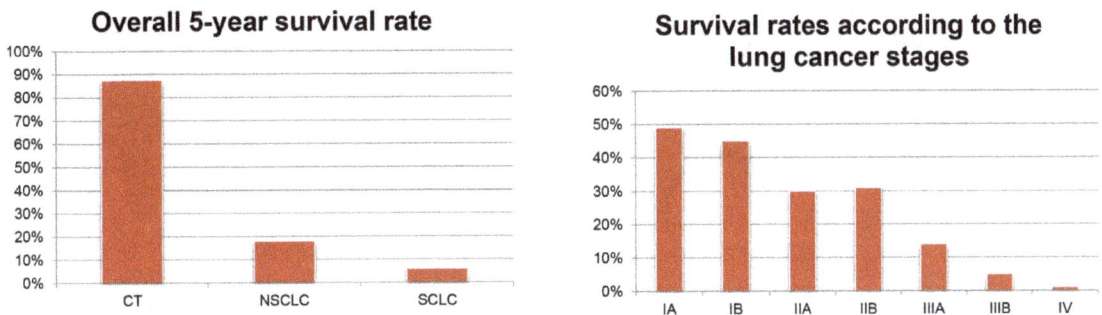

Figure 2. The overall survival rates associated with different lung cancer subtypes (NSCLC, SCLC) and the 5-year survival rate based on lung cancer stages.

3. Angiogenesis—beyond hallmarks of lung cancer

Nowadays, the cancer hallmarks are at the center of carcinogenesis: prolonged proliferation signals, escaping of growth inhibitors, apoptosis inhibition, indefinite replicative potential, vascular network development (angiogenesis) and activation of cell invasion, and thus metastasis (**Figure 3**) [31]. Although all of these hallmarks represent key elements without which tumorigenesis could not more or less advance, angiogenesis surpasses this listing of malignant processes: without the ability to receive oxygen and nutrients and evacuate waste products, the spreading of the tumor is naturally restricted. Moreover, the vessel network is one of the invasion routes used by transformed mesenchymal cell in order to evade from the original carcinogenic site and invade other tissues [31]. All these features stand at the base of the therapeutic concept, where angiogenesis is one of the main signaling pathway targeted in the treatment of cancer patients, including individuals with lung cancer. Inhibition of this malignant progression pathway through exogenous administration of targeted agents in the form of ncRNAs/anti-ncRNAs will enable the proper management of tumor spreading and will serve as a feasible therapeutic strategy for lung cancer [33].

The most promising proangiogenic target in lung cancer is VEGF (vascular endothelial growth factor), more precisely the interaction of VEGF with the transmembrane receptors or receptors downstream the signaling pathways. However, prolonged exposure to VEGF/VEGFR inhibitors may force tumor cells to find alternative pathways for vascular

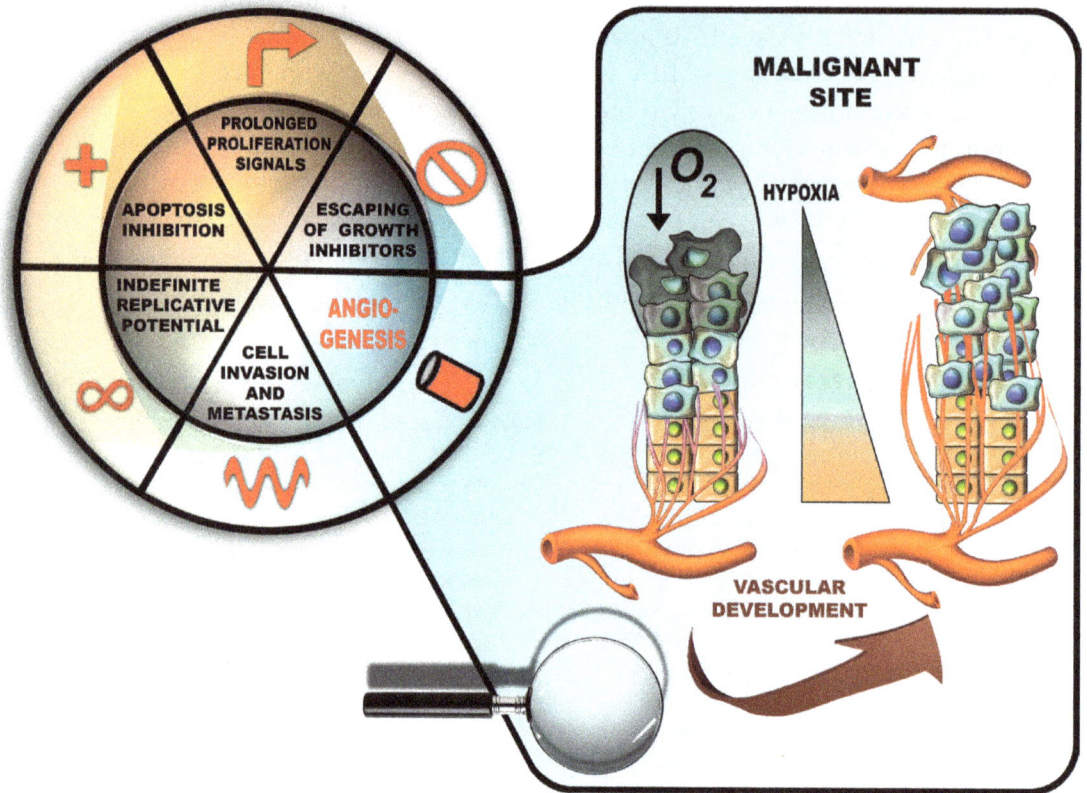

Figure 3. Lung cancer hallmarks with focus on angiogenesis.

development [34]. Additionally, some other angiogenic pathways have been explored with the same purpose, where FGFRs (fibroblast growth factor receptors), angiopoietin, PDGFRs (platelet-derived growth factor receptors), and, in the last few years, semaphorins and the related receptors captured the attention [32, 34]. The metastatic cascade, a multievent process that leads to the spreading of the tumor cells to numerous sites in the organism and causes death, represents the main challenge in cancer treatment and angiogenesis plays a major role in this progression [35].

3.1. Implication of ncRNAs in regulation of lung cancer angiogenesis

As a result of the limited success of the classical antiangiogenic therapies targeting VEGF and its related receptors [35, 36], researchers have deepened their knowledge by analyzing the expression of ncRNAs sequences in this pathology (**Figure 4**) [37, 38]. The mechanism of lung cancer angiogenesis is far from being completely deciphered and implicit the process of therapeutic inhibition via ncRNAs remains to be further investigated. Targeting ncRNAs will enable a more precise treatment and will avoid compensatory mechanisms retrieved in lung cancer [2, 37, 38].

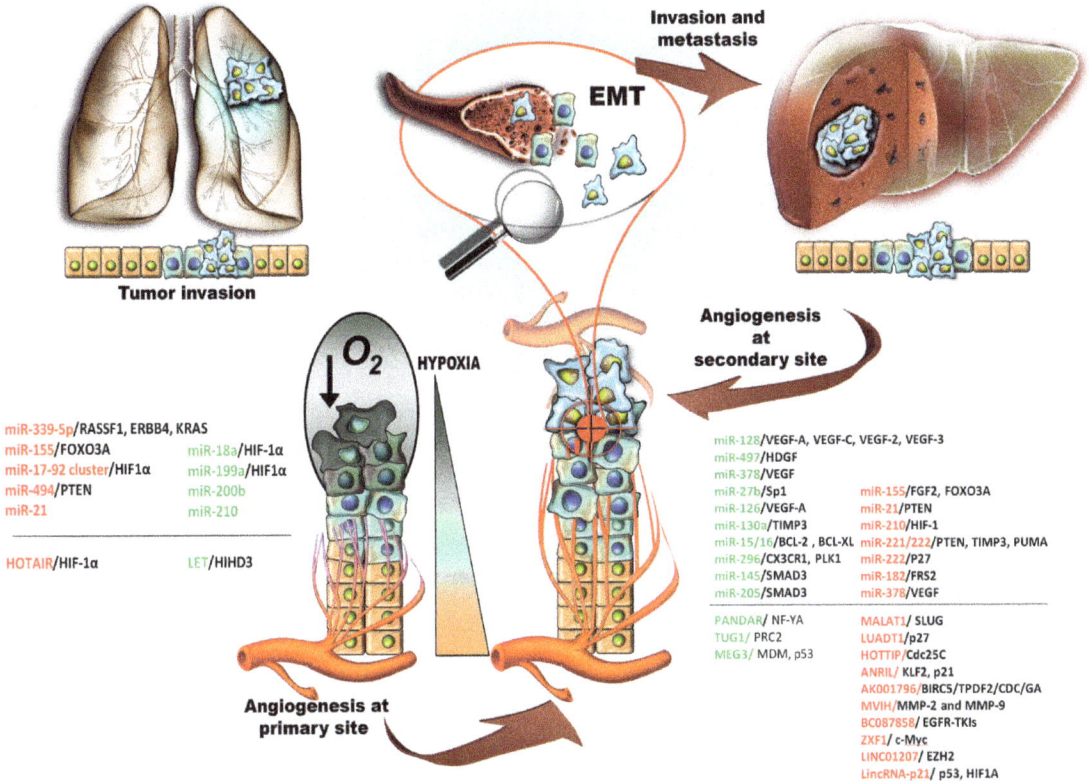

Figure 4. Evolution of vascular network within lung cancer. Malignant cells lacking nutrients and oxygen enter in hypoxic stress, state that promotes the signaling pathways related to angiogenesis in order to sustain cell proliferation. The same process is present at the metastatic sites, where mesenchymal cells that went through epithelial to mesenchymal transition are establishing new malignant formations. The complex malignant scheme is strictly regulated by noncoding RNAs (miRNAs and lncRNAs). Red - overexpressed ncRNAs; Green- downregulated ncRNAs.

3.2. miRNAs related to lung cancer angiogenesis

Among all types of ncRNAs, miRNAs molecules are the most intensive studied in what regards novel cancer therapies. Although the majority of the studies are concentrated on oncogenic miRNA inhibition via exogenous delivery of complementary (antisense) sequences through different vectors, it seems that another therapeutic alternative consists in miRNA replacement. This last type of targeted treatment may be even more effective due to the fact that the predominant pathological model consists more in dowregulated tumor suppressor sequences than overexpressed oncogenic genes [5, 21, 39].

Until this moment, several miRNA patterns involved in different lung cancer processes such as cell proliferation, resistance to therapy, invasion, metastasis, and angiogenesis have been identified. We will focus on some important miRNAs that presented the most aberrant expression related to lung cancer angiogenesis (**Tables 1** and **2**).

No.	Name	Location	Length (nucleotides)	Expression level	Target gene	Activity	Possible role in lung cancer angiogenesis	Clinical potential	References
1	miR-27b	9q22.32	22	▲	Sp1	Possible key miRNA regarding the development of lung cancer; ectopic expression reduced the cell growth and invasion	Sp1, a target gene of miR-27b, was associated with the angiogenic phenotype in gastric cancer, with key roles in the manipulation of this process; patients with high levels of Sp1 presented a more vascularized phenotype	Therapeutic target	[40, 41]
2	miR-126	9q34.3	22	▲	VEGF-A	Low expression of this miRNA is associated with high vascular density in NSCLC; this data were also observed in vitro	Due to direct targeting of miR-126 on VEGF-A, overexpression of this miRNA could be suitable for anti-angiogenic therapies	Therapeutic target and also prognosis tool	[42]
3	miR-130a	11q12.1	21	▲	MET	miR-130a downregulates the expression levels of two oncogenic miRNAs, miR-221 and miR-222; MET suppression	MET represents a key factor for vascular development and miR-221/222 cluster could also play an important role in angiogenesis due to the direct down regulation of TIMP3, an inhibitor of MET; miR-130 is able to reduce the levels of both this systems	Important therapeutic potential	[43, 44]
4	miR-15/16	13q14.3	–	▲	BCL-2 and BCL-XL	MiR-15/16 cluster was found as downregulated in NSCLCs; miR-15 directly targets BCL-2 and BCL-XL	BCL-2 has a suppressive action on VEGF and TP in lung cancer, both strongly implicated in angiogenesis development	Contradictory results; further studies needed	[45–47]
5	miR-378	5q32	21	▲	VEGF	Inhibition of lung cancer angiogenesis through VEGF targeting	Regulator of a central element in lung cancer angiogenesis	*In vivo* demonstrated therapeutic target	[48, 49]
6	miR-296	20q13.32	21	▲	CX3CR1, PLK1	Tumor suppressor role in lung cancer development targeting chemosensitivity and cell viability	MIR-296 has been associated with angiogenesis	Potential therapeutic target	[50–52]

No.	Name	Location	Length (nucleotides)	Expression level	Target gene	Activity	Possible role in lung cancer angiogenesis	Clinical potential	References
7	miR-128	2q21.3	23	▼	VEGF-A, VEGF-C, VEGF-2, VEGF-3	*In vitro* and *in vivo* overexpression of miR-128 led to significant suppression of angiogenesis due to down regulation of the target genes; furthermore miR-128 expression is correlated with the development stages of lung cancer	Current data shows that miR-128 could be used effectively as therapeutic target or prognostic tool	Therapeutic target for enhanced expression and prognosis tool	[53]
8	miR-497	17p13.1	20	▼	HDGF	Ectopic expression of this sequence in an animal model demonstrated positive effects through inhibition of cell proliferation and angiogenesis	Experimental data shows that miR-497 could be used with success as an antiangiogenic agent for lung cancer	Therapeutic target	[54]
9	let-7b	22q13.31	21	▼	RAS	Lung cancer tumors tissue revealed a downregulated pattern and was associated with increased vascular density	The collected data suggest a possible role for miR-7b as antiangiogenic tool in the moment of ectopic expression	Prognosis and therapeutic tool	[55]
10	miR-145	5q32	22	▼	SMAD3	Implicated in EMT and invasion	Enhancement of this miR expression could serve as a therapeutic strategy for lung cancer	Possible therapeutic target	[56]
11	miR-205	1q32.2	20	▼	VEGF	Implicated in EMT and invasion	Enhancement of this miR expression could serve as a therapeutic strategy for lung cancer	Possible therapeutic target	[57]

Table 1. The main tumor suppressor altered miRNAs implicated in lung cancer angiogenesis.

No	Name	Location	Length (nucleotides)	Expression level	Target gene	Activity	Possible role in lung cancer angiogenesis	Clinical potential	References
1	miR-221 miR-222	Xp11.3	23	▲	PTEN, TIMP3	Highly expressed in lung cancer cells; promotes invasion and migration	miR-221/222 cluster could have a role in angiogenesis promotion through down regulation of TIMP3, an inhibitor of MET, an angiogenesis promoter	Therapeutic target and patients stratification toll	[58]
					PUMA	Co-modulation of the two miRNAs on PUMA promotes cell proliferation and inhibits apoptosis			[59]
2	miR-222	Xp11.3	23	▲	P27	Increased miR-221/222 expression promotes H460 cells viability and proliferation	Considering the possible in vivo role of p27, where the overexpression of this gene impaired angiogenesis, miR-222 that inhibits the expression of p27 could become a potent therapeutic target regarding antiangiogenic strategies	Therapeutic target for inhibition	[60, 61]
3	miR-210	11p15.5	22	▲		Significantly up-regulated in lung cancer tissues and associated with angiogenic potential in other types of cancers	Due to the regulation by HIF-1 involved in hypoxia (event that triggers angiogenesis development), miR-210 could also become a therapeutic target	Still limited data	[62, 63]
4	miR-155	21q21.3	22	▲/▼	FGF2	MIR-155 expression is correlated with FGF2 levels, an important molecule for lung cancer angiogenesis. Also, mimR-155 was correlated with VEGF-A in the N+ subgroup of NSCLC	Several studies have investigated the role of this miR in angiogenesis	Prognosis and therapeutic tool	[64, 65]
					FOXO3A, SOCS1, SOCS6, and PTEN	Hypoxia promotes miR-155 increased expression concomitant with the downregulation of FOXO3A target			[65, 66]

No	Name	Location	Length (nucleotides)	Expression level	Target gene	Activity	Possible role in lung cancer angiogenesis	Clinical potential	References
5	miR-21	17q23.1	21	▲	PTEN, SOCS1, and, SOCS6	After antiangiogenic therapy this miR was observed as downregulated	Possible role in lung cancer angiogenesis observed after the post-antiangiogenic down regulation	Possible therapeutic target	[66]
6	miR-182	7q32.2	23	▲	FRS2	miR-182 directly targets FRS2 in lung cancer, gene that represents a key molecule for NSLC progression and antigenesis	N/A	Therapeutic and diagnosis tool	[67]
7	miR-106a	Xq26.2	22	▲	–	Augmented expression of miR-106 in NSCLC was reported in several studies	Previously associated with hypoxia progression in colon and breast cancer that could enable a possible role in lung cancer hypoxia/angiogenesis	Possible therapeutic target	[67–69]

Table 2. The main oncogenic miRNAs involved in lung cancer angiogenesis.

3.3. LncRNAs related to lung cancer angiogenesis

The number of lncRNAs has significantly increased due to the progresses offered by sequencing methods in genomic research. Long noncoding transcripts act as gene regulators via a wide range of mechanism [70], those related to lung cancer being summarized in **Table 3**. The first long noncoding sequence associated with lung cancer was MALAT1 that through increased expression and gene targeting (caspase-8, caspase-3, BCL-XL, BCL-2, and BAX) promotes the proliferation and invasiveness of cancer cells. Recently it was emphasized to target SLUG gene via a competitively "sponging" miR-204 [71]. Following this initial lncRNA, a significant list of lncRNA was associated with lung cancer progression or inhibition through modulation of key mechanisms involved in the hallmarks of lung pathology. The regulatory process is complex, lncRNAs being able to escort chromatin modifying enzymes to target loci within the genome, to bind the promoter of genes and modify the transcription process, to be processed into miRNAs and further act as short noncoding transcripts, and finally to modify the stability of specific mRNAs through direct binding [70].

Recent evidences suggested the role of PANDAR in lung cancer cell proliferation through p53/PANDAR/NF-YA/Bcl-2 axis [72]. Another lncRNA positively regulated by p53 is TUG1, whose downregulation is associated with increased cell proliferation and poor survival rate in lung cancer patients [73]. Also, considering the antiangiogenetic role of the p53 gene and the positive correlation between the two sequences, there is a possible role for TUG1 in angiogenesis suppression, however further investigations are necessary. HOTTIP is a long noncoding transcript that is associated with tumor growth [74], process that involves the formation of new blood vessel network, fact that could transform HOTTIP into a new target for antiangiogenetic therapies. MVIH is associated with microvascular invasion in HCC, being upregulated in this type of cancer with an increased oncogenic potential. Further studies have investigated the possible role of the same lncRNA in lung cancer and the results were increasingly similar with the previous pathology, MVIH representing a biomarker for poor prognosis and associated tumor cell proliferation [75]. There are also other lncRNAs with tumor suppressor or tumor promoting roles in lung cancer malignancies, like MEG3 (tumor suppressor), ANRIL, and AK001796 (oncogenic role) that are involved in cell proliferation and cell viability, processes that go hand in hand with the angiogenetic transformation [76–78]. lnRNA BC087858 is overexpressed in NSCLC and was demonstrated to be connected with drug resistance via EGFR-TKIs axis [80]. MEG3 was proved to be downregulated in tumoral tissue, and directly related with high tumoral stage. Preclinical studies demonstrated a reduced proliferation rate in the case of MEG3 overexpression, by targeting MDM2 and p53 proteins. MEG3 is presented not only as prognostic marker but also as important therapeutic target [76]. ANRIL is overexpressed in lung cancer tissue, being correlated with tumor-node-metastasis stages and tumor size, but until now there are not presented data with a direct connection with angiogenesis [78].

3.4. Ultraconserved regions (UCRs)

Ultraconserved regions (UCRs) are genome sequences longer than 200 bp and, as the name suggests, are conserved within humans, rats, and mouse, preserving their nucleotide

lncRNA	Target gene	Biological role	Reference
TUG1	PRC2	Tumor suppressor lncRNA regulated by p53, gene that promotes the expression of TUG1	[73]
MEG3	MDM and p53	Tumor suppressor role through cell proliferation reduction and increased survival. P53 expression is frequently correlated with the expression of the MEG3, with possible cumulative role in angiogenesis suppression	[76]
MALAT1	SLUG	Promoter of EMT and metastasis, via miR-204	[71]
PANDAR	NF-YA	Inhibits tumor cell proliferation in the moment of overexpression through p53/PANDAR/NF-YA/ Bcl-2 axis	[72]
LUADT1	p27	Oncogenic role through promotion of cell proliferation; knockdown of the target gene significantly contribute to the reduced tumor size by inhibition of cell expansion	[79]
HOTTIP	Cdc25C	Promotes tumor growth and is overexpressed in lung cancers	[74]
ANRIL	KLF2 and p21	Oncogenic role; knockdown of this lncRNA reduced proliferation and increased apoptosis	[78]
MEG3	MDM and p53	Tumor suppressor role exercised through cell proliferation reduction and increased survival. P53 expression is frequently correlated with the expression of the MEG3, with possible cumulative role in angiogenesis suppression	[76]
AK001796	BIRC5/TPDF2/CDC/GA	Oncogenic role; involved in maintaining the tumor cell viability through complex mechanisms	[77]
MVIH	MMP-2 and MMP-9	Overexpressed in lung malignancies, being associated with increased cell proliferation and poor prognosis; previously recognized as angiogenesis promoter in HCCs	[75]
BC087858	EGFR-TKIs	Promotes cells invasion and induces drug resistance to EGFR-TKIs by activating PI3K/AKT and MEK/ ERK pathways and EMT via up-regulating ZEB1 and Snail	[80]
ZXF1	c-Myc	LncRNA ZXF1overexpression was connected with a relatively poor prognosis; Knockdown by siRNA has no effect on cell proliferation, but decreased the migration and invasion of lung cancer cells	[81, 82]
LINC01207	EZH2	Cancer initiation and progression	[83]
LincRNA-p21	p53 and HIF1A	Regulation of TP53-dependent apoptosis and Warburg effect and angiogenesis	[84]

Table 3. The main lncRNAs involved in lung cancer angiogenesis and possible therapeutic targets for inhibiting lung cancers.

succession during the evolution [85, 86]. Until this moment there are a number of 481 conserved sequences, a part of them being situated at sensitive sites regarding cancer susceptibility and are further transcribed (T-UCR) into pathological expression patterns. Considering this recent discovery, it has been postulated that the differential expression pattern could serve as stratification tool in the oncology domain, being able to differentiate between human cancers and possible between molecular subtypes of carcinomas [85, 86].

The exact mechanism that leads to aberrant expression of T-UCR is not fully deciphered, although it is thought that the primary regulation models are represented by miRNAs interactions and epigenetic modifications in CpG islands hypermethylation [85].

Calin et. al. were the first to discover the T-UCR spectrum in malignant cells compared with healthy ones and found significant differences between the two states [85]. So far, molecular analysis have revealed different T-UCR signatures in a number of carcinomas, including prostate, hepatocellular, and colorectal cancer, as well as in chronic lymphocytic leukemia and neuroblastoma. Presently was observed upregulation of several T-UCRs and demonstrated by multiple investigations to be related with increased risks for tumour occurrence and a high metastatic rate. Therefore, the main investigation area is focused on integration of synthetic antisense oligonucleotides (ASOs) to inhibit T-UCR functions [85]. In lung cancer, an important number of T-UCRs need to be characterized and then used for developing novel therapies. In spite of the interest on the T-UCR, there are only few investigations on T-UCR therapy.

4. ncRNAs related to hypoxia in lung cancer

Hypoxia is a preangiogenetic process driven by specific gene modifications, alterations that are able to induce the installation of the mesenchymal phenotype through epithelial to mesenchymal transition (EMT), acquisition of drug and radiation resistance, and propagation of lung cancer stem cells [87, 88]. Compared to other cancers, lung malignancy is severely sustained by the installation of hypoxia through complex interactions between specific molecules (HIF1α and miRNAs or other ncRNAs, as displayed in **Tables 4** and **5**) and establishment of noncoding regulatory networks related to connection with the cell cycle regulation, apoptosis or autophagy [88].

In terms of lung cancer hypoxia, miRNAs play a pivotal role through the ability to orchestrate extensive signaling networks involved in this carcinogenic step. MiR-200 family has been extensively characterized in numerous malignant scenarios and miR-200b member seems to have a role that could be exploited in the context of the clinical area regarding hypoxia induced EMT where cells acquire motility characteristic and are able to invade secondary sites within the organism promoting lung cancer metastasis [89]. Reinforced expression of the tumor suppressor miRNAs inhibited EMT through regulation of key genes involved in this pathway [88]. Another possible therapeutic target is represented by miR-21, that is elevated in NSCLC-derived cells grown under hypoxic conditions [90]. Hypoxic conditions also triggered miR-155 overexpression and downregulation of FOXO3A target gene, and protects lung cancer cells to irradiation, elucidating a possible course of treatment through inhibition of miR-155 combined with radiotherapy [65].

Type of miRNA	Expression level	Name	Target gene	miRNA role in lung cancer hypoxia	Possible clinical role of miRNAs in lung cancer	References
Tumor suppressor miRNAs	▼	miR-200b	–	Hypoxia-induced EMT in lung cancer, influencing the activity of key genes involved in mesenchymal transition miR-200 mimic blocks hypoxia-induced EMT	Novel therapeutic strategy via Nobiletin delivery	[89]
	▼	miR-210	–	Regulate cellular response under hypoxic conditions High levels connected with a positive outcome in NSCLC patients	Biomarker for prognosis and patient stratification	[63, 91]
	▼	miR-18a	HIF-1α	Connected with lung metastasis of breast cancer cells ability to decrease the hypoxic stress *in vitro* and reduce cell invasiveness	Possible prognosis factor of lung metastasis in breast cancer	[92]
	▼	miR-199a	HIF1α	Inhibition of cancer cell hypoxia induced proliferation in NSCLC cells	Possible prognosis factor	[93]
Oncogenic miRNAs	▲	miR-21	–	NSCLC derived cell lines grown under hypoxic condition showed an elevated miR-21 expression; modulates radiation resistance via hypoxic mechanism	Possible therapeutic and prognosis role	[87, 90]
	▲	miR-339	RASSF1, ERBB4, KRAS	Activity correlated with the process of response to hypoxia	Possible target for therapeutic strategies	[94]
	▲	miR-155	FOXO3A	Correlates with poor prognosis and protects hypoxic lung cancer cells to irradiation and conversely	Therapeutic potential for radio sensitization of hypoxic lung cancer cells	[65]
	▲	miR-17-92 cluster	HIF1α	Downregulation of HIF1α does not affect the cellular adaptation to hypoxia	Possible prognosis factor	[95]
	▲	miR-494	PTEN	Promotes angiogenesis through direct targeting of PTEN and activation of Akt/eNOS pathway; expression is induced during hypoxia	Possible prognosis and therapeutic tool	[96]

Table 4. Tumor suppressor and oncogenic miRNAs involved in lung cancer hypoxia with possible roles in diagnosis, prognosis, and therapy.

Type of lncRNA	Expression level	Name	Target gene	lncRNA role in lung cancer hypoxia	Possible clinical role of lncRNAs in lung cancer	References
Tumor supressor lncRNAs	▼	lncRNA-LET (Low expression in tumor)	HIHD3; hypoxia-induced histone deacetylase 3	Squamous-cell lung carcinomas downregulated by HIHD3 promotes hypoxia-induced cancer cell invasion	New methods for therapeutic intervention	[97]
	▼	GAS5-AS1	–	Downregulation of GAS5-AS1 contributes to hypoxia tumor metastasis in non-small cell lung cancer	Prognosis and therapeutic marker	[98]
	▼	LincRNA-p21	TP53 and HIF-1α	Target angiogenic mechanisms	Prognosis marker	[84]
Oncogenic lncRNAs	▲	HOTAIR (HOX transcript antisense intergenic RNA)	HIF-1α	HOTAIR is upregulated in hypoxic conditions and is a direct target of HIF-1α; Promotion of cancer cell proliferation and ability to migrate and invade other sites	Novel therapeutic target	[99, 100]
	▲	H19	HIF-1α	Possess oncogenic properties triggered by hypoxic stress Correlates with p53 tumor suppressor status	Prognosis/ Diagnosis marker	[101]

Table 5. LncRNAs involved in lung cancer hypoxia with possible roles in diagnosis, prognosis, and therapy.

Hypoxia management has led to reduced angiogenesis and thus obtuse the malignant cell proliferation and survival due to deprivation of nutrients and oxygen via various molecules including the noncoding transcripts represented by miRNAs and lncRNAs. Multiple targeting through ncRNAs that are able to influence the fate of the hypoxic microenvironment will bring new insights into the pathogenesis of lung cancer, permitting the development of new clinical tools for cancer management, improving the concerning survival rate of this pathology. The list of miRNAs and lncRNAs implicated in the vascular invasion of the pulmonary malignancy is presented in **Tables 4** and **5**.

LncRNAs have recently emerged as important prognosis and therapeutic tolls in different malignancies and even for specific carcinogenic processes as lung cancer hypoxia. One of the main studied lncRNAs is HOTAIR, pathological expressed in numerous malignant scenarios, being associated with tumor promoting roles and a negative outcome in oncological patients. It was demonstrated that this lncRNA is a direct target for HIF-1α that act as an enhancer of expression and contribute together to the securitization of hypoxia followed by cell proliferation, migration, and metastasis. This information could transform HOTAIR in a possible therapeutic target under hypoxic conditions for NSCLC, that is limited in what regards the therapeutic options [99, 100]. Another newly discovered lncRNAs in lung cancer hypoxia that is lncRNA-LET targeted by HIHDR. The interaction between these two molecules ends with reduction of histone acetylation at the promoter region of the noncoding transcripts and thus decreased expression. Moreover, the downregulation process secures the expression of nuclear factor 90 proteins, a key element for cell migration induced by hypoxia. This data suggest that lncRNA-LET can be used as a clinical tool against cancer promotion [97].

LincRNA-p21 impacts prognosis in resected nonsmall-cell lung cancer patients through angiogenesis regulation. LincRNA-p21 was proved to be activated by TP53 and HIF1A [84]. It was proved to target the apoptosis pathway via regulation by p53 and the Warburg effect. LincRNA-p21 is downregulated in tumor tissue, and has effect on the lung cancer patients via angiogenesis regulation [84].

Other important ncRNA structures with a significant role in the development of novel molecular therapies are represented by PIWI-interacting RNAs (piRNAs). piRNAs are recognized to be involved in transposon silencing and gene expression during development and the complete role on the somatic cells remains to be deciphered [8]. In a recent paper were emphases a different piRNASs expression profiles between normal bronchial epithelial cells and lung cancer cells. The most downregulated piRNAs in lung cancer cells was piRNA-like-163 (piR-L-163) having as direct target the phosphorylated ERM (p-ERM) [102]. S100A4-small interfering RNA (S100A4-siRNA) was proved to activate the apoptosis and increase the radiosensitivity of A549 lung cells. S100A4 may promote A549 cell proliferation but also invasion, and metastasis by regulating the expression of E-cadherin and p53 protein [103].

5. ncRNAs targeting semaphorines and its related receptors in lung cancer

Semaphorins are guidance molecules which were characterized initially as directing elements for axon outgrowth; however advances in genomic and translational medicine revealed a more complex role for these proteins, being involved in cell migration, vascular network, and tissue development [32, 104]. Considering their vital role in physiological processes is not surprising that these guidance proteins are also involved in similar pathological processes especially from the oncologic area, where they exercise the same functions, but in a negative manner [32]. Therefore, semaphorins are implicated in carcinogenic establishment, metastasis, and especially angiogenesis in numerous cancers, including lung cancer. Regarding their role in angiogenesis, the family of semaphorins is divided into two main pathological classes: tumor suppressors inhibiting the angiogenic process and onco-genes through promotion of vascular invasion. Therefore, loss of expression in the case of antiangiogenic semaphorins and/or increased expression pattern for the procarcinogenic ones translates into sustaining of the malignant cells [106]. Immediately after the estab-lishment of their newly discovered role, *in vitro* and *in vivo* studies confirmed the ability of semaphorins to serve as therapeutic targets in the form of suppression or enhancement [32]. Despite the fact that their role in pulmonary malignant processes is quite extensively studied, little is known about the ncRNAs regulatory action on the expression pattern of semaphorins. Deciphering the regulatory noncoding sequence panel for these proteins will enable a more advanced and specific molecular management of lung cancer, especially in angiogenesis that has a vital role regarding the maintenance of tumor cells integrity and proliferation.

The process of angiogenesis, can also occur through semaphorin receptors, neuropilins, and plexins (**Figure 5**). In the case of neuropilins, we encounter a multiple ligation system, this membrane proteins being able to bind both class-3 semaphorins, VEGF and growth factors. Also, this type of receptors that are essential to proper vascular development during organ-ism development are generally mutated in lung cancer. On the other hand, *in vivo* suppres-sion of neuropilins led to improper vascular network.

Among the first studies that elucidated the role of neuropilins in vascular development is the research where the authors observed that overexpressing of *Nrp1* was lethal for embryos due to extensive vascular defects like overdevelopment of blood vessel network and deformed hearts [107]. This discovery paved the way for further research in the area of cancer manage-ment with focus on targeted therapy. Therefore, it has been proven that a combined form of therapy represented by neuropilins inhibitors (semaphorin, anti-NRP, soluble NRP - B domain, and VEGF mimetics) administrated concomitant with anti-VEGF signaling mole-cules (kinase inhibitors, anti-VEGF, anti-VEGFR-2, and soluble VEGFR for VEGF) is more efficient than the classical antiangiogenic therapeutic strategy targeted towards VEGF alone [104]. Research studies demonstrated a role for NRP1 and NRP2 in lung cancer progression and angiogenesis where these two molecules were observed as normally expressed in bron-chial basal cells, and as it progressed in the severity of the cell lesions, the level of neuropilins increased significantly, concomitant with VEGF expression [104]. NRP1 has been previously associated with cancer angiogenesis: overexpression of NRP1 in AT2.1 cells (*in vitro* model of prostate cancer) resulted in advanced vascular density, cell proliferation, and also inhibited apoptosis [108]; rat estrogen-induced pituitary tumors presented increased levels of NRP1, level that was also correlated in a positive manner with the aggressiveness of angiogenesis development [109].

The competitive binding of class-3 semaphorins and VEGF that in physiological conditions leads to the proper development of the vascular platform is changed during malignant sce-narios where proangiogenic VEGF takes the lead due to mutations in the structure of the bind-ing domain that decreases the complementarity with semaphorins or enhances the expression of receptors. Therefore, an alternative therapeutic pathway could be represented by the

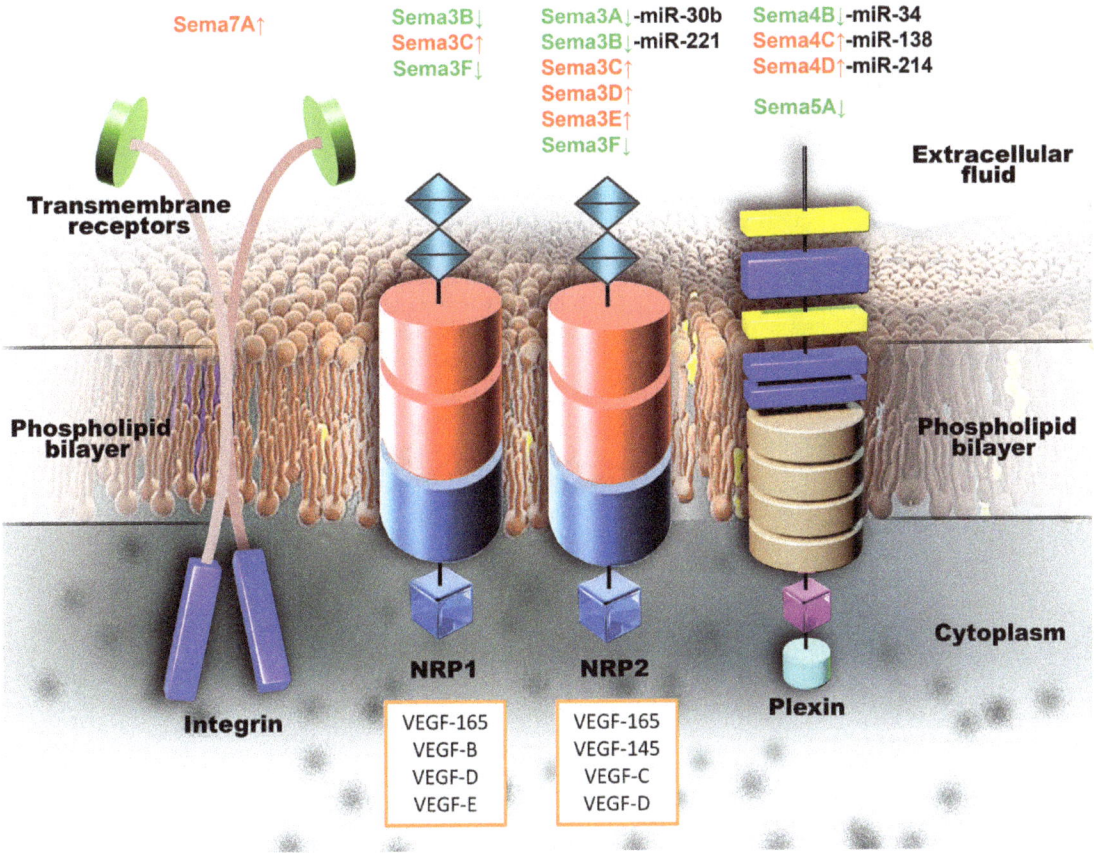

Figure 5. Semaphorin receptors and ncRNAs regulation. Green – downregulated genes; Red – overexpressed genes.

modulation of neuropilins (NRPs) expression. Furthermore, the specific malignant expression is most likely influenced by other molecules such as miRNAs and lncRNAs (**Table 6**).

Lung cancer therapies focused on semaphorins and their receptors are still an insufficiently explored domain that could hold great promises regarding the inhibition of cancer spreading. Considering the competitive binding between class-3 semaphorins and VEGF in vascular development, antiangiogenic strategies as antibodies for VEGF or NRP inhibition, soluble NRP or NRP blocking peptides have been tested with effective results [104, 106]. A more recent treatment compromising both VEGF and SEMA3A inhibitors have been applied *in vitro* and *in vivo* for colon cancer [105]. Another type of action could be represented by the induced internalization of the neuropilins through administration of dextran sulfate and fucoidan that significantly decreased the number of endothelial surface receptors, including VEGFR [131]. Although anti-VEGF molecules are well-known as efficient angiogenesis inhibitors, combining the modulation of VEGF/VEGFR with SEMA/NRP may hold significant clinical usage. Moreover, extension of the molecular insight regarding noncoding RNAs regulation of semaphorins and their receptor could improve even more the inhibition of angiogenesis if we take in consideration the ability of noncoding RNAs to regulate waste singling networks that involve more than one target gene.

Semaphorin	Regulatory miRNAs	Predicted targeting miRNAs	Role in lung cancer	Potential clinical role in lung cancer	Ref.
Semaphorin 3A (SEMA 3A)	miR-30b	miR-95-3p miR-589-5p	NSCLC-anticarcinogenic activity; low expression of SEMA 3A correlates with lymph node metastasis	Biomarker for prognosis	[104, 110]
Semaphorin 3B (SEMA 3B)	miR-221	miR-155-5p miR-107 miR-187-5p miR-18a-3p miR-708 miR-3074-5p miR-106b-3p miR-340-3p miR-3074-5p	Cell proliferation and invasion Small-cell lung cancer-tumor suppressor role via induction of apoptosis and inhibition of angiogenesis	Marker for cancer progression	[111, 112]
Semaphorin 3C (SEMA 3C)	–	miR-4746-5p miR-500a-5p miR-187-5p miR-301a-5p miR-21-3p miR-106a-3p miR-4677-3p miR-3074-5p let-7g-3p miR-183-3p miR-29a-3p miR-519a-5p miR-200c-5p miR-4668-3p miR-16-2-3p miR-193a-3p miR-4326 miR-4417 miR-3664-3p miR-155-5p miR-590-5p miR-616-3p miR-3182 miR-103a-2-5p miR-501-5p miR-362-3p miR-330-5p miR-30e-5p	A549 lung cancer cells -p65-SEMA3C (cleaved SEMA3C) – protumorigenic activities	Novel antitumorigenic drug	[113]
Semaphorin 3D (SEMA 3D)	–	miR-484 miR-15b-3p miR-16-2-3pmiR-32-3p miR-32-5p miR-33a-5p miR-33b-3p miR-340-5p miR-4668-3p miR-345-5p miR-629-5p miR-18a-5p miR-1306-5p	Proangiogenic and metastatic role	Prediction of response and survival	[114, 115]

Semaphorin	Regulatory miRNAs	Predicted targeting miRNAs	Role in lung cancer	Potential clinical role in lung cancer	Ref.
		let-7a-3p miR-183-3p miR-21-3p miR-21-5p miR-4742-5p miR-425-5p miR-200a-5p miR-301a-5p miR-3619-3p miR-589-5p miR-3614-3p miR-141-5p miR-106a-3p miR-93-3p			
Semaphorin 3E (SEMA 3E)	–	miR-340-5p miR-1306-5p miR-15b-3p let-7d-5p miR-1307-3p miR-629-5p miR-629-3p miR-4677-3p let-7g-3p miR-301a-5p miR-15b-5p miR-19a-3p miR-16-2-3p miR-105-3p miR-18a-5p miR-1306-5p miR-19a-3p miR-1307-5p miR-505-5p	*In vivo* promotion of lung metastasis and tumor progression	Possible target for therapeutic strategies	[116]
Semaphoring 3F (SEMA 3F)	–	miR-29c-3p miR-191-3p miR-29b-1-5p miR-18a-5p miR-20a-5p miR-29b-2-5p miR-200c-5p let-7g-3p let-7a-3p let-7d-5p miR-7-5p miR-3619-3p miR-590-5p miR-29b-2-5p miR-30e-5p miR-676-3p miR-135b-3p miR-30c-1-3p miR-140-3p miR-135b-3p miR-140-3p	Role in TGF-beta1-induced EMT Antitumor role; Downregulated in lung cancer Targets HIF-1 and VEGF	Possible prognosis biomarker and therapeutic target	[117, 118]

Semaphorin	Regulatory miRNAs	Predicted targeting miRNAs	Role in lung cancer	Potential clinical role in lung cancer	Ref.
Semaphorin 4B (SEMA 4B)	miR-34	miR-34	NSCLC—inhibition of invasion and growth—prevention of metastasis-direct target of hypoxia-inducible factor 1 (HIF-1) miR-34/p53 axis	Novel therapeutic target for inhibition of metastasis and growth -Novel therapeutic target through inhibition of HIF-1	[119–121]
Semaphorin 4C (SEMA 4C)	miR-138	miR-138	NSCLC-cell proliferation and EMT	New target or prognosis marker for lung cancer treatment	[122]
Semaphorin 4D (SEMA 4D)	miR-214	miR-199b-3p miR-127-3p miR-185-5p miR-421 miR-500a-5p miR-22-3p miR-500a-5p miR-22-3p miR-505-5p let-7g-3p miR-1269a miR-18a-5p miR-3614-3p miR-331-3p miR-18a-5p miR-18a-3p	Highly expressed in lung cancer; promotion of angiogenesis; NSCLC-*in vitro* inhibition of cell proliferation, migration, and invasion	Possible early prognosis tool and therapeutic target	[124–126]
Semaphorin 5A (SEMA 5A)	-	miR-3677-3p miR-3200-3p miR-32-5p miR-29b-1-5p miR-183-3p miR-345-5p miR-454-5p miR-3614-3p miR-18a-3p miR-500a-5p miR-106b-3p miR-27b-5p let-7g-3p miR-660-5p miR-135b-3p miR-1306-5p miR-29a-3p miR-29b-2-5p miR-425-3p miR-365a-5p miR-3136-3p miR-93-3p miR-4787-3p miR-19a-3p	NSCLC-tumor suppressor role; low levels associated with poor survival rate	New biomarker for NSCLC	[127]

Semaphorin	Regulatory miRNAs	Predicted targeting miRNAs	Role in lung cancer	Potential clinical role in lung cancer	Ref.
Semaphorin 6A (SEMA 6A)	miR-27a/b	miR-1307-3p miR-940 miR-3187-3p miR-33a-5p miR-425-3p miR-99b-5p miR-99b-3p miR-183-3p miR-3176 miR-760 miR-345-5p miR-4461	Endothelial cell repulsion	New therapeutic target through manipulation of miR-27a/b expression	[128, 129]
Semaphorin 7A (SEMA 7A)	–	22_40957679_40957783 (novel miRNA)	Promotion of tumor microenvironment and metastasis through regulation of prototypic chitinase-like protein (Chi3l1)	Possible role as therapeutic target	[130]

Table 6. Semaphorin and the targeting miRNAs with implication in lung cancer.

6. ncRNAs therapies targeting lung cancer angiogenesis

Once considered the "trash" of the genome, the noncoding RNA sequences are now emerging as important therapeutic targets (Table 7). Due to the complex regulatory network involving ncRNAs and also because of the personalized pathological expression pattern among cancer types, subtypes and malignant stages, ncRNAs are subjected to numerous preclinical studies regarding their silencing or induced expression [2]. A lipid-based delivery vehicle for tumor suppressor miR-34 was developed in order to enhance the expression of the specific molecule in a mouse model of non-small-cell lung cancer [132]. This approach has demonstrated to be efficient in both locally and systemically administration, being observed a reinforced miR expression concomitant with downregulation of the specific targets. Moreover, the intravenous delivery of miR-34 mimic did not produce an immune reaction in mice, but unfortunately this was not the case in humans. Very recently, MRX34, the miR-34 mimic, was stopped to be administrated in a cancer clinical trial due to major immune reactions [133].

Another therapeutic alternative that is currently on the scientific spotlight consist in the manipulation of the ciRNAs that can function as microRNA sponges, modulating their oncogenic or tumor suppressor activity [136]. Despite the fact that there is a number of research studies focused on this type of noncoding RNAs, relatively little is known about the regulatory mechanism of circRNAs in cancer development. Future perspectives imply ciRNAs-based therapy that can stand as "super-sponges" and modulate the activity of extended regulatory miRNA networks, influencing at a superior level the carcinoma progression [136].

miRNAs	Lung cancer subtype	Experimental model	Therapeutic approach	Delivery system	Target gene	Obtained results	References
miR-128	NSCLC	NSCLC cells	Ectopic miR-128 overexpression		VEGF-C	Inhibition of VEGF-C expression concomitant with angiogenesis restriction	[53]
		HUVECs and NSCLC cells			VEGF-A, VEGFR-2 and VEGFR-3	Low expression of the target genes that are critical factors for angiogenesis	
		Nude mice (A549 cells)	In vivo replacement therapy			Inhibition of lymphangiogenesis	
miR-497	NSCLC	NSCLC cells	Over expression of the miRNA		VEGF-A	Decreases in the levels of VEGF-A protein with no significant changes for the VEGF-A mRNA; inhibition of cell invasion	[123]
			miRNA inhibition			Increased levels of VEGF-A protein with no significant changes for the VEGF-A mRNA; increased cell invasion	
		NSCLC cells SCID mouse xenograft model	Ectopic expression of the miRNA sequence		HDGF	Restoration of the miR-497 levels reduced tumor development and angiogenesis in both in vitro and in vivo experimental models	[54]
miR-378	NSCLC	Swiss nude immunodeficient murine model (NCI-H292-Luc cells overexpressing miR-378 — subcutaneous xenografts)	Overexpression of miR-378	Lentiviral vectors particles (pEZX-MR03 backbone)	HMOX1	mir-378 over expression models presented tumors with decreased vascularisation compared to the models with HMOX1 induced over expression; increased oxygen partial pressure; increased MUC5AC, Ang-1,MMP12 levels and decreased TNF-α and IL-1β levels - all essential genes for angiogenesis	[48]
miR-126	NSCLC	A549, Y-90 and SPC-A1 cells	Overexpression of miR-126	mir-126 expression vector (LV-miR-126)	VEGF-A	Dowregulation of VEGF-A gene correlated with inhibited cell growth	[42]
		Tumor xenograft model (A549 infected with LV-miR-126)	mir-126 expression vector (LV-miR-126)				

miRNAs	Lung cancer subtype	Experimental model	Therapeutic approach	Delivery system	Target gene	Obtained results	References
miR-222	NSCLC	H460 cells	Inhibition of miR-222 expression	miR-222 inhibitor	p27 (*in vivo* over expression of p27 impaired angiogenesis)	Inhibition of oncogenic miR expression resulted in decreased cell viability and proliferation	[60, 61]
miR-27b	NSCLC	HEK293 cells	Cotransfection of miR-27b mimics and WT Sp1 in order to express both miRNA and target gene	psiCHECK-2 vector	Sp1	Expression of miR-27b resulted in suppression of cell growth and reduced invasion	[128]
miR-130a	NSCLC	A549, CALU-1, H1299 and A459 cells	Transfection with miR-130a in order to increase the endogenous levels of this sequence	pre-miR 130a	MET	Strong reduction of MET (angiogenesis promoter) mRNA and protein levels; down regulation of miR-221 and miR-222, that are able to inhibit TIMP3 expression, molecule that in turn inhibits MET	[44]
miR-210	Adenocarcinoma	A549 cells	Knocked down of miR-210 in hypoxic parameters	antimiR-210	SDHD (positive-regulatory loop between miR-210 and HIF-1α)	Decreased cell survival and alteration of mitochondrial phenotype	[63]
miR-155	Adenocarcinoma	A549 and H460 cells	Inhibition of miR-155 levels in cells preserved in hypoxic conditions	Synthetic antimiR-155	FOXO3A (associated with roles in angiogenesis)	miR-155 inhibition exercise a positive role through radiosensitization of the cells	[65, 134]
miR-21	NSCLC	A549	*In vitro* inhibition of miR-21	miR-21-sponge	PDCD4 (associated with angiogenesis development)	Inhibition of miR-21 ameliorates cell proliferation, migration, and invasion through PDCD4 modulation; knockdown of PDCD4 has been demonstrated to stimulate angiogenesis through positive regulation of Ang-2 (negative prognostic factor in lung cancer)	[66, 135]

Table 7. Some relevant miRNAs tested on cell culture and animal models as potential therapeutic agents in lung cancer.

The discovery of lncRNAs as regulators of cancer development has naturally conducted towards potential therapeutic alternatives using these long fragments as direct targets. The expression pattern of these sequences has been also investigated in lung cancer and the list of oncogenic and tumor suppressor pathological expressed lncRNAs is continuously growing. Administration of siRNA, shRNA, and miRNAs or antisense oligonucleotides in order to inhibit oncogenic lncRNAs is currently under investigation [137]. HOTAIR has been on the spotlight of artificial knockdown via siRNA delivery with great rates of success in lung cancer and also breast and pancreatic malignancies [100].

Moreover, the same approaches have been shown to be effective for the reverse of cisplatin resistance through reduced expression of p21 [138]. Downregulation of MALAT1 through shRNA delivery is also a potent therapeutic approach for lung cancer as it was shown reduced cell viability after this type of treatment [71]. MALAT1 has been also inhibited by exogenous antisense oligonucleotides, approach that induced reduced cancer progression through cell cycle arrest [151]. Considering that in lung cancer there are also downregulated tumor suppressor lncRNAs, the replacement therapy could also stand as an effective therapeutic approach for this type of carcinoma, but nonetheless the scientific information are quite limited regarding this area.

The discovery that miRNA sequences can act as key regulators in cancer pathways through aberrant expression has led to the idea that these fragments could serve as potent therapeutic targets [139]. In this sense, several strategies have been implemented until now: inhibition strategies—inhibitory antisense oligonucleotides and delivery vectors (miRNA sponges) and enhancement strategies—miRNA replacement therapy (**Figure 6**) [139, 140].

For the case of therapeutics that follow an antagonistic pattern, the activity of tumor promoting miRNAs that are hazardous expressed is inhibited via administration of single stranded oligonucleotides complementary with the specific molecule or with the target binding site on the mRNA molecule; in either situation, the interaction between miRNAs and mRNA molecules is blocked and the downstream pathological pathway is strongly affected [140].

Delivery of anti-miRNA oligonucleotides (AMOs) in the context of preclinical studies is still a problematic area considering the necessity of target administration, prolonged stability, and increased pharmacokinetic properties [140]. In this means, there is an urgent need for efficient delivery vectors/vehicles that are able to fulfill the reminded request in order to accomplish the treatment purpose. The majority of the freely administrated oligonucleotides is retrieved in the liver and kidneys and then eliminated through the urine. Also, the necessary dose of synthetic sequences is usually very high and the chance for off-target delivery is also increasing. Establishment of an effective delivery system will break the grounds of miRNAs therapeutics and also other noncoding treatment strategies [139]. The current strategy for *in vivo* administration implies conjugation-based methods, where miRNA sequences are conjugated with different molecules like cholesterol [141] and α-tocopherol [142]. Although these studies have demonstrated promising results, the efficiency of miRNA targeting is still limited. Another type of delivery method consists in liposome-mediated delivery of siRNAs, where the first attempt [143] was to inhibit the replication of hepatitis B virus (HBV) in an animal model through administration of siRNAs integrated in as polyethylene glycol (PEG)–lipid conjugate (SNALP). Since then, different liposome-based vehicles have been tested and the results are encouraging considering that the administration dose is significantly decreased

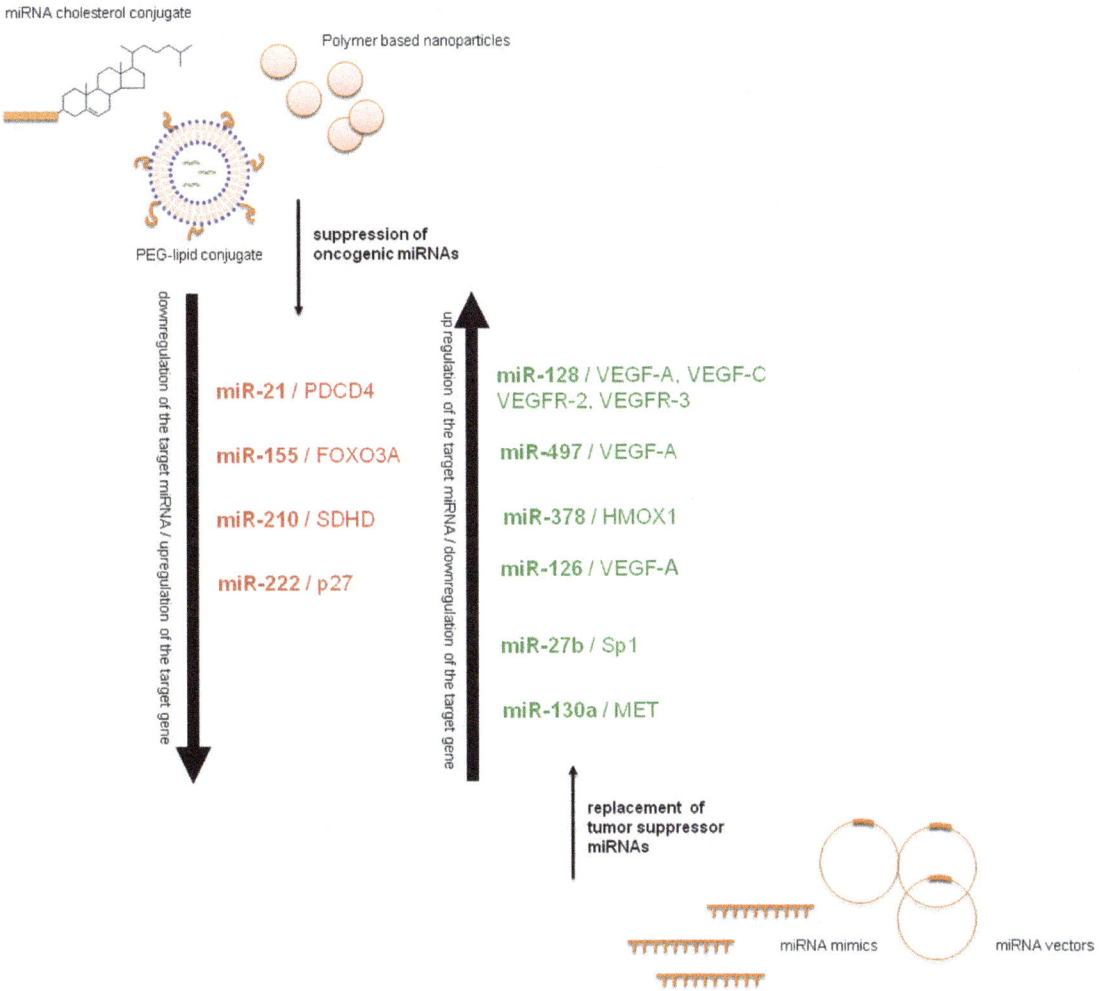

Figure 6. MicroRNAs have emerged as important regulators of lung cancer angiogenesis and also as key therapeutic targets regarding inhibition or enhancement strategies. MiRNAs sequences that are marked with green composed the tumor suppressor group that have been tested in the context of replacement therapies; the genes marked with the same color represent the target genes that have been downregulated after therapeutic modulation of miRNAs. Inversely, miRNAs sequences marked with red are oncogenic ones proposed for inhibition in what regards antiangiogenic programs; the genes marked with the same color also represent the target genes, but in this case their expression has been augmented.

comparing to the naked oligonucleotides [144–147]. Progresses in the area of material science produced a promising *in vivo* delivery system in the form of polymer-based nanoparticles that are more flexible than liposomes and also can be produced in a more homogenous manner regarding their size and form [139]. In respect of siRNAs and anti-miRs delivery, the size of the vehicle is very important in order to permit the passing through cellular compartments, where nanoparticles can fulfill this request having a size between 10 and 100 nm [139]. Moreover, in order to avoid the stimulation of the immune system, cyclodextrin–PEG conjugated nanoparticles have been developed and tested for the inhibition of EWS–FLI1 in an *in vivo* model of Ewing's sarcoma [148]. Attracting strategies for targeted therapies consist in the conjugation of siRNAs or anti-miR sequences with specific antibodies able to conduct the small fragments towards distinctive cells expressing the desired antigen [147, 149, 150].

MiRNA replacement therapy is more limited regarding the current attempts and results, although it seems to emerge as a more efficient form of treatment considering that the majority of pathological expressed miRNAs consist in downregulated or inhibited tumor suppressor sequences [140]. Even if the success of this therapeutic strategy could be greater than miRNA inhibition workflows, the requirements for the structure and composition of the replacement fragment are much more stringent considering the necessity of RISC uptake. Furthermore, the impediments regarding the delivery system for these oligonucleotides are the same as in the case of inhibitory antisense attempts.

7. Conclusions and future perspectives

Lung cancer remains the most deadly disease from the oncological field, being an aggressive form of cancer that is usually diagnosed in late stages with minimal therapeutic alternatives. Even in the case of early discovery, the classical treatments have failed numerous times due to compensatory mechanisms developed within the tumor environment leading to the same negative outcome. Therefore, we face a crisis situation where we need to develop new thera-peutic tools for lung cancer management able to target key elements/pathways, but avoid in the same time the possibility of alternative carcinogenic pathways activation. One of the hallmarks of cancer is represented by angiogenesis, process that is in the sight of research-ers for some time, but the classical inhibition of central molecules like VEGF has failed to deliver long-lasting results. Therefore, ncRNAs have emerged as potential lifesaving agents due to the capacity of extensive modulation, where the same ncRNA is able to target multiple genes and regulate their function. Also the same microRNA, or more recently discovered, the lncRNA can be encounter in different consecutive processes in pulmonary carcinogenesis, as in the case of hypoxia and angiogenesis. Development of novel therapeutic tools able to transform the pathological expression of ncRNAs, mainly through silencing of upregulated patterns, will enable a more extensive, and in the same time, specific approach that will prob-ably excludes the installation of compensatory mechanism and significantly contribute to a better outcome in lung cancer patients. The concept of noncoding RNAs as therapeutic tar-gets in the clinical context is now more feasible than ever, being supported by numerous preclinical studies. One of the main approaches should involve manipulation of miRNAs that are actively implicated in the regulation of VEGF genes expression, genes that hold a key role in the vascular development process. Even more, a heterogeneous approach that implies the administration of different miRNA sequences able to target multiple genes and naturally multiple pathological pathways within the angiogenic process will represent a more extended form of therapy that could modify extensive regulatory networks. This type of tar-geting will also minimize the compensatory mechanisms that are usually encountered after the implementation of classical therapeutic strategies due to concomitant regulation of mul-tiple signaling pathways. Additionally, some other approaches may be used for the inhibi-tion of angiogenesis. For example, semaphorins are now emerging as important regulators of vascular density in malignancies, with possible roles as prognostic tools or even therapeutic targets. Inhibition of procarcinogenic semaphorins would represent a novel course of action regarding cancer treatment considering their central role in vascular density. Moreover, the receptors associated with semaphorins contain binding sites for both semaphorins and VEGF molecules, engaging the competitive binding between these types of molecules. Managing the expression of VEGF via miRNA therapy concomitant with the levels of neuropilins (semaphorins receptors) will enable a more dramatic approach that could have more drastic results for cancer development.

Current therapeutic programs are promoting the effectiveness of specific sequence inhibition or enhancement through administration of antisense oligonucleotides or supplementation of the same sequence through exogenous enhancement. Development of chemically modified oligonucleotides under the form of medication for individuals diagnosed with cancer is now at the close horizon. Administration of synthetic oligonucleotides for noncoding RNAs inhibition or upregulation will enhance the effect of the current therapeutic strategies by modulation of specific gene expression able to influence the carcinogenic process or even reverse the malignant installation. In this sense, it is now clearly understood that the major strategy towards cancer treatment is focused on taking advantage of the key roles of noncoding sequences regarding the modulation of entire aberrant regulatory networks through manipulation of central molecules.

Acknowledgments

This work was supported by the POC-P_37_796 grant, entitled "Clinical and economical impact of personalized targeted anti-microRNA therapies in reconverting lung cancer chemoresistance"-CANTEMIR.

Author details

Ioana Berindan-Neagoe[1,2,3]*, Cornelia Braicu[1], Diana Gulei[2], Ciprian Tomuleasa[1,4] and George Adrian Calin[5]

*Address all correspondence to: ioana.neagoe@umfcluj.ro

1 Research Center for Functional Genomics, Biomedicine and Translational Medicine, "Iuliu Hatieganu", University of Medicine and Pharmacy Iuliu-Hatieganu, Cluj-Napoca, Romania

2 Medfuture—Research Center for Advanced Medicine, University of Medicine and Pharmacy Iuliu-Hatieganu, Cluj-Napoca, Romania

3 Department of Functional Genomics and Experimental Pathology, The Oncological Institute "Prof. Dr. Ion Chiricuta", Cluj-Napoca, Romania

4 Department of Hematology, The Oncological Institute "Prof. Dr. Ion Chiricuta", Cluj-Napoca, Romania

5 Department of Experimental Therapeutics, The University of Texas M.D. Anderson Cancer Center, Houston, TX, USA

References

[1] Mattick, J.S. and I.V. Makunin, *Non-coding RNA*. Hum Mol Genet, 2006. **15 Spec No 1**: pp. R17–29.

[2] Braicu, C., et al., *NCRNA combined therapy as future treatment option for cancer*. Curr Pharm Des, 2014. **20**(42): pp. 6565–74.

[3] Choudhuri, S., *Small noncoding RNAs: biogenesis, function, and emerging significance in toxicology*. J Biochem Mol Toxicol, 2010. **24**(3): pp. 195–216.

[4] Berindan-Neagoe, I., et al., *MicroRNAome genome: a treasure for cancer diagnosis and therapy*. CA Cancer J Clin, 2014. **64**(5): pp. 311–36.

[5] Berindan-Neagoe, I. and G.A. Calin, *Molecular pathways: microRNAs, cancer cells, and microenvironment*. Clin Cancer Res, 2014. **20**(24): pp. 6247–53.

[6] Kung, J.T., D. Colognori, and J.T. Lee, *Long noncoding RNAs: past, present, and future*. Genetics, 2013. **193**(3): pp. 651–69.

[7] Liu, Y. *MicroRNAs and PIWI-interacting RNAs in oncology*. Oncol Lett, 2016. **12**(4): pp. 2289–2292.

[8] Ng, K.W., C. Anderson, E.A. Marshall, B.C. Minatel, K.S. Enfield, H.L. Saprunoff, W.L. Lam, and V.D. Martinez, *Piwi-interacting RNAs in cancer: emerging functions and clinical utility*. Mol Cancer, 2016. **15**: p. 5.

[9] Hansen, T.B., J. Kjems, and C.K. Damgaard, *Circular RNA and miR-7 in cancer*. Cancer Res, 2013. **73**(18): pp. 5609–12.

[10] Peng, L., X.Q. Yuan, and G.C. Li, *The emerging landscape of circular RNA ciRS-7 in cancer (Review)*. Oncol Rep, 2015. **33**(6): pp. 2669–74.

[11] Ebbesen, K.K., T.B. Hansen, and J. Kjems, *Insights into circular RNA biology*. RNA Biol, 2016 Dec 16:0. [Epub ahead of print]

[12] Hansen, T.B., et al., *Natural RNA circles function as efficient microRNA sponges*. Nature, 2013. **495**(7441): pp. 384–8.

[13] Shao, T., et al., *Identification of module biomarkers from the dysregulated ceRNA-ceRNA interaction network in lung adenocarcinoma*. Mol Biosyst, 2015. **11**(11): pp. 3048–58.

[14] Taft, R.J., et al., *Non-coding RNAs: regulators of disease*. J Pathol, 2010. **220**(2): pp. 126–39.

[15] Malone, C.D. and G.J. Hannon, *Small RNAs as guardians of the genome*. Cell, 2009. **136**(4): pp. 656–68.

[16] Carthew, R.W. and E.J. Sontheimer, *Origins and mechanisms of miRNAs and siRNAs*. Cell, 2009. **136**(4): pp. 642–55.

[17] Ghildiyal, M. and P.D. Zamore, *Small silencing RNAs: an expanding universe*. Nat Rev Genet, 2009. **10**(2): pp. 94–108.

[18] Sobecka, A., W. Barczak, and W.M. Suchorska. *RNA interference in head and neck oncology.* Oncol Lett., 2016. **12**(5): pp. 3035–3040.

[19] Meister, G. *Argonaute proteins: functional insights and emerging roles.* Nat Rev Genet, 2013. 14(7): pp. 447–59.

[20] Tordonato, C., P.P. Di Fiore, and F. Nicassio, *The role of non-coding RNAs in the regulation of stem cells and progenitors in the normal mammary gland and in breast tumors.* Front Genet, 2015. **6**: p. 72.

[21] Kilgoz, H.O., et al., *KRAS and the reality of personalized medicine in non-small cell lung cancer.* Mol Med, 2016. **22**.

[22] Nicholson, S.A., et al., *Small cell lung carcinoma (SCLC): a clinicopathologic study of 100 cases with surgical specimens.* Am J Surg Pathol, 2002. **26**(9): pp. 1184–97.

[23] Nicholson, A.G., et al., *The international association for the study of lung cancer lung cancer staging project: proposals for the revision of the clinical and pathologic staging of small cell lung cancer in the forthcoming eighth edition of the TNM classification for lung cancer.* J Thorac Oncol, 2016. **11**(3): pp. 300–11.

[24] Cheng, T.D., et al., *The international epidemiology of lung cancer: latest trends, disparities, and tumor characteristics.* J Thorac Oncol, 2016. 11(10):1653–71.

[25] Okereke, I.C., et al., *Outcomes after surgical resection of pulmonary carcinoid tumors.* J Cardiothorac Surg, 2016. **11**: p. 35.

[26] Govindan, R., et al., *Changing epidemiology of small-cell lung cancer in the United States over the last 30 years: analysis of the surveillance, epidemiologic, and end results database.* J Clin Oncol, 2006. **24**(28): pp. 4539–44.

[27] Urman, A. and H.D. Hosgood, *Curbing the burden of lung cancer.* Front Med, 2016. **10**(2): pp. 228–32.

[28] Landrigan, P.J., *Comments on the 2014 Helsinki Consensus Report on Asbestos.* Ann Glob Health, 2016. **82**(1): pp. 217–20.

[29] http://www.cancer.org/cancer/lungcancer-non-smallcell/detailedguide/non-small-cell-lung-cancer-survival-rates, accessed, august 2016

[30] http://globocan.iarc.fr/old/FactSheets/cancers/lung-new.asp, accessed, august 2016

[31] Hanahan, D. and R.A. Weinberg, *Hallmarks of cancer: the next generation.* Cell, 2011. **144**(5): pp. 646–74.

[32] Neufeld, G., N. Shraga-Heled, T. Lange, N. Guttmann-Raviv, Y. Herzog, and O. Kessler, *Semaphorins in cancer.* Front Biosci, 2005. **10**: pp. 751–60.

[33] Piperdi, B., A. Merla, and R. Perez-Soler, *Targeting angiogenesis in squamous non-small cell lung cancer.* Drugs, 2014. **74**(4): pp. 403–13.

[34] Cabebe, E. and H. Wakelee, *Role of anti-angiogenesis agents in treating NSCLC: focus on bevacizumab and VEGFR tyrosine kinase inhibitors.* Curr Treat Options Oncol, 2007. **8**(1): pp. 15–27.

[35] Lee, S.M., et al., *Anti-angiogenic therapy using thalidomide combined with chemotherapy in small cell lung cancer: a randomized, double-blind, placebo-controlled trial.* J Natl Cancer Inst, 2009. **101**(15): pp. 1049–57.

[36] Arnedos, M., et al., *Personalized treatments of cancer patients: a reality in daily practice, a costly dream or a shared vision of the future from the oncology community?* Cancer Treat Rev, 2014. **40**(10): pp. 1192–8.

[37] Li, H. and X. Lv, *Functional annotation of noncoding variants and prioritization of cancer-associated lncRNAs in lung cancer.* Oncol Lett, 2016. **12**(1): pp. 222–230.

[38] Stenvang, J., M. Lindow, and S. Kauppinen, *Targeting of microRNAs for therapeutics.* Biochem Soc Trans, 2008. **36**(Pt 6): pp. 1197–200.

[39] Zhang, B., X. Pan, G.P. Cobb and T.A. Anderson, *microRNAs as oncogenes and tumor suppressors.* Dev Biol, 2007 Feb 1. **302**(1): pp. 1–12.

[40] Wang, L., et al., *Altered expression of transcription factor Sp1 critically impacts the angiogenic phenotype of human gastric cancer.* Clin Exp Metastasis, 2005. **22**(3): pp. 205–13.

[41] Safe S. *MicroRNA-Specificity Protein (Sp) Transcription factor interactions and significance in carcinogenesis.* Curr Pharmacol Rep, 2015. **1**(2): pp. 73–78.

[42] Liu, B., et al., *MiR-126 restoration down-regulate VEGF and inhibit the growth of lung cancer cell lines in vitro and in vivo.* Lung Cancer, 2009. **66**(2): pp. 169–75.

[43] Zhou, Y.M., J. Liu, and W. Sun, *MiR-130a overcomes gefitinib resistance by targeting met in non-small cell lung cancer cell lines.* Asian Pac J Cancer Prev, 2014. **15**(3): pp. 1391–6.

[44] Acunzo, M., et al., *miR-130a targets MET and induces TRAIL-sensitivity in NSCLC by down-regulating miR-221 and 222.* Oncogene, 2012. **31**(5): pp. 634–42.

[45] Sun, C.Y., X.M. She, Y. Qin, Z.B. Chu, L. Chen, L.S. Ai, L. Zhang, and Y. Hu. *miR-15a and miR-16 affect the angiogenesis of multiple myeloma by targeting VEGF.* Carcinogenesis, 2013. **34**(2): pp. 426–35.

[46] Tafsiri, E., et al., *Expression of miRNAs in non-small-cell lung carcinomas and their association with clinicopathological features.* Tumour Biol, 2015. **36**(3): pp. 1603–12.

[47] Koukourakis, M.I., et al., *bcl-2 and c-erbB-2 proteins are involved in the regulation of VEGF and of thymidine phosphorylase angiogenic activity in non-small-cell lung cancer.* Clin Exp Metastasis, 1999. **17**(7): pp. 545–54.

[48] Skrzypek, K., et al., *Interplay between heme oxygenase-1 and miR-378 affects non-small cell lung carcinoma growth, vascularization, and metastasis.* Antioxid Redox Signal, 2013. **19**(7): pp. 644–60.

[49] Chen, L.T., et al., *MicroRNA-378 is associated with non-small cell lung cancer brain metastasis by promoting cell migration, invasion and tumor angiogenesis.* Med Oncol, 2012. **29**(3): pp. 1673–80.

[50] Luo, W., et al., *miRNA-296-3p modulates chemosensitivity of lung cancer cells by targeting CX3CR1*. Am J Transl Res, 2016. **8**(4): pp. 1848–56.

[51] Xu, C., et al., *miR-296-5p suppresses cell viability by directly targeting PLK1 in non-small cell lung cancer*. Oncol Rep, 2016. **35**(1): pp. 497–503.

[52] Suarez, Y. and W.C. Sessa, *MicroRNAs as novel regulators of angiogenesis*. Circ Res, 2009. **104**(4): pp. 442–54.

[53] Hu, J., et al., *microRNA-128 plays a critical role in human non-small cell lung cancer tumourigenesis, angiogenesis and lymphangiogenesis by directly targeting vascular endothelial growth factor-C*. Eur J Cancer, 2014. **50**(13): pp. 2336–50.

[54] Zhao, W.Y., et al., *Downregulation of miR-497 promotes tumor growth and angiogenesis by targeting HDGF in non-small cell lung cancer*. Biochem Biophys Res Commun, 2013. **435**(3): pp. 466–71.

[55] Xia, X.M., W.Y. Jin, R.Z. Shi, Y.F. Zhang, and J. Chen. *Clinical significance and the correlation of expression between Let-7 and K-ras in non-small cell lung cancer*. Oncol Lett, 2010. **1**(6): pp. 1045–1047.

[56] Hu, H., et al., *MiR-145 and miR-203 represses TGF-beta-induced epithelial-mesenchymal transition and invasion by inhibiting SMAD3 in non-small cell lung cancer cells*. Lung Cancer, 2016. **97**: pp. 87–94.

[57] Li, J., et al., *The role of miR-205 in the VEGF-mediated promotion of human ovarian cancer cell invasion*. Gynecol Oncol. 2015. **137**: pp. 125–133.

[58] Garofalo, M., et al., *miR-221&222 regulate TRAIL resistance and enhance tumorigenicity through PTEN and TIMP3 downregulation*. Cancer Cell, 2009. **16**(6): pp. 498–509.

[59] Zhang, C., et al., *PUMA is a novel target of miR-221/222 in human epithelial cancers*. Int J Oncol, 2010. **37**(6): pp. 1621–6.

[60] Zhong, C., et al., *MicroRNA-222 promotes human non-small cell lung cancer H460 growth by targeting p27*. Int J Clin Exp Med, 2015. **8**(4): pp. 5534–40.

[61] Goukassian, D., et al., *Overexpression of p27(Kip1) by doxycycline-regulated adenoviral vectors inhibits endothelial cell proliferation and migration and impairs angiogenesis*. FASEB J, 2001. **15**(11): pp. 1877–85.

[62] Devlin, C., et al., *miR-210: More than a silent player in hypoxia*. IUBMB Life, 2011. **63**(2): pp. 94–100.

[63] Puissegur, M.P., et al., *miR-210 is overexpressed in late stages of lung cancer and mediates mitochondrial alterations associated with modulation of HIF-1 activity*. Cell Death Differ, 2011. **18**(3): pp. 465–78.

[64] Donnem, T., et al., *Prognostic impact of MiR-155 in non-small cell lung cancer evaluated by in situ hybridization*. J Transl Med, 2011. **9**: p. 6.

[65] Babar, I.A., et al., *Inhibition of hypoxia-induced miR-155 radiosensitizes hypoxic lung cancer cells.* Cancer Biol Ther, 2011. **12**(10): pp. 908–14.

[66] Xue, X., Y. Liu, Y. Wang, M. Meng, K. Wang, X. Zang, et al. MiR-21 and MiR-155 promote non-small cell lung cancer progression by downregulating SOCS1, SOCS6, and PTEN. Oncotarget, 2016.

[67] Yanaihara, N., et al., *Unique microRNA molecular profiles in lung cancer diagnosis and prognosis.* Cancer Cell, 2006. **9**(3): pp. 189–98.

[68] Donnem, T., et al., *MicroRNA signatures in tumor tissue related to angiogenesis in non-small cell lung cancer.* PLoS One, 2012. **7**(1): pp. e29671.

[69] Patnaik, S.K., et al., *Evaluation of microRNA expression profiles that may predict recurrence of localized stage I non-small cell lung cancer after surgical resection.* Cancer Res, 2010. **70**(1): pp. 36–45.

[70] Sang, H., et al., *Long non-coding RNA functions in lung cancer.* Tumour Biol, 2015. **36**(6): pp. 4027–37.

[71] Li, J., et al., *LncRNA MALAT1 exerts oncogenic functions in lung adenocarcinoma by targeting miR-204.* Am J Cancer Res, 2016. **6**(5): pp. 1099–107.

[72] Han, L., et al., *Low expression of long noncoding RNA PANDAR predicts a poor prognosis of non-small cell lung cancer and affects cell apoptosis by regulating Bcl-2.* Cell Death Dis, 2015. **6**: p. e1665.

[73] Zhang, E.B., et al., *P53-regulated long non-coding RNA TUG1 affects cell proliferation in human non-small cell lung cancer, partly through epigenetically regulating HOXB7 expression.* Cell Death Dis, 2014. **5**: p. e1243

[74] Deng, H.P., et al., *Long non-coding RNA HOTTIP promotes tumor growth and inhibits cell apoptosis in lung cancer.* Cell Mol Biol (Noisy-le-grand), 2015. **61**(4): pp. 34–40.

[75] Nie, F.Q., et al., *Long non-coding RNA MVIH indicates a poor prognosis for non-small cell lung cancer and promotes cell proliferation and invasion.* Tumour Biol, 2014. **35**(8): pp. 7587–94.

[76] Lu, K.H., et al., *Long non-coding RNA MEG3 inhibits NSCLC cells proliferation and induces apoptosis by affecting p53 expression.* BMC Cancer, 2013. **13**: pp. 461.

[77] Yang, Q., et al., *A novel long noncoding RNA AK001796 acts as an oncogene and is involved in cell growth inhibition by resveratrol in lung cancer.* Toxicol Appl Pharmacol, 2015. **285**(2): pp. 79–88.

[78] Nie, F.Q., et al., *Long noncoding RNA ANRIL promotes non-small cell lung cancer cell proliferation and inhibits apoptosis by silencing KLF2 and P21 expression.* Mol Cancer Ther, 2015. **14**(1): pp. 268–77.

[79] Qiu, M., et al., *A novel lncRNA, LUADT1, promotes lung adenocarcinoma proliferation via the epigenetic suppression of p27.* Cell Death Dis, 2015. **6**: pp. e1858.

[80] Pan, H., et al., *Long non-coding RNA BC087858 induces non-T790M mutation acquired resistance to EGFR-TKIs by activating PI3K/AKT and MEK/ERK pathways and EMT in non-small-cell lung cancer.* Oncotarget, 2016. **7**(31): pp. 49948–60.

[81] Zhang, L., et al., *Enhanced expression of long non-coding RNA ZXF1 promoted the invasion and metastasis in lung adenocarcinoma.* Biomed Pharmacother, 2014. **68**(4): pp. 401–7.

[82] Yang, Z.T., et al., *Overexpression of Long Non-Coding RNA ZXF2 Promotes Lung Adenocarcinoma Progression Through c-Myc Pathway.* Cell Physiol Biochem, 2015. **35**(6): pp. 2360–70.

[83] Wang, G., H. Chen, and J. Liu, *The long noncoding RNA LINC01207 promotes proliferation of lung adenocarcinoma.* Am J Cancer Res, 2015. **5**(10): pp. 3162–73.

[84] Castellano, J.J., et al., *LincRNA-p21 impacts prognosis in resected non-small-cell lung cancer patients through angiogenesis regulation.* J Thorac Oncol, 2016. **11**(12):2173–82

[85] Calin, G.A., et al., *Ultraconserved regions encoding ncRNAs are altered in human leukemias and carcinomas.* Cancer Cell. **12**(3): pp. 215–229.

[86] Peng, J.C., J. Shen, and Z.H. Ran, *Transcribed ultraconserved region in human cancers.* RNA Biol, 2013. **10**(12): pp. 1771–7

[87] Jiang, S., et al., *MicroRNA-21 modulates radiation resistance through upregulation of hypoxia-inducible factor-1alpha-promoted glycolysis in non-small cell lung cancer cells.* Mol Med Rep, 2016. **13**(5): pp. 4101–7.

[88] Kenneth, Niall S. and S. Rocha, *Regulation of gene expression by hypoxia.* Biochem J, 2008. **414**(1): pp. 19–29.

[89] Gao, X.J., et al., *Nobiletin inhibited hypoxia-induced epithelial-mesenchymal transition of lung cancer cells by inactivating of Notch-1 signaling and switching on miR-200b.* Pharmazie, 2015. **70**(4): pp. 256–62.

[90] Haigl, B., et al., *Expression of microRNA-21 in non-small cell lung cancer tissue increases with disease progression and is likely caused by growth conditional changes during malignant transformation.* Int J Oncol, 2014. **44**(4): pp. 1325–34.

[91] Eilertsen, M., et al., *Positive prognostic impact of miR-210 in non-small cell lung cancer.* Lung Cancer, 2014. **83**(2): pp. 272–8.

[92] Krutilina, R., et al., *MicroRNA-18a inhibits hypoxia-inducible factor 1alpha activity and lung metastasis in basal breast cancers.* Breast Cancer Res, 2014. **16**(4): p. R78.

[93] Ding, G., et al., *MiR-199a suppresses the hypoxia-induced proliferation of non-small cell lung cancer cells through targeting HIF1alpha.* Mol Cell Biochem, 2013. **384**(1–2): pp. 173–80.

[94] Guo, W.G., et al., *Bioinformatics analyses combined microarray identify the desregulated microRNAs in lung cancer.* Eur Rev Med Pharmacol Sci, 2013. **17**(11): pp. 1509–16.

[95] Taguchi, A., et al., *Identification of hypoxia-inducible factor-1 alpha as a novel target for miR-17-92 microRNA cluster*. Cancer Res, 2008. **68**(14): pp. 5540–5.

[96] Mao, G., et al., *Tumor-derived microRNA-494 promotes angiogenesis in non-small cell lung cancer*. Angiogenesis, 2015. **18**(3): pp. 373–82.

[97] Yang, F., et al., *Repression of the long noncoding RNA-LET by histone deacetylase 3 contributes to hypoxia-mediated metastasis*. Mol Cell, 2013. **49**(6): pp. 1083–96.

[98] Wu, Y., et al., *Downregulation of the long noncoding RNA GAS5-AS1 contributes to tumor metastasis in non-small cell lung cancer*. Sci Rep, 2016, **6**: p. 31093.

[99] Zhou, C., et al., *Long noncoding RNA HOTAIR, a hypoxia-inducible factor-1alpha activated driver of malignancy, enhances hypoxic cancer cell proliferation, migration, and invasion in non-small cell lung cancer*. Tumour Biol, 2015. **36**(12): pp. 9179–88.

[100] Yao, Y., J. Li, and L. Wang, *Large intervening non-coding RNA HOTAIR is an indicator of poor prognosis and a therapeutic target in human cancers*. Int J Mol Sci, 2014. **15**(10): pp. 18985–99.

[101] Matouk, I.J., et al., *The oncofetal H19 RNA connection: hypoxia, p53 and cancer*. Biochim Biophys Acta, 2010. **1803**(4): pp. 443–51.

[102] Mei, Y., et al., *A piRNA-like small RNA interacts with and modulates p-ERM proteins in human somatic cells*. Nat Commun, 2015. **6**: p. 7316.

[103] Qi, R., T. Qiao, and X. Zhuang, *Small interfering RNA targeting S100A4 sensitizes non-small-cell lung cancer cells (A549) to radiation treatment*. Onco Targets Ther, 2016. **9**: pp. 3753–62.

[104] Geretti, E. and M. Klagsbrun, *Neuropilins: novel targets for anti-angiogenesis therapies*. Cell Adh Migr, 2007. **1**(2): pp. 56–61.

[105] Nguyen, Q.D., et al., *Inhibition of vascular endothelial growth factor (VEGF)-165 and semaphorin 3A-mediated cellular invasion and tumor growth by the VEGF signaling inhibitor ZD4190 in human colon cancer cells and xenografts*. Mol Cancer Ther, 2006. **5**(8): pp. 2070–7.

[106] Geretti, E., A. Shimizu, and M. Klagsbrun, *Neuropilin structure governs VEGF and semaphorin binding and regulates angiogenesis*. Angiogenesis, 2008. **11**(1): pp. 31–9.

[107] Kitsukawa, T., et al., *Overexpression of a membrane protein, neuropilin, in chimeric mice causes anomalies in the cardiovascular system, nervous system and limbs*. Development, 1995. **121**(12): pp. 4309–18.

[108] Miao, H.Q., et al., *Neuropilin-1 expression by tumor cells promotes tumor angiogenesis and progression*. FASEB J, 2000. **14**(15): pp. 2532–9.

[109] Banerjee, S.K., et al., *Overexpression of vascular endothelial growth factor164 and its co-receptor neuropilin-1 in estrogen-induced rat pituitary tumors and GH3 rat pituitary tumor cells*. Int J Oncol, 2000. **16**(2): pp. 253–60.

[110] Han, F., et al., *MicroRNA-30b promotes axon outgrowth of retinal ganglion cells by inhibiting Semaphorin3A expression.* Brain Res, 2015. **1611**: pp. 65–73.

[111] Loginov, V.I., et al., *Tumor suppressor function of the SEMA3B gene in human lung and renal cancers.* PLoS One, 2015. **10**(5): pp. e0123369.

[112] Cai, G., S. Qiao, and K. Chen, *Suppression of miR-221 inhibits glioma cells proliferation and invasion via targeting SEMA3B.* Biol Res, 2015. **48**: p. 37.

[113] Mumblat, Y., et al., *Full-length semaphorin-3C is an inhibitor of tumor lymphangiogenesis and metastasis.* Cancer Res, 2015. **75**(11): pp. 2177–86.

[114] Meert, A.P., et al., *[Difficulties and limitations in conducting translational research in thoracic oncology. A practical example].* Rev Mal Respir, 2016. **33**(7): pp. 594–9.

[115] Foley, K., et al., *Semaphorin 3D autocrine signaling mediates the metastatic role of annexin A2 in pancreatic cancer.* Sci Signal, 2015. **8**(388): p. ra77.

[116] Christensen, C., et al., *Proteolytic processing converts the repelling signal Sema3E into an inducer of invasive growth and lung metastasis.* Cancer Res, 2005. **65**(14): pp. 6167–77.

[117] Nasarre, P., et al., *Neuropilin-2 Is upregulated in lung cancer cells during TGF-beta1-induced epithelial-mesenchymal transition.* Cancer Res, 2013. **73**(23): pp. 7111–21.

[118] Clarhaut, J., et al., *ZEB-1, a repressor of the semaphorin 3F tumor suppressor gene in lung cancer cells.* Neoplasia, 2009. **11**(2): pp. 157–66.

[119] Jian, H., et al., *SEMA4B inhibits growth of non-small cell lung cancer in vitro and in vivo.* Cell Signal, 2015. **27**(6): pp. 1208–13.

[120] Jian, H., B. Liu, and J. Zhang, *Hypoxia and hypoxia-inducible factor 1 repress SEMA4B expression to promote non-small cell lung cancer invasion.* Tumour Biol, 2014. **35**(5): pp. 4949–55.

[121] Jian, H., et al., *SEMA4b inhibits MMP9 to prevent metastasis of non-small cell lung cancer.* Tumour Biol, 2014. **35**(11): pp. 11051–6.

[122] Li, J., Q. Wang, R. Wen, J. Liang, X. Zhong, W. Yang, et al. *MiR-138 inhibits cell proliferation and reverses epithelial-mesenchymal transition in non-small cell lung cancer cells by targeting GIT1 and SEMA4C.* J Cell Mol Med, 2015. **19**(12): pp. 2793–805.

[123] Gu, A., J. Lu, W. Wang, C. Shi, B. Han, M. Yao. *Role of miR-497 in VEGF-A-mediated cancer cell growth and invasion in non-small cell lung cancer.* Int J Biochem Cell Biol, 2016. **70**: pp. 118–25.

[124] Ruan, S.S., et al., *Expression and clinical significance of Semaphorin4D in non-small cell lung cancer and its impact on malignant behaviors of A549 lung cancer cells.* J Huazhong Univ Sci Technolog Med Sci, 2014. **34**(4): pp. 491–6.

[125] Liu, Y., et al., *MiR-214 suppressed ovarian cancer and negatively regulated semaphorin 4D.* Tumour Biol, 2016. **37**(6): pp. 8239–48.

[126] Fazzari, P., et al., *Plexin-B1 plays a redundant role during mouse development and in tumour angiogenesis.* BMC Dev Biol, 2007. **7**: p. 55.

[127] Lu, T.P., et al., *Identification of a novel biomarker, SEMA5A, for non-small cell lung carcinoma in nonsmoking women.* Cancer Epidemiol Biomarkers Prev, 2010. **19**(10): pp. 2590–7.

[128] Veliceasa, D., et al., *Therapeutic manipulation of angiogenesis with miR-27b.* Vasc Cell, 2015. **7**: p. 6.

[129] Urbich, C., et al., *MicroRNA-27a/b controls endothelial cell repulsion and angiogenesis by targeting semaphorin 6A.* Blood, 2012. **119**(6): pp. 1607–16.

[130] Ma, B., et al., *Role of chitinase 3-like-1 and semaphorin 7a in pulmonary melanoma metastasis.* Cancer Res, 2015. **75**(3): pp. 487–96.

[131] Narazaki, M., M. Segarra, and G. Tosato, *Sulfated polysaccharides identified as inducers of neuropilin-1 internalization and functional inhibition of VEGF165 and semaphorin3A.* Blood, 2008. **111**(8): pp. 4126-36.

[132] Wiggins, J.F., et al., *Development of a lung cancer therapeutic based on the tumor suppressor microRNA-34.* Cancer Res, 2010. **70**(14): pp. 5923–30.

[133] AUSTIN, Texas, BUSINESS WIRE - *Mirna Therapeutics*, Inc. (Nasdaq:MIRN) September 20, 2016

[134] Potente, M., et al., *Involvement of Foxo transcription factors in angiogenesis and postnatal neovascularization.* J Clin Invest, 2005. **115**(9): pp. 2382–92.

[135] Krug, S., et al., *Knock-down of Pdcd4 stimulates angiogenesis via up-regulation of angiopoietin-2.* Biochim Biophys Acta, 2012. **1823**(4): pp. 789–99.

[136] Wang, F., A.J. Nazarali, and S. Ji, *Circular RNAs as potential biomarkers for cancer diagnosis and therapy.* Am J Cancer Res, 2016. **6**(6): pp. 1167–76.

[137] Ricciuti, B., et al., *Long noncoding RNAs: new insights into non-small cell lung cancer biology, diagnosis and therapy.* Med Oncol, 2016. **33**(2): p. 18.

[138] Liu, Z., M. Sun, K. Lu, J. Liu, M. Zhang, W. Wu, et al. *The long noncoding RNA HOTAIR contributes to cisplatin resistance of human lung adenocarcinoma cells via downregualtion of p21(WAF1/CIP1) expression.* PLoS One, 2013. **8**(10): p. e77293.

[139] Li, Z. and T.M. Rana. *Therapeutic targeting of microRNAs: current status and future challenges.* Nat Rev Drug Discov, 2014. **13**(8): pp. 622–38.

[140] Roberts, T.C. and M.J. Wood. *Therapeutic targeting of non-coding RNAs.* Essays Biochem, 2013. **54**: pp. 127–45.

[141] Krutzfeldt, J., N. Rajewsky, R. Braich, K.G. Rajeev, T. Tuschl, M. Manoharan, et al. *Silencing of microRNAs in vivo with 'antagomirs'.* Nature, 2005. **438**(7068): pp. 685–9.

[142] Bagga, S., J. Bracht, S. Hunter, K. Massirer, J. Holtz, R. Eachus, et al. *Regulation by let-7 and lin-4 miRNAs results in target mRNA degradation.* Cell, 2005. **122**(4): pp. 553–63.

[143] Morrissey, D.V., J.A. Lockridge, L. Shaw, K. Blanchard, K. Jensen, W. Breen, et al. *Potent and persistent in vivo anti-HBV activity of chemically modified siRNAs*. Nat Biotechnol, 2005. **23**(8): pp. 1002–7.

[144] Akinc, A., et al., *A combinatorial library of lipid-like materials for delivery of RNAi therapeutics*. Nat Biotechnol, 2008. **26**(5): pp. 561–9.

[145] Peer, D., et al., *Systemic leukocyte-directed siRNA delivery revealing cyclin D1 as an anti-inflammatory target*. Science, 2008. **319**(5863): pp. 627–30.

[146] Palliser, D., et al., *An siRNA-based microbicide protects mice from lethal herpes simplex virus 2 infection*. Nature, 2006. **439**(7072): pp. 89–94.

[147] Kumar, P., et al., *A single siRNA suppresses fatal encephalitis induced by two different flaviviruses*. PLoS Med, 2006. **3**(4): pp. e96.

[148] Hu-Lieskovan, S., et al., *Sequence-specific knockdown of EWS-FLI1 by targeted, nonviral delivery of small interfering RNA inhibits tumor growth in a murine model of metastatic Ewing's sarcoma*. Cancer Res, 2005. **65**(19): pp. 8984–92.

[149] Song, E., et al., *Antibody mediated in vivo delivery of small interfering RNAs via cell-surface receptors*. Nat Biotechnol, 2005. **23**(6): pp. 709–17.

[150] Yao, Y.D., et al., *Targeted delivery of PLK1-siRNA by ScFv suppresses Her2+ breast cancer growth and metastasis*. Sci Transl Med, 2012. **4**(130): p. 130ra48.

[151] Gutschner, T., et al., *The noncoding RNA MALAT1 is a critical regulator of the metastasis phenotype of lung cancer cells*. Cancer Res, 2013. **73**(3): pp. 1180–9.

7

Anti-VEGF Therapy in Cancer: A Double-Edged Sword

Victor Gardner, Chikezie O. Madu and Yi Lu

Abstract

Vascular endothelial growth factor (VEGF) is a mitogen that plays a crucial role in angiogenesis and lymphangiogenesis. It is involved in tumor survival through inducing tumor angiogenesis and by increasing chemoresistance through autocrine signaling. Because of its importance in tumor formation and survival, several medications have been developed to inhibit VEGF and reduce blood vessel formation in cancer. Although these medications have proven to be effective for late-stage and metastatic cancers, they have been shown to cause side effects such as hypertension, artery clots, complications in wound healing, and, more rarely, gastrointestinal perforation and fistulas. Current research in using anti-VEGF medication as a part of cancer treatments is focusing on elucidating the mechanisms of tumor resistance to VEGF medication, developing predictive biomarkers that assess whether a patient will respond to VEGF therapy and creating novel treatments and techniques that increase the efficacy of antiangiogenic medication. This chapter aims to review the role of VEGF in tumor angiogenesis and metastasis, the structure and function of VEGF and its receptors, and VEGF's role in cancer are discussed. Furthermore, tumor therapies targeting VEGF along with their side effects are presented and, finally, new directions in anti-VEGF therapy are considered along with the challenges.

Keywords: VEGF, angiogenesis, side effect, medication

1. Introduction

Oxygen and nutrients are critical to the functioning and survival of cells in the body. This need is met through the creation of an extensive vascular system, which is maintained through the process of angiogenesis, and the creation of blood vessels from the existing vasculature [1]. In the angiogenesis process, endothelial cells initially respond to changes in the local environment and migrate toward the growing tumor. The endothelial cells then migrate together forming tubular structures that are ultimately encapsulated by recruiting periendo-thelial support cells to establish a vascular network that facilitates tumor growth and metas-tasis. Angiogenesis is subject to a complex regulatory system of both pro- and antiangiogenic factors after a tissue is fashioned [1–3] and deregulating angiogenesis–a classic trademark of cancer–leads to an aberrant microenvironment and promotion of tumor progression. Angiogenesis is initiated by the binding actions of vascular endothelial growth factor (VEGF) and fibroblast growth factors (FGF1/2) [4].

VEGF is an essential proangiogenic factor whose production is itself extensively regulated by a plethora of growth factors, cytokines, and other extracellular molecules produced in response to the various metabolic and mechanical conditions present in the cell's environ-ment [2–6]. VEGF plays a pivotal role in tumor angiogenesis. The overexpression of VEGF is one of the central factors that leads to the onset and progression of cancer. In order to sustain their growth beyond any current size, tumors require an increased supply of blood, and this is achieved through the expression and secretion of VEGF, which stimu-lates the induction of new blood vessels around the tumor. Furthermore, the cancer cells, through the action of this subfamily of growth factors, invade other organs and areas of the body (metastasis) [4]. Consequently, VEGF and the resulting tumor angiogenesis present an attractive therapeutic target in the treatment of cancer. Inhibitors of VEGF/angiogenesis have been garnering interest and studied for their therapeutic application in most solid tumors [7, 8]. Moreover, a series of preclinical studies have revealed that anti-VEGF com-pounds increase the efficacy of ensuing antitumor treatment, although the mechanism of this effect is unclear [9].

2. Structure and function of VEGF and VEGFRs

VEGF is a dimeric glycoprotein secreted by cells that is able to induce permeability of blood vessels and promotes angiogenesis. The VEGF family contains seven members, all part of the platelet-derived growth factor (PDGF) supergene family: VEGF-A, VEGF-B, VEGF-C, VEGF-D, VEGF-E, VEGF-F, and PlGF [10, 11]. All members contain a core region comprised of eight cysteine residues forming a cysteine knot motif. These residues are involved in both inter- and intramolecular disulfide bonds at one end of a central four-stranded β-sheet within each monomer, which dimerizes in antiparallel fashion [11]. VEGFs A–D and PlGF are all produced in humans, whereas VEGF-E is produced in the Orf virus, has a 25% amino acid homology to mammalian VEGF, and lacks a heparin-binding domain [12]. VEGF-F is pro-duced in snake venom and varies its structure and function by species, helping to produce a variety of venom [13].

The VEGF-A gene contains eight different exons that create six different isoforms through alternative splicing. These isoforms have lengths (in amino acids) of 121, 145, 165, 183, 189, and 206 that are produced by the alternate splicing of a single gene containing eight exons, and they all contain exons 1–5 and 8. All forms of VEGF-A except for VEGF-A$_{121}$ can bind to heparin [11]. VEGF$_{165}$ is the one most commonly secreted by tumor cells and acts most strongly on endothelial cells to lead them to form new capillaries. VEGF-B exists as two isoforms of lengths 167 and 186 amino acids and has been shown to act as a cell survival factor while exhibiting little proangiogenic effect [14]. VEGF-C and VEGF-D are resealed proteolytically from their respective precursor proteins and play important roles in regulating lymphangiogenesis [10, 11]. PlGF upregulates angiogenesis through binding to VEGFR-1 (thereby freeing VEGF-A to bind to VEGFR-2) and exists in four isoforms of amino acid lengths 131, 152, 203, and 224 [15]. It has also been shown to induce a specific phosphorylation and activation of c-Jun N-terminal kinase (JNK) and p38 [16].

VEGF signaling pathway plays a major role in angiogenesis. VEGF receptors (VEGFRs) are type V receptor tyrosine kinases (RTKs) activated upon ligand-mediated dimerization [17]. Two high-affinity VEGF receptors, VEGFR-1 (Flt-1) and VEGFR-2 (Flk-1/KDR), have been identified in endothelial cells. Flk-1 (R2) has been shown to play a major role in tumor angiogenesis. In all, there are three types of receptors, with VEGFR-3 only binding to VEGFs –C and –D. Each of the three types of receptor (VEGFR-1, -2, and -3) is composed of seven immunoglobulin-like domains in the extracellular region, a transmembrane region, and a tyrosine kinase sequence with a kinase insert domain [11].

Signaling of VEGF is initiated via binding to its receptors, which are tyrosine kinases that are able to transphosphorylate tyrosine residues of SH2 domain-containing signaling molecules, thus activating kinase-dependent transcription factors known as STAT proteins, to modulate cell responses induced by VEGF. VEGFR-1 and -2 are both involved in endothelial cell function and angiogenesis [18], while VEGFR-3, to which only VEGFs –C and –D can bind, plays a critical role in lymphangiogenesis and primarily involved in normal embryonic development [11]. VEGF-1 has also been shown to be required in inducing the migration of monocytes and macrophages [19]. Neuropilins-1 and -2 are important coreceptors for VEGF signaling and increase the affinity of VEGF-A$_{165}$ for its receptors [5]. Refer to **Figure 1** for a summary of how each VEGF pairs with each VEGF receptor.

VEGF is heavily involved in promoting angiogenesis and research suggests that it also plays a role in regulating intussusceptive angiogenesis as well. In sprouting angiogenesis, hypoxia induces parenchymal cells to release VEGF-A into the extracellular matrix (ECM). VEGF-A then causes tip cells to produce the Delta-like-4 (Dll4) ligand, which is a membrane-bound ligand that serves to activate the Notch receptor, a highly conserved transmembrane receptor that regulates cell proliferation, cell fate, and cell death in metazoans on neighboring cells through cell to cell contact [20]. Dll4 then inhibits migratory behavior through activating the Notch receptor on neighboring stalk cells. Tip cell filopodia, actin-rich protrusions on the cell membrane that serve as a mechanism for a cell to explore its environment, sense a gradient in VEGF-A and align their sprouting to this gradient. The tip cell then anchors itself onto the substratum while actin microfilaments in the filopodia contract, pulling the tip cell toward the VEGF-A source while stalk cells proliferate. When the tip cells from different sprouts meet, they fuse to become a functional capillary through which blood can flow [1]. The function of VEGF in sprouting angiogenesis is less well understood, although it is suspected that VEGF cooperating with angiopoietin-1 (Ang-1) plays a role in stimulating the process [21, 22].

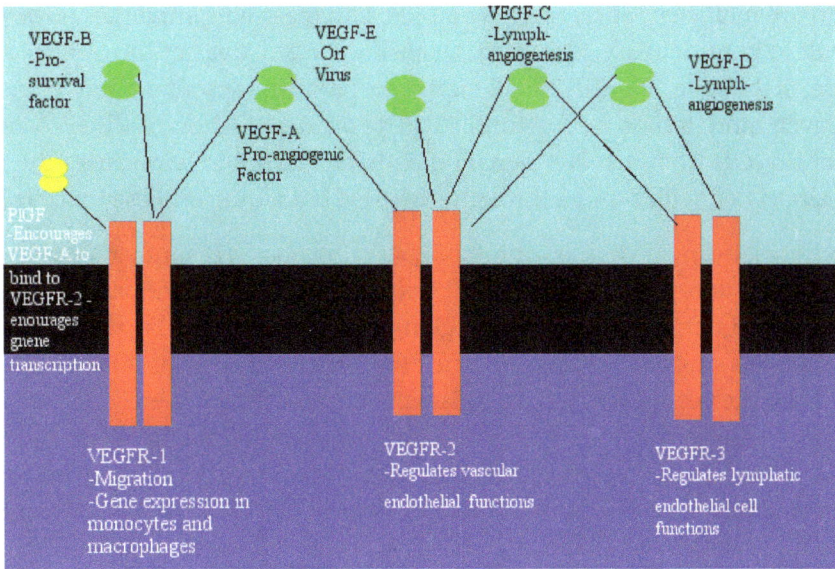

Figure 1. A summary of the functions of each form of VEGF and PlGF and each VEGF receptor. VEGFR-1 regulates cell migration and gene expression in monocytes and macrophages; VEGFR-2 regulates vascular endothelial functions; and VEGFR-3 regulates lymphatic endothelial functions. VEGF-A is a proangiogenic factor; VEGF-B is a prosurvival factor; VEGF-C and –D regulate lymphangiogenesis; VEGF-E is found in the Orf virus; and PlGF encourages VEGF-A to bind to VEGFR-2, thereby stimulating angiogenesis, and encourages the transcription of JNK and p38.

3. The role of VEGF in cancer

Tumors need oxygen to survive. At first, they are able to obtain enough oxygen by coopting the surrounding vasculature, altering its morphology, physiology, and response to therapy in the process. However, when a tumor becomes too large to be sufficiently supplied by existing vasculature, an "angiogenic switch" is turned on, and the tumor begins the process of tumor angiogenesis, thereby creating its own vasculature for an oxygen supply [23–26].

The angiogenic switch is triggered by hypoxia occurring when the tumor becomes too large for oxygen to diffuse from existing vasculature to tumor cells [27]. Hypoxia induces the production of VEGF in tumor cells through hypoxia-inducible factor-1α (HIF-1α) [25, 27], a master transcriptional factor that regulates a group of downstream genes including VEGF that promote angiogenesis and metastasis, while inhibitors of angiogenesis such as angiostatin and interferon are downregulated [23]. A suite of other proangiogenic genes (such as Ang-1 and -2) and regulatory mechanisms (such as micro-RNAs) are also regulated by the hypoxia-induced HIF pathway [25]. Tumor cells then release VEGF into the surrounding extracellular space, which binds to VEGF R of surrounding or nearby endothelial cells, promoting local angiogenesis and forming tumor-associated microvessels in order to delivering oxygen-carrying blood to the tumor.

Compared with normal vasculature, tumor vessels are highly irregular and inefficient at delivering nutrients. They branch irregularly, follow a tortuous path, are far larger than their normal counterparts, are unusually permeable to large molecules, have a high interstitial pressure, and are inefficient at carrying blood [26, 28]; these abnormalities of the tumor vasculature result in poor delivery of nutrients, causing certain areas of the tumor to be chronically hypoxic, stabilizing the HIF/VEGF signaling pathway described above and therefore resulting in even more tumor vasculature [25]. The overproduction of VEGF-A results in an abundance of tip cells from the Dll4 signaling pathway, which in part causes the malformed vasculature associated with tumors through excessive branching of these tip cells [25, 29].

Tumor blood vessel can be divided into six general classes: (1) mother vessels, which are enlarged, tortuous, thin-walled, lacking in pericytes, and highly permeable; (2) capillaries, which are similar to normal capillaries; (3) glomeruloid microvascular proliferations, which are tangles of vessels situated within a mixture of disordered pericytes; (4) vascular malformations, which are large vessels with an irregular coat of smooth muscle cells; (5) feeder arteries; and (6) draining vessels, which are enlarged, serpentine smooth muscle cell-coated vessels that supply and drain the blood vessels within the tumor [30]. The irregular pericyte and smooth muscle cell formations on these vessels, which in normal vasculature serve to enhance tight junctions and decrease leakiness, serve to decrease vessel efficacy in tumor angiogenesis [31].

Oncogenes play a prominent role in triggering the angiogenic switch. Expression of the H-Ras oncogene in the immortalized rat intestinal epithelial cell line IEC-18 led to the upregulation of VEGF and a significant increase of *in vivo* vascularization [32]. Ras signaling also results in the stabilization of the resulting mRNAs and possible enhancement of their transcription [33]. The p53 suppressor gene normally serves to downregulate VEGF while upregulating thrombospondin-1, an antiangiogenic factor; mutations in these genes serve to increase the activity of VEGF [34, 35]. p53 acts as a foil to C-Myc, a gene that triggers the expression of VEGF while downregulating thrombospondin-1. In tumors, mutations in p53 serve to increase the activity of c-Myc, thereby increasing the activity of VEGF [34].

Compared to VEGF-A, VEGF-B plays an insignificant role in angiogenesis. Rather, it acts as a potent survival factor, inhibiting the production of several proapoptotic factors such as BH-3-related proteins. The prosurvival effects of VEGF-B are mediated by both VEGFR-1 and the coreceptor NP-1 [36, 37]. More recent research suggests that VEGF-B may trigger tumor angiogenesis through a VEGF-A-independent pathway and that it may even be a prognostic marker for cancer metastasis [38].

VEGF-C and VEGF-D are both heavily involved in lymphangiogenesis. In tumors, these two forms of VEGF are overexpressed and activate VEGFR-3 by means of a paracrine signaling loop, thereby encouraging lymphatic growth within the tumor [39, 40]. Lymphatic vessels created through tumor angiogenesis tend to be larger than normal, enhancing the delivery of tumor cells to the lymph nodes, from which metastasis can occur (while VEGFR-3 activation causes lymphatic vessels to sprout, it should be noted that VEGFR-2 causes the vessels to become dilated) [41]. For example, metastasis of breast cancer occurs primarily through the lymphatic system, and VEGF-C has been shown to enhance tumor metastasis in this disease [42]. Because both lymphatic vessels and blood vessels provide nutrients and a metastatic pathway for a tumor, vascular density (lymphatic vessels density or blood vessel density) within the tumor may be a prognostic factor of metastatic potential [41, 43].

4. Anti-VEGF medications

Because of tumor dependence on VEGF for growth and survival, much work has been put into developing VEGF inhibitors for use in the clinic. Most of these inhibitors fall under two broad categories that differ in structure and mechanism of action: small-molecule inhibitors (SMIs) and monoclonal antibodies (mAbs). **Table 1** contains a list of the anti-VEGF medications mentioned in this chapter, their types, FDA approval dates, the forms of cancer they are approved to treat, and some common side effects associated with their use.

Some SMIs targeting VEGF signaling pathway are able to pass through the cellular membrane and interact with the cytoplasmic domain of receptor tyrosine kinases (RTKs) [44, 45]. Most act as competitive inhibitors with ATP. As the ATP binding site is common to all RTKs, specificity in the SMI is created by engineering the part of the molecule not similar to ATP [44]. Small molecule tyrosine kinase inhibitors (SMTKIs) can be divided into three broad categories: those that hydrogen bond with the ATP binding site of the enzyme's active conformation (type I), those that hydrogen bond with the hydrophobic pocket directly next to the ATP binding site in the enzyme's inactive conformation (type II), and those that bond covalently and irreversibly with specific cysteine residues on the kinase (type III) [44].

Sunitinib is a type I SMTKI [44] that is able to inhibit RTKs containing a split-kinase domain, such as VEGFRs -1, -2, and -3; PDGFRs –A and –B; cKIT; FLT3; CSF-1R; and RET [46]. The inhibition of the RTKs blocks signal transduction, thereby preventing tumor growth and angiogenesis among other processes. Sunitinib is administered orally in a recommended dose of 50 mg once daily for 4 weeks followed by a 2-week rest [47]. The medicine is currently FDA approved for use in progressive well-differentiated pancreatic neuroendocrine tumors in patients with unresectable, locally advanced, or metastatic disease; metastatic renal cell carcinoma; and gastrointestinal stromal tumors after intolerance to imatinib mesylate [46].

Sorafenib is a type II SMTKI [45]. Sorafenib inhibits VEGFR-2, VEGFR-3, PDGFR-β, and Kit; therefore, it operates through a dual mechanism of action, inhibiting both tumor growth and angiogenesis [48]. Sorafenib is administered in a recommended dose of 400 mg twice daily around mealtimes [47]. The medicine is FDA approved for use in recurrent or metastatic progressive differentiated thyroid carcinoma, advanced renal cell carcinoma, and unresectable hepatocellular carcinoma [49].

Vandetanib is a type III SMTKI [44]. It inhibits VEGFR-2, EGFR, and RET, blocking several signal transduction pathways that control tumor growth and angiogenesis [50]. Vandetanib was approved in 2011 for use against unresectable, locally advanced, or metastatic medullary thyroid cancer. The recommended daily dose of the medicine is 300 mg per day, administered orally [51].

In contrast to small molecule inhibitors, monoclonal antibodies (mAbs) cannot translocate through the plasma membrane to interact with the cytoplasmic domains of RTKs; they are, however, more specific in action than SMIs [45]. mAbs used in antiangiogenic therapies can be divided into two broad categories: those that bind to VEGF and inhibit VEGF's ability to bind with its receptors, and those that bind to VEGFRs and inhibit ligand-receptor interaction and activate immune responses.

Medicine	Type of medication	FDA approval date	Types of cancers approved for to date	Common Grade 3-4 side effects
Apatinib [114]	SMI	N/A	N/A	N/A
Bevacizumab [125]	mAb	26-Feb-04	Metastatic colorectal cancer, nonsmall cell lung cancer, glioblastoma, metastatic renal cell carcinoma, cervical cancer (in combination with chemotherapy), platinum-resistant recurrent epithelial ovarian, fallopian tube, or primary peritoneal cancer in combination with chemotherapy FDA approval for the use of bevacizumab in metastatic HER2-negative breast cancer was revoked on 18 Nov. 2011 on account of potentially life-threatening side effects and the few benefits associated with its use	Sensory neuropathy, hypertension, fatigue, neutropenia, vomiting, diarrhea
Cabozantinib [116]	SMI	25-Apr-16	Renal cell carcinoma in patients who have received prior antiangiogenic therapy	Abdominal pain, pleural effusion, diarrhea, and nausea
Pazopanib [126]	SMI	Oct-09	Advanced renal cell carcinoma, advanced soft tissue sarcoma	Diarrhea, hypertension, and proteinuria
Ramucirumab [96]	mAb	21-Apr-14	Gastric/gastroesophageal junction adenocarcinoma (with and without paclitaxel), with docetaxel for platinum-resistant metastatic nonsmall cell lung cancer, with FOLFIRI for metastatic colorectal cancer	Hypertension, hyponatremia, neutropenia, pneumonia
Sorafenib [50]	SMI	20-Dec-05	Advanced renal cell carcinoma, unresectable hepatocellular carcinoma, progressive differentiated thyroid carcinoma	Diarrhea, hand-foot syndrome
Sunitinib [46]	SMI	26-Jan-06	Gastrointestinal stromal tumor, advanced kidney cancer, pancreatic neuroendocrine tumors	Hypertension, diarrhea, nausea, vomiting
Vandetanib [52]	SMI	6-Apr-11	Medullary thyroid cancer in patients with unresectable, locally advanced, or metastatic disease	Diarrhea/colitis, hypertension and hypertensive crisis, QT prolongation, fatigue, and rash
Zif-Aflibercept [127]	VEGF-Trap (hybrid of VEGFR-1 binding domain and VEGFR-2 domain 3)	3-Aug-12	Metastatic colorectal cancer that is resistant to an oxaliplatin-containing regimen	Neutropenia, diarrhea, hypertension, leukopenia, stomatitis, fatigue, proteinuria, and asthenia
33C3 [57]	mAb	N/A	N/A	N/A

Table 1. FDA approvals for antiangiogenic drugs.

Perhaps the most well-known mAb targeting VEGF is bevacizumab, first approved in the EU in January 2005 [52]. The medicine targets all forms of VEGF-A, thereby inhibiting its ability to activate angiogenesis [53]. 2C3 is another mAb that binds to VEGF, preventing it from interacting with VEGFR-2, but not VEGFR-1; it blocks the growth of blood vessels in tumors and inhibits increases in vascular permeability [54]. IMC1121B (ramucirumab) binds to the ligand binding site of VEGFR-2 [55]. 33C3 is an antibody that binds to Ig domains 4-7 of VEGFR-2 and therefore, on account of binding to VEGFR-2 as opposed to a VEGF molecule, has the potential to act independently of VEGF concentration [56].

A type of VEGF inhibitor that defies simple classification into one of these two categories was developed recently as VGEF-trap, otherwise known as aflibercept. Aflibercept is a fusion protein consisting of the VEGFR-1 and VEGFR-2 binding domains and the Fc region of the IgG1 antibody [57, 58]. The protein binds to VEGF-A, VEGF-B, and PlGF, inhibiting activation of VEGFR-1 and VEGFR-2 and thereby inhibiting angiogenesis [57, 58]. Aflibercept was approved as Zaltrap on 3 August 2012 for use in combination with a FOLFIRI (folinic acid, fluorouracil, and irinotecan) chemotherapy regimen in adults with colorectal cancer [59], and has been shown to provide significant benefits in OS and PFS [60].

5. Side effects of anti-VEGF medications

No metabolically active tissue in the human body is more than a few hundred micrometers away from a capillary vesicle. The extensive nature of the vascular system in humans is produced and maintained through angiogenesis; changes in metabolic activity lead to changes in demand for oxygen which in turn regulate angiogenesis [1]. Therefore, angiogenesis inhibitors are bound to have adverse side effects. These side effects are generally less severe than those encountered from chemotherapy, although they can still be life-threatening [61]. Common side effects include hypertension, arterial thromboembolic events (ATEs), cardiotoxicity, and problems with bleeding, gastrointestinal perforation, and wound healing. See **Table 2** for a description of grades of adverse events.

Perhaps the most well documented side effect of angiogenesis inhibitors is hypertension. VEGF has been shown to decrease blood pressure; for example, in a phase I clinical trial (the VIVA trial, a double-blind placebo-controlled study), recombinant VEGF was shown to decrease systolic blood pressure by as much as 22% [62]. This decrease in blood pressure is caused by the generation of blood capillaries, which increases the total cross-sectional surface area available for blood to flow and thereby reduces blood pressure, and VEGF-induced vasodilation, which occurs when VEGF induces the production of nitric oxide and PGI_2 as part of its signal transduction pathway [63]. VEGF inhibitors therefore cause hypertension by inhibiting the production of nitric oxide and PGI_2, leading to vasoconstriction and an increase in blood pressure [64, 65]. Hypertension caused from VEGF inhibition can be managed using standard therapies, such as angiotensin-converting enzyme inhibitors, beta blockers, calcium channel blockers, diuretics, and angiotensin II receptor blockers [66].

VEGF-dependent interactions between the glomeruli and endothelial cells are also inhibited through anti-VEGF therapies (such as bevacizumab, sunitinib, and sorafenib [67]), leading to proteinuria, a common side effect in anti-VEGF treatment [65, 68]. Inhibition of the VEGF signaling pathway leads to the suppression of nephrin, which in turn leads to a decrease in maintenance of the glomerular slit diaphragm [68]. Luckily, most instances of proteinuria are mild, presenting as only grades I and II, although more severe proteinuria has been reported in a share of cases [67, 68].

Treatment with VGEF inhibitors is also associated with an increased risk of arterial thrombo-embolic events (ATEs) [65, 69, 70]. This increased risk is caused by a reduction in the regenerative capacity of endothelial cells and can diminish antiapoptotic factors while encouraging procoagulant changes in the blood vessels [70]. The rate of venous thromboembolic events does not seem to be affected by VEGF inhibition, at least when comparing bevacizumab with chemotherapy and chemotherapy alone [69]. It is recommended that patients on anti-VEGF therapy who develop an ATE be taken off the therapy immediately [65]. The use of aspirin during therapy has been shown to increase the likelihood of grade 3 and 4 bleeding events, although no significant difference has been found between aspirin users in control and bevacizumab-treated groups [69]. Patients with a history of ATEs and older patients are at greater risk in developing a thromboembolic event when using VEGF inhibitors such as bevacizumab [69].

Cardiotoxicity is also a common side effect of VEGF inhibition, and has been observed in patients on bevacizumab, sunitinib, and sorafenib. The exact mechanisms of this toxicity are often unclear, and they may either have to do with inhibition of VEGF, inhibition of other signaling pathways concomitantly with VEGF, or both. Cardiomyopathy has been observed in sunitinib monotherapy in a phase I/II trial in which 11% of all participants (8/75) had a cardiovascular event [71]. Another study found evidence that sunitinib induces cardiotoxocity through the inhibition of the AMPK signal transduction pathway [72]. Moreover, bevacizumab given after acute myelogenous leukemia chemotherapy resulted in an increase in cardiovascular toxicity, although the mechanisms for this toxicity remain unknown [73]. Sorafenib has also been demonstrated to cause cardiotoxicity in mice due to myocyte necrosis [74].

Grade	Description	Example with gastric fistula
I	Mild with few or no symptoms; no interventions required	Asymptomatic; clinical or diagnostic observations only; intervention not indicated
II	Moderate, with minimal intervention needed; some limitation of activities	Symptomatic; altered GI function
III	Severe but not life threatening; hospitalization required; limitation of patient's ability to care for him or herself	Severely altered GI function; bowel rest tube feeding; TPN or hospitalization indicated
IV	Life threatening; urgent intervention required	Life-threatening consequences; urgent operative intervention indicated
V	Death related to adverse event	death

Table 2. Explanation of grades of adverse events [76].

Some side effects are caused by the fact that VEGF impairment impairs wound healing on account of its antiangiogenic properties [65]. Gastrointestinal perforation has been known to occur in patients on anti-VEGF therapy. In the AVOREN trial, three patients receiving bevacizumab in combination with IFN-α experienced grade 4 gastrointestinal perforations, while one patient experienced grade 3 gastrointestinal perorations [66]. Sorafenib and sunitinib have also been shown to cause gastrointestinal perforations [65]. These perforations are caused by tumors, often metastatic, and the healing of these perforations is impaired because angiogenesis is itself prevented. Moreover, a significantly increased risk of hemorrhagic events of all grades is observed in patients on sorafenib, sunitinib, pazopanib, bevacizumab, and aflibercept [65, 75].

6. New directions

Although much progress has been made in angiogenesis inhibition therapy, research in the field is still ongoing. The following section reviews (i) how does tumor resistance against anti-VEGF mediation grow? (ii) what are the challenges in assessing biomarkers for the efficacy of antiangiogenic therapies in specific cases? and (iii) how can treatment methodologies and new treatments improve overall survival (OS)?

6.1. How does tumor resistance against anti-VEGF medication grow?

Tumor resistance to antiangiogenic therapies can be classified into two broad categories: intrinsic and acquired [65, 77]. Acquired antiangiogenic resistance, in contrast to normal methods of acquired drug resistance in which mutational alteration of the drug target prevent the drug from working, consists of tumors initiating alternative methods to cope with hypoxia [77]. There are at least four distinct mechanisms through which this acquired resistance operates: (1) through the activation and upregulation of alternative proangiogenic pathways; (2) through the recruitment of bone marrow-derived proangiogenic cells including increased pericyte coverage of tumor vasculature; (3) through increased tumor aggressiveness resulting in metastasis to provide vasculature through widespread vessel cooption as opposed to tumor angiogenesis; and (4) through the adoption of alternative angiogenic mechanisms [77].

6.1.1. Proangiogenic pathways not involving VEGF

Several proangiogenic molecular pathways are upregulated when the VEGF/VEGFR pathway is inhibited. This often results in a return of tumor vascularization after a period of refractoriness [65, 78]. Some examples of alternative proangiogenic pathways include fibroblast growth factors (FGFs), platelet-derived growth factors (PDGFs), tumor necrosis factor-α (TNF-α), placenta growth factor (PlGF), angiogenin, stromal-derived factor 1α (SDF-1α), and interleukins-1α and -1β (IL-1α, IL-1β) [79–81]. Several of these molecules are regulated through HIF-1 expression, which in turn is controlled by hypoxia [79]. Therefore, through inducing the regression of tumor vasculature, anti-VEGF therapies can induce the expression of other proangiogenic pathways that reduce their own efficacy.

Several therapies are being developed that target both VEGF and alternative angiogenic pathways at the same time. For example, blockage of both VEGF and bFGF with brivanib resulted in prolonged tumor stasis following previous angiogenic inhibition in mouse neuroendocrine tumors [82]. Another study reported that inhibiting SDF-1α after irradiating mice with implanted human U251 GBM tumors prevented the revascularization of irradiated tumors more effectively than inhibiting VEGF, thereby suggesting that SDF-1α may be involved in acquired resistance to anti-VEGF therapies as well [81]. It has also been suggested that synergism between FGF-2 and PDGF-bb could induce angiogenesis, even if they are only present at low concentrations within the cytoplasm [79]. Taken together, these results suggest that inhibition of alternative angiogenic pathways in addition to inhibiting VEGF could increase the efficacy of antiangiogenic therapy.

6.1.2. BMDCs

Bone marrow–derived cells (BMDCs) such as pericytes and macrophages play important roles in both normal and pathological angiogenesis [1, 83, 84]. Tumor-associated macrophages (TAMs) are attracted to hypoxic regions of tumors through the upregulation of chemoattractants caused by hypoxia. Following extravasation into the tumor region, monocytes migrate into hypoxic areas of the tumor, following a chemoattractant gradient [85]. Monocyte chemoattractant protein-1 (MCP-1) has been shown to be an important chemoattractant in this process [86]. Once in the hypoxic region of the tumor, macrophages will promote tumor progression and metastasis through their trophic role (breaking down the ECM and encouraging tumor cell motility) and through excreting compound such as mutagenic oxygen, nitrogen radicals, and several proangiogenic factors such as VEGF and angiopoietin-2 [83, 87].

The process through which pericytes contribute to cancer progression and metastasis is poorly understood. Normally, pericytes are associated with newly formed blood vessels, creating a single, often discontinuous, layer around the endothelial cell tube that serves to support a mature vessel. However, in tumor angiogenesis, pericyte coverage can be greater than, or less than normal tissue vasculature depending on the tumor type; for example, glioblastoma exhibits lower than normal pericytes coverage, while islet carcinomas exhibit higher than normal coverage. This aberrant pericyte coverage can result in tumor growth and metastasis [88]. Current pericytes-targeted cancer therapies aim to reach a balance between pro-and antiangiogenic factors, encouraging vascular normalization [89].

6.1.3. Increased tumor aggressiveness

In most cancers, the appearance of a proinvasive phenotype following antiangiogenic therapy is in question; however, in glioblastoma it is relatively undisputed [78], and there is evidence suggesting its occurrence in pancreatic cancer [90]. The proinvasive phenotype allows tumors from these cancers to circumvent the need for a blood supply, obviating the necessity of tumor angiogenesis. The mechanisms underlying this increased tumor aggressiveness are not fully known. HIFs have been widely accepted as playing a role in increased tumor aggressiveness and metastasis [90]. Moreover, increased collagen signaling in the presence of VEGF inhibition, including activation of discoidin domain receptor 1, protein tyrosine kinase 2, and pseudopodium-enriched atypical kinase 1, has been shown to increase tumor progression and aggressiveness in murine models of pancreatic ductal adenocarcinoma [91]. In glioblastoma, VEGF inhibition creates hypoxic conditions in the tumor, which in turn causes increased expression of c-Met, an HGF receptor tyrosine kinase, through HIF-1α; this increase in c-Met expression correlates with increased invasion and poorer survival [80]. When both VEGF and c-Met are blocked, the increased tumor invasiveness and aggressiveness associated with anti-VEGF medications is suppressed in murine GBM and PNET, suggesting new routes for research in antiangiogenic therapies [80, 92].

6.1.4. Alternative angiogenic mechanisms

Another method through which tumors can circumvent angiogenic inhibition is though alternative angiogenic mechanisms such as intussusceptive angiogenesis, glomeruloid angiogenesis, vasculogenic mimicry, looping angiogenesis, and vessel cooption [78, 83]. These forms of angiogenesis occur through other signaling pathways that do not involve VEGF, and are upregulated when VEGF signaling is inhibited. One such alternative angiogenic pathway is vasculogenic mimicry (VM), which may be encouraged when anti-VEGF medications provide selective pressure for stem-like cancer cells that participate in the process. This phenomenon highlights the need for novel therapeutic methods that target the signaling pathways that control VM in addition to VEGF [93]. Similar combination therapies could be used to increase the efficacy of antiangiogenic medication in general by restricting the tumor's ability to acquire resistance to antiangiogenic therapies.

6.2. Challenges in biomarkers

Unfortunately, no validated biomarkers are currently available for determining which patients will respond best to antiangiogenic therapy [93, 94]. An array of biomarkers has been studied in hope to find effective biomarkers, including systemic measurements, gene analysis, circulating biomarkers, tissue markers, and imaging parameters [95]. Various challenges stand in the way of establishing effective biomarkers, such as the inability to perform repeated biopsies (inhibiting researchers' ability to assess dynamic biomarkers), the unpredictability of response and toxicity, the expensive and complex nature of human trials, the unpredictability of toxicity and response to therapies, and the specificity of each biomarker to disease [95].

The degree of hypertension experienced by a patient has been proposed as a potential systemic biomarker of tumor response, although more research is needed to establish the validity of this measurement [95, 96, 97]. Because hypertension is dependent on the VEGF-signaling pathway, it is possible that patients who do not develop hypertension are not responding to VEGF treatment at the current dose. In fact, the degree of hypertension correlates with survival, with patients who develop more severe hypertension experiencing better cancer remission than patients who develop no hypertension [97]. Interestingly, VEGF polymorphisms may play a role in determining the degree of hypertension, of anti-VEGF medications, which certain polymorphisms being more susceptible to inhibition than others. For example, VEGF-634 SNP (single nucleotide polymorphism) G/G is correlated with higher hypertension in suninitib-treated patients with mRCC than either VEGF-634 C/G or VEGF-634 C/C [98].

Several circulating biomarkers have been proposed that circulate in the bloodstream of patients. For example, high levels of soluble VEGF-R1 (sVEGFR1) correlate with decreased efficacy of bevacizumab in GBM, rectal carcinoma, breast cancer, hepatocellular carcinoma, and metastatic colorectal carcinoma. This correlation is probably caused by sVEGFR1 acting as an endogenous VEGF-trap, so adding a VEGF-specific monoclonal antibody does little to further inhibit VEGF signaling pathways [94]. Another potential circulating biomarker is SDF1α, as levels of this chemokine correlate with evasion of anti-VEGF therapies, although further study is needed to assess this potential biomarker [94]. Pretreatment levels of circulating VEGF-A has been shown to be prognostic in metastatic colorectal, lung, and renal cell cancers, but it is not predictive for bevacizumab treatment [99]. Moreover, a phase II study presented evidence that plasma concentrations of VEGF-A and IL-8 are prognostic for OS in MRCC, with high levels being unfavorable, while low plasma levels or sVEGFR-3 are may be predictive for a positive outcome in patients with mRCC receiving sunitinib [100]. Another phase II trial found that serum levels of Ang-2 and MMP-2, along with tumor levels of HIF-1α, are potential baseline efficacy biomarkers for sunitinib in advanced RCC [101]. Finally, low circulating endothelial cell levels (<65 CEC/4 mL blood) have been found to correlate with longer median PFS and OS in patients with colorectal cancer receiving bevacizumab [102].

Imaging techniques provide potential of imaging parameters as biomarkers as well. For example, MRI- and CT-based tissue vascular measured such as blood flow, blood volume, and permeability have been shown to occur after bevacizumab administration, although more research is needed to assess the efficacy of these measures as biomarkers [95]. Moreover, pretreatment ADC histogram analysis has been shown to be a possible predictive biomarker for bevacizumab treatment in recurrent glioblastoma [103]. Imaging studies can also be used to augment other biomarker studies, and can be used in cooperation with systems pharmacology to create multilevel computational models that predict the efficacy of treatment in patients, as well as suggesting dosing schedules that could be more efficacious than current practices [104]. Another potential biomarker could be patient genotype. As discussed above, some VEGF SNPs may be more receptive to treatment than others. However, some genes show little or no correlation with the efficacy of antiangiogenic therapies. For example, the mutation status of KRAS, a common oncogene, does not correlate with VEGF therapy efficacy [105]. More research must be done to establish which genes can and cannot be considered biomarkers.

6.3. Treatment methodologies and new treatments

According to the normalization hypothesis, during the course of antiangiogenic therapy, there is a dose-dependent window of time during which aberrant tumor vasculature is normalized. In this state, it is easier to deliver cytotoxic drugs from conventional chemotherapy to the tumor in a treatment schedule that takes advantage of the window presented by antiangiogenic agents given in low doses [106]. However, there are two important considerations to take into account when scheduling chemotherapy with antiangiogenic agents: first, the dose of antiangiogenic agents affects the normalization window during which chemotherapy can be delivered effectively. Second, the size of the chemotherapeutic agents matters, as vascular normalization causes the pores in aberrant tumor vessels to shrink, limiting the ability of large molecules to pass through to the tumor [94]. Vascular normalization has also been shown to improve the outcome of immunotherapy, making delivery of immune cells to the tumor easier, and can even decrease the intravasation of cancer cells, limiting the possibility of metastasis [94].

Most of the time, resistance to chemotherapy occurs through heritable changes in the tumor genotype. However, because resistance to VEGF inhibitors does not occur through natural selection, as discussed above, it is possible that rechallenging after disease progression following an intervening interval of time during which VEGF therapy is suspended may allow for a return of efficacy in antiangiogenic VEGF inhibitors. For example, patients with metastatic renal cell carcinoma (mRCC) who experience disease progression after initial response to sunitinib can eventually respond to the drug upon rechallenge after an intervening period on alternative therapies, such as sorafenib (patients with more than 6 months off sunitinib experienced greater PFS than patients with less than 6 months off sunitinib, although in each case the second PFS was shorter than the original) [99]. Moreover, in a randomized phase III trial, patients with unresectable metastatic colorectal cancer progressing up to 3 months after discontinuing bevacizumab plus chemotherapy experienced moderate survival benefits when bevacizumab plus chemotherapy was given as a second line treatment as compared to chemotherapy alone [107].

More research must be done to assess the efficacy of antiangiogenic agents in the adjuvant and neoadjuvant settings. In the neoadjuvant setting, VEGF inhibition may cause tumor regression, converting an unresectable tumor to a resectable one [82], with 12 of 30 patients in one single-arm phase II study who received oxaliplatin plus bevacizumab having initial nonsynchronous unresectable CLM become resectable [108]. However, antiangiogenic neoadjuvant treatment in mouse models of metastatic disease has been shown not to correlate with postsurgical survival [109]. In the adjuvant setting, it is possible that antiangiogenic therapies may prevent relapse by preventing the reestablishment of tumor vasculature. However, bevacizumab has delivered poor results in OS when used in combination with chemotherapy for adjuvant colorectal cancer, although PFS is improved [78].

Some work is also being put into developing novel VEGF and VEGFR inhibitors. For example, ramucirumab, a monoclonal antibody that inhibits VEGFR-2, was given FDA approval in 2014 for use as a single agent in the treatment of patients with gastroesophageal carcinoma; it has since been given approval for use in combination with paclitaxel, docetaxel, and FOLFIRI [110]. Ramucirumab is the first biological treatment to show moderate survival benefits as a single agent after gatroesophageal adenocarcinoma progression following first-line chemotherapy in a phase 3 trial (ramucirumab vs. placebo, OS = 5.2 months vs. 3.8 months, respectively) [111]. The drug has also shown moderate OS benefits when used in combination with docetaxel for second-line treatment of stage IV NNSCLS compared with docetaxel alone after progression on platinum-based chemotherapy (10.5 months vs. 9.1 months, ramucirumab plus docetaxel vs. docetaxel alone, respectively) [112]. Apatinib is another novel VEGFR-2 inhibitor, a small molecule not yet given FDA approval (although it is approved for use in China in treating metastatic gastric or gastroesophageal adenocarcinoma after second-line chemotherapy) [113]. The drug thus far has shown only moderate survival benefits of 1.8 months, and several trials are ongoing to assess its efficacy in different settings [114].

Yet another new small molecule VEGF inhibitor, cabozantinib (Cabometyx, Exelixis, Inc.) was given FDA approval on 25 April, 2016, for the treatment of renal cell carcinoma in patients who have received prior antiangiogenic therapy. Approval was given based on improved progression-free survival (7.4 months vs. 3.8 months in the cabozantinib and everolimus arms, respectively), improved overall survival (21.4 months vs. 16.5 months) and improved confirmed response rate (17 vs. 3%). The drug exhibits the standard side effects associated with VEGF inhibition; 40% of patients who received cabozantinib experienced a serious adverse event such as abdominal pain, pleural effusion, diarrhea, and nausea [115].

Another potential target for anticancer therapy has also been found in lymphangiogenesis. Several studies are examining the potential of inhibiting the VEGFR-3/VEGF-C/VEGF-D signaling axis in preventing lymph-node-mediated metastasis and disease progression. Inhibition of VEGF-C/-D with soluble VEGFR-3 has been shown to reduce tumor metastasis in mouse models, as has blocking VEGF-C/-D proteolysis or blocking VEGF-C from binding with the Nrp-2 receptor [116]. Moreover, foretinib, a multiple kinase inhibitor currently undergoing clinical trials, has shown promise in inhibiting the activity of VEGFR-3 and lymphangiogenesis and could potentially be used to inhibit lymph-node-mediated metastasis [117]. Corosolic acid has also been shown to induce apoptosis in CT-26 colon carcinoma in a mouse model, in addition to inhibiting lymphangiogenesis, but more study is needed before this substance becomes useable as a cancer therapy [118].

PlGF inhibition is another potential novel therapeutic approach in the fight against cancer, and preclinical studies have shown that inhibiting PlGF using genetic inhibition or anti-PlGF antibodies slows tumor growth and metastasis, and can even induce tumor regression in preexisting medulloblastoma [119]. However, the efficacy of inhibiting PlGF in tumors has come under question, with some preclinical studies showing that inhibiting PlGF does not significantly inhibit tumor grows [120, 121]. More research is needed to assess whether PlGF inhibition could be an efficacious cancer therapy.

7. Conclusion

Ever since its discovery, VEGF has been at the center of attention in new and developing cancer therapies. Since its early successes, however, antiangiogenic therapy has often presented only modest improvements in overall survival and progression-free survival [122]. Researchers have not given up hope that this therapeutic technique contains promise in the arsenal against cancer. Therefore, much recent research has been done in pushing the frontier of antiangiogenic therapies, trying to improve patient outcome.

Because the biology of VEGF and its receptors is well understood, current research focuses on why some tumors become resistant to antiangiogenic therapies and others are intrinsically resistant, how to circumvent this intrinsic or acquired resistance, and how to best utilize these expensive therapies by developing predictive biomarkers for treatment outcome. More research is also being done to develop novel VEGF inhibition techniques, and in characterizing the rare yet serious toxicities associated with these drugs.

As they stand now, antiangiogenic therapies face a set of limitations that severally impacts their efficacy. Tumors can acquire resistance to the drugs (if they do not already have intrinsic resistance) and demonstrate an increase in aggressiveness. Moreover, antiangiogenic therapies may cause a decrease in chemotherapy perfusion, lowering the efficacy of chemotherapies given in combination with antiangiogenic medicine [123]. These difficulties suggest that, at least when given alone, antiangiogenic therapies may face severe limitations in survival benefits. Therefore, future research should focus on more than simply inhibiting VEGF on a continuous schedule. Rather, it should focus on increasing the efficacy of chemotherapy through utilizing antiangiogenic therapy to induce vascular normalization, allowing for more efficient delivery of chemotherapeutic agents [123, 124]. Moreover, research should also find ways to decrease resistance to these therapies through inhibiting proangiogenic factors that are upregulated in response to the inhibition of VEGF and through developing predictive biomarkers for the efficacy of these expensive treatments [123, 124].

Author details

Victor Gardner[1], Chikezie O. Madu[1, 2] and Yi Lu[2]*

*Address all correspondence to: ylu@uthsc.edu

1 White Station High School, Memphis, TN, USA

2 Department of Pathology and Laboratory Medicine, University of Tennessee Health Science Center, Memphis, TN, USA

References

[1] Adair TH, Montani JP. Angiogenesis. San Rafael (CA): Morgan & Claypool Life Sciences; 2010. Chapter 1, Overview of Angiogenesis. Available from: http://www.ncbi.nlm.nih.gov/books/NBK53238/

[2] Adair TH, Montani JP. Angiogenesis. San Rafael (CA): Morgan & Claypool Life Sciences; 2010. Chapter 3, Regulation: Metabolic Factors. Available from: http://www.ncbi.nlm.nih.gov/books/NBK53243/

[3] Adair TH, Montani JP. Angiogenesis. San Rafael (CA): Morgan & Claypool Life Sciences; 2010. Chapter 4, Regulation: Mechanical Factors. Available from: http://www.ncbi.nlm.nih.gov/books/NBK53240/

[4] Hanahan D, Weinberg RA. Hallmarks of cancer: the next generation. Cell. 2011;144(5):646–74. DOI: 10.1016/j.cell.2011.02.013

[5] Neufeld G, Cohen TG, Poltorak Z. Vascular endothelial growth factor (VEGF) and its receptors. The FASEB Journal. 1999;13(1):9–22. DOI: 10.1016/j.cell.2011.02.013

[6] Groothuis A, DudaGN, Wilson CJ, Thompson, MS, Hunter MR, Simon P, Bail HJ, van Scherpenzeel KM, Kasper G. Mechanical stimulation of the pro-angiogenic capacity

of human fracture haematoma: involvement of VEGF mechano-regulation. Bone. 2010;**47**(2):438–44. DOI: 10.1016/j.bone.2010.05.026

[7] Heath VL, Bicknell R. Anticancer strategies involving the vasculature. Nature Reviews Clinical Oncology. 2009;**6**(7):395–404. DOI: 10.1038/nrclinonc.2009.52

[8] Cesca M, Bizzaro F, Zucchetti M, Giavazzi R. Tumor delivery of chemotherapy combined with inhibitors of angiogenesis and vascular targeting agents. Frontiers in Oncology. 2013;**3**:259. DOI: 10.3389/fonc.2013.00259

[9] Fuso Nerini I, Cesca M, Bizzaro F, Giavazzi R. Combination therapy in cancer: effects of angiogenesis inhibitors on drug pharmacokinetics and pharmacodynamics. Chinese Journal of Cancer. 2016;**35**:61. DOI:10.1186/s40880-016-0123-1

[10] Shibuya M. Vascular endothelial growth factor (VEGF) and its receptor (VEGFR) signaling in angiogenesis: a crucial target for anti- and pro-angiogenic therapies. Genes & Cancer 2011;**2**(12):1097–105. DOI: 10.1177/1947601911423031

[11] Hoeben A, Landuyt B, Highley MS, Wildiers H, Van Oosterom AT, De Brujin EA. Vascular endothelial growth factor and angiogenesis. Pharmacological Reviews 2004;**56**(4):549–80. DOI: 10.1124/pr.56.4.3

[12] Ogawa S, Oku A, Sawano A, Yamaguchi S, Yazaki Y, Shibuya M. A novel type of vascular endothelial growth factor, VEGF-E (NZ-7 VEGF), preferentially utilizes KDR/Flk-1 receptor and carries a potent mitotic activity without heparin-binding domain. The Journal of Biological Chemistry. 1998;**273**(43):31273–82.

[13] Yamazaki Y, Matsunaga Y, Tokunaga Y, Obayashi S, Saito M, Morita T. Snake venom vascular endothelial growth factors (VEGF-Fs) exclusively vary their structures and functions among species. The Journal of Biological Chemistry. 2009;**284**(15):9885–91. DOI: 10.1074/jbc.M809071200

[14] Li X, Lee C, Tang Z, et al. VEGF-B: a survival, or an angiogenic factor? Cell Adhesion & Migration 2009;**3**(4):322–7.

[15] De Falco S. The discovery of placental growth factor and its biological activity. Experimental and Molecular Medicine 2012;**44**:1–9. DOI: 10.3858/emm.2012.44.1.025

[16] "The biochemistry and role of placenta growth factor (PlGF)" (Application Note), ParkinElmer, Inc., 2009. Available from: https://shop.perkinelmer.com/Content/ApplicationNotes/APP_BiochemistryAndRoleOfPlGF.pdf

[17] Stuttfeld E, Ballmer-Hofer K. Structure and function of VEGF receptors. IUBMB Life. 2009;**61**:915–22. DOI: 10.1002/iub.234

[18] Rahimi N. VEGFR-1 and VEGFR-2: two non-identical twins with a unique physiognomy. Frontiers in Bioscience?: A Journal and Virtual Library. 2006;**11**:818–29.

[19] Holmes K, Robert OL, Thomas AM, Cross MJ. Vascular endothelial growth factor receptor-2: structure, function, intracellular signaling and therapeutic inhibition. Cell Signal. 2007;**10**:2003–12. DOI: 10.1016/j.cellsig.2007.05.013

[20] Kopan R. Notch signaling. Cold Spring Harbor Perspectives in Biology. 2016;8(7). DOI: 10.1101/cshperspect.a011213

[21] Makanya AN, Hushchuk R, DjnovVG. Intussuseptive angiogenesis and its role in vascular morphogenesis, patterning, and remodeling. Angiogenesis. 2009;12(2):113–23. DOI: 10.1007/s10456-009-9129-5

[22] Burri PH, Hlushchuk R, Djonov V. Intussusceptive angiogenesis: its emergence, its characteristics, and its significance. Developmental Dynamucs. 2004;231:474–88. DOI: 10.1002/dvdy.20184

[23] Nishida N, Yano H, Nishida T, Kamura T, Kojiro M. Angiogenesis in cancer. Vascular Health and Risk Management. 2006;2(3):213–9.

[24] Carmeliet P. VEGF as a key mediator of angiogenesis in cancer. Oncology. 2005;69(31):4–10. DOI: 10.1159/000088478

[25] Krock BL, Skuli N, Simon MC. Hypoxia-induced angiogenesis: good and evil. Genes & Cancer. 2011;2(12):1117–33. DOI: 10.1177/1947601911423654

[26] Leendders WPJ, Kusters B, de Waal RMW. Vessel co-option: how tumors obtain blood suppl in the absence of sprouting angiogenesis. Endothelium: Journal of Endothelial Cell Research. 2002;9(2):83–7.

[27] Cavallaro U, Christofori G. Molecular mechanisms of tumor angiogenesis and tumor progression. Journal of Neuro-Oncology. 2000;50(1):63–70.

[28] Nagy JA, Chang S-H, Shih S-C, Dvorak AM, Dvorak HF. Heterogeneity of the tumor vasculature. Seminars in Thrombosis and Hemostasis. 2010;36(3):321–31. DOI: 10.1055/s-0030-1253454

[29] Dudley AC. Tumor endothelial cells. Cold Spring Harbor Perspectives in Medicine. 2012;2(3): a006536. DOI: 10.1101/cshperspect.a006536.

[30] Nagy JA, Chang S-H, Dvorak AM, Dvorak HF. Why are tumour blood vessels abnormal and why is it important to know? British Journal of Cancer. 2009;100:865–9. DOI: 10.1038/sj.bjc.6604929

[31] Bergers G, Song S. The role of pericytes in blood-vessel formation and maintenance. Neuro-Oncology. 2005;7:452–64. DOI: 10.1215/S1152851705000232

[32] Rak J. Oncogenes and angiogenesis: signaling three-dimensional tumor growth. Journal of Investigative Dermatology Symposium Proceedings. 2000;5(1):24–33. DOI: 10.1046/j.1087-0024.2000.00012.x

[33] Onno K, Martijn F.B.G, Emile EV. Stimulation of angiogenesis by Ras proteins. Biochimica et Biophysica Acta (BBA) – Reviews on Cancer. 2004;1654(1):23–37. DOI: 10.1016/j.bbcan.2003.09.004

[34] Bottos A, Bardelli A. Oncogenes and angiogenesis: a way to personalize anti-angiogenic therapy? Cellular and Molecular Life Sciences. 2013;70(21):4131–40. DOI: 10.1007/s00018-013-1331-3

[35] Rak J, Filmus J, Finkenzeller G, Grugel S, Marme D, Kerbel RS. Oncogenes as indicators of tumor angiogenesis. Cancer and Metastasis Reviews. 1995;14(4):263–77. DOI: 10.1007/BF00690598

[36] Zhang F, Tang Z, Hou X, et al. VEGF-B is dispensable for blood vessel growth but critical for their survival, and VEGF-B targeting inhibits pathological angiogenesis. Proceedings of the National Academy of Sciences of the United States of America. 2009;106(15):6152–7. DOI: 10.1073/pnas.0813061106

[37] Li Y, et al. VEGF-B inhibits apoptosis via VEGFR-1–mediated suppression of the expression of BH3-only protein genes in mice and rats. Journal of Clinical Investigation. 2008;118(3):913–23. DOI: 10.1172/JCI33673

[38] Yang X, Zhang Y, Hosaka K, Andersson P, et al. VEGF-B promotes cancer metastasis through a VEGF-A-independent mechanism and serves as a marker of poor prognosis for cancer patients. Proceedings of the National Academy of Sciences of the United States of America. 2015;112(22):E2900–9. DOI: 10.1073/pnas.1503500112

[39] Yonemura Y, Endo Y, Tabata K, Kawamura T, Yun HY, Bandou E, Sasaki T, Miura M. Role of VEGF-C and VEGF-D in lymphangiogenesis in gastric cancer. International Journal of Clinical Oncology 2005;10(5):316–27. DOI: 10.1007/s10147-005-0508-7

[40] Achen MG, Williams RA, Baldwin ME, Lai P, Roufail S, Alitalo K, Stacker SA. The angiogenic and lymphangiogenic factor vascular endothelial growth factor-D exhibits a paracrine mode of action in cancer. Growth Factors 2002;20(2):99–107.

[41] Christiansen A, Detmar M. Lymphangiogenesis and cancer. Genes and Cancer. 2011;2(12):1146–58. DOI: 10.1177/1947601911423028

[42] Skobe M, Hawighorst T, Jackson DG, et al. Induction of tumor lymphangiogenesis by VEGF-C promotes breast cancer metastasis. Nature Medicine. 2001;7:192–8. DOI: 10.1038/84643

[43] Liu W, Xu J, Wang M, Wang Q, Bi Y, Han M. Tumor-derived vascular endothelial growth factor (VEGF)-a facilitates tumor metastasis through the VEGF-VEGFR1 signaling pathway. International Journal of Oncology. 2011;39:1213–20. DOI: 10.3892/ijo.2011.1138

[44] Gotink KJ, Verheul HMW. Anti-angiogenic tyrosine kinase inhibitors: what is their mechanism of action? Angiogenesis. 2010;13(1):1–14. DOI: 10.1007/s10456-009-9160-6

[45] Imai K, Takaoka A. Comparing antibody and small-molecule therapies for cancer. Nature Reviews Cancer 2006;6:714–27. DOI 10.1007/s10456-009-9160-6

[46] National Cancer Institute: FDA Approval for Sunitinib Malate [Internet]. 2011. http://www.cancer.gov/about-cancer/treatment/drugs/fda-sunitinib-malate [Accessed 2016-06-22].

[47] Kim A, Balis FM, Widemann BC. Sorafenib and sunitinib. Oncologist. 2009;8:800–5. DOI: 10.1634/theoncologist.2009-0088

[48] Adnane L, Trail PA, Taylor I, Wilhelm SM. Sorafenib (BAY 43-9006, Nexavar), a dual-action inhibitor that targets RAF/MEK/ERK pathway in tumor cells and tyrosine kinases

VEGFR/PDGFR in tumor vasculature. Methods Enzymol. 2006;**407**:597–612. DOI: 10.1016/S0076-6879(05)07047-3

[49] National Cancer Institute: FDA Approval for Sorafenib Tosylate [Internet]. 2013. Available from: http://www.cancer.gov/about-cancer/treatment/drugs/fda-sorafenib-tosylate [Accessed 2016-06-23].

[50] Morabito A, Piccirillo MC, Falasconi F, De Feo G, Del Giudice A, Bryce J, Di Maio M, De Maio E, Normanno N, Perrone F. Vandetanib (ZD6474), a dual inhibitor of vascular endothelial growth factor receptor (VEGFR) and epidermal growth factor receptor (EGFR) tyrosine kinases: current status and future directions. Oncologist. 2009;**4**:378–90. DOI: 10.1634/theoncologist.2008-0261

[51] National Cancer Institute: FDA Approval for Vandetanib [Internet]. 2013. Available from: http://www.cancer.gov/about-cancer/treatment/drugs/fda-vandetanib [Accessed 2016-06-23].

[52] European Medicines Agency: Avastin [Internet]. 2016. Available from: http://www.ema.europa.eu/ema/index.jsp?curl=pages/medicines/human/medicines/000582/human_med_000663.jsp [Accessed 2016-06-26].

[53] Keating GM. Bevacizumab: a review of its role in advanced cancer. Drugs. 2014;**74**(16):1891–925. DOI: 10.1007/s40265-014-0302-9

[54] Sullivan LA, Brekken RA. The VEGF family in cancer and antibody-based strategies for their inhibition. mAbs. 2010;**2**(2):165–175.

[55] Lilly R. CYRAMZA is a human, monoclonal antibody that specifically blocks activation of vascular endothelial growth factor (VEGF) Receptor 2 [Internet]. 2015. Available from: http://www.cyramzahcp.com/lung/mechanism-of-action.html [Accessed 2016-06-25].

[56] Kendrew J, Eberlein C, Hedberg B, McDaid K, Smith NR, Weir HM, Wedge SR, Blakey DC, Foltz I, Zhou J, Kang JS, Barry ST. An antibody targeted to VEGFR-2 Ig domains 4-7 inhibits VEGFR-2 activation and VEGFR-2-dependent angiogenesis without affecting ligand binding. Molecular Cancer Therapeutics. 2011;**10**(5):770–83. DOI: 10.1158/1535-7163

[57] Regeneron Pharmeceuticals: Multiple Angiogenic Factor Trap [Internet]. 2016. Available from: http://www.zaltrap.com/hcp/about/mechanism-of-action [Accessed 2016-07-01].

[58] Holash J, Davis S, Papadopoulos N, et al. VEGF-trap: a VEGF blocker with potent anti-tumor effects. Proceedings of the National Academy of Sciences of the United States of America. 2002;**99**(17):11393–8. DOI: 10.1073/pnas.172398299

[59] U.S. Food and Drug Administration: FDA approves Zaltrap for metastatic colorectal cancer [Internet]. 2012. Available from: http://www.fda.gov/NewsEvents/Newsroom/PressAnnouncements/ucm314372.htm [Accessed 2016-03-04].

[60] Al-Husein B, Abdalla M, et al. Anti-angiogenic therapy for cancer: an update. Pharmacotherapy. 2012;**32**(12):1095–111. DOI: 10.1002/phar.1147

[61] "Anti-Angiogenesis Treatment", American Cancer Society [Internet]. 2009. Available from: http://www.cancer.org/acs/groups/cid/documents/webcontent/002988-pdf.pdf [Accessed 2016-03-15].

[62] Henry TD, Annex BH, McKendall GR, Azrin MA, Lopez JJ, Giordano FJ, Shah PK, Willerson JT, Benza RL, Berman DS, et al. The VIVA trial: vascular endothelial growth factor in Ischemia for Vascular Angiogenesis. Circulation. 2003;107:1359–65.

[63] Sane DC, Anton L, Brosnihan KB. Angiogenic growth factors and hypertension. Angiogenesis. 2004;7(3):193–201. DOI: 10.1007/s10456-004-2699-3

[64] van Heeckeren WJ, Ortiz J, Cooney MM, Remick SC. Hypertension, proteinuria, and antagonism of vascular endothelial growth factor signaling: clinical toxicity, therapeutic target, or novel biomarker? Journal of Clinical Oncology. 2007;25:2993–5. DOI: 10.1200/JCO.2007.11.5113

[65] Chen HX, Cleck JN: Adverse effects of anticancer agents that target the VEGF pathway. Nature Reviews Clinical Oncology. 2009;6(8):465–77. DOI: 10.1038/nrclinonc.2009.94

[66] Hutson T, Figlin R, Kuhn J, Motzer R. Targeted therapies for metastatic renal cell carcinoma: an overview of toxicity and dosing strategies. Oncologist. 2008;13:1084–96. DOI: 10.1634/theoncologist.2008-0120

[67] Tesarova P, Tesar V. Proteinuria and hypertension in patients treated with inhibitors of the VEGF signalling pathway–incidence, mechanisms and management. Folia Biol (Praha). 2013;59:15–25.

[68] Izzedine H, Massard C, Spano JP. VEGF signalling inhibition-induced proteinuria: mechanisms, significance and management. European Journal of Cancer. 2010;46:439–48. DOI: 10.1016/j.ejca.2009.11.001

[69] Scappaticci FA, Skillings JR, Holden SN, et al. Arterial thromboembolic events in patients with metastatic carcinoma treated with chemotherapy and bevacizumab. Journal of the National Cancer Institute. 2007;99:1232–9. DOI: 10.1093/jnci/djm086

[70] Kamba T, McDonald DM. Mechanisms of adverse effects of anti-VEGF therapy for cancer. British Journal of Cancer. 2007;96(12):1788–95. DOI: 10.1038/sj.bjc.6603813

[71] Chu TF, Jeffrey A, et al. Cardiotoxicity associated with tyrosine kinase inhibitor sunitinib. The Lancet 2007;370(9604):2011–9. DOI: 10.1016/S0140-6736(07)61865-0

[72] Kerkela R, Woulfe KC, Durand J-B, et al. Sunitinib-induced cardiotoxicity is mediated by off-target inhibition of AMP-activated protein kinase. Clinical and Translational Science. 2009;2(1):15–25. DOI: 10.1111/j.1752-8062.2008.00090.x

[73] Karp JE, Gojo I, Pili R, Gocke CD, Greer J, Guo C, et al. Targeting vascular endothelial growth factor for relapsed and refractory adult acute myelogenous leukemias: therapy with sequential 1-beta-d-arabinofuranosylcytosine, mitoxantrone, and bevacizumab. Clinical Cancer Research. 2004;10:3577–85. DOI: 10.1158/1078-0432. CCR-03-0627

[74] Duran JM, Makarewich CA, Trappanese D, et al. Sorafenib cardiotoxicity increases mortality after myocardial infarction. Circulation Research. 2014;**114**(11):1700–12. DOI: 10.1161/CIRCRESAHA.114.303200

[75] Qi WX, Tang LN, Sun YJ, et al. Incidence and risk of hemorrhagic events with vascular endothelial growth factor receptor tyrosine-kinase inhibitors: an up-to-date meta-analysis of 27 randomized controlled trials. Annals of Oncology. 2013;**24**(12):2943–52. DOI: 10.1093/annonc/mdt292

[76] Common Terminology Criteria for Adverse Events. Version 4.0, National Institutes of Health, National Cancer Institute, 14 June 2010. Available from: http://evs.nci.nih.gov/ftp1/CTCAE/CTCAE_4.03_2010-06-14_QuickReference_5x7.pdf

[77] Bergers G, Hanahan D. Modes of resistance to anti-angiogenic therapy. Nature Reviews Cancer. 2008;**8**(8):592–603. DOI: 10.1038/nrc2442

[78] Vasudev NS, Reynolds AR. Anti-angiogenic therapy for cancer: current progress, unresolved questions and future directions. Angiogenesis. 2014;**17**(3):471–94. DOI: 10.1007/s10456-014-9420-y

[79] Renaud G, Gilles P. Molecular mechanisms of resistance to tumour anti-angiogenic strategies. Journal of Oncology. 2010;2010:8 p. Article ID 835680, DOI:10.1155/2010/835680

[80] Lu KV, Bergers G. Mechanisms of evasive resistance to anti-VEGF therapy in glioblastoma. CNS Oncology. 2013;**2**(1):49–65. DOI: 10.2217/cns.12.36

[81] Kioi M, Vogel H, Schultz G, Hoffman RM, Harsh GR, Brown JM. Inhibition of vasculogenesis, but not angiogenesis, prevents the recurrence of glioblastoma after irradiation in mice. The Journal of Clinical Investigation. 2010;**120**(3):694–705. DOI: 10.1172/JCI40283

[82] Allen E, Walters IB, Hanahan D. Brivanib: a dual FGF/VEGF inhibitor, is active both 1st and 2nd line against mouse pancreatic neuroendocrine tumors (PNET) developing adaptive/evasive resistance to VEGF inhibition. Clinical Cancer Research: An Official Journal of the American Association for Cancer Research. 2011;**17**(16):5299–310. DOI: 10.1158/1078-0432

[83] Newman AC, Hughes CW. Macrophages and angiogenesis: a role for Wnt signaling. Vascular Cell. 2012;**4**(1):13. DOI: 10.1186/2045-824X-4-13

[84] Ding Y, Song N, Luo Y. Role of bone marrow-derived cells in angiogenesis: focus on macrophages and pericytes. Cancer Microenvironment. 2012;**5**(3):225–36. DOI: 10.1007/s12307-012-0106-y

[85] Murdoch C, Giannoudis A, Lewis CE. Mechanisms regulating the recruitment of macrophages into hypoxic areas of tumors and other ischemic tissues. Blood. 2004;**104**(8):2224–34. DOI: 10.1182/blood-2004-03-1109

[86] Deshmane SL, Kremlev S, Amini S, Sawaya BE. Monocyte chemoattractant protein-1 (MCP-1): an overview. Journal of Interferon & Cytokine Research. 2009;**29**(6):313–26 DOI: 10.1089/jir.2008.0027

[87] Lal A, Peters H, St Croix B, Haroon ZA, Dewhirst MW, Strausberg RL, et al. Transcriptional response to hypoxia in human tumors. Journal of National Cancer Institute. 2001;**93**:1337–43.

[88] Hall AP. Review of the pericyte during angiogenesis and its role in cancer and diabetic retinopathy. Toxicology Pathology. 2006;**34**(6):763–75. DOI: 10.1080/01926230600936290

[89] Meng MB, Zaorsky NG, Deng L, Wang HH, Chao J, Zhao LJ, Yuan ZY, Ping W. Pericytes: a double-edged sword in cancer therapy. Future Oncology. 2015;**11**(1):169–79. DOI: 10.2217/fon.14.123

[90] Bao B, et al. Hypoxia-induced aggressiveness of pancreatic cancer cells is due to increased expression of VEGF, IL-6 and miR-21, which can be attenuated by CDF treatment. PLoS One. 2012;**7**(12). DOI: 10.1371/journal.pone.0050165

[91] Aguilera KY, Rivera LB, Hur H, et al. Collagen signaling enhances tumor progression after anti-VEGF therapy in a murine model of pancreatic ductal adenocarcinoma. Cancer Research. 2014;**74**(4):1032–44. DOI: 10.1158/0008-5472

[92] Sennino B, Ishiguro-Oonuma T, Wei Y, et al. Suppression of tumor invasion and metastasis by concurrent inhibition of c-Met and VEGF signaling in pancreatic neuroendocrine tumors. Cancer Discovery. 2012;**2**(3):270–87. DOI: 10.1158/2159-8290.CD-11-0240

[93] Schnegg CI, Yang MH, Ghosh SK, Hsu M-Y. Induction of vasculogenic mimicry overrides VEGF-A silencing and enriches stem-like cancer cells in melanoma. Cancer Research. 2015;**75**(8):1682–90. DOI: 10.1158/0008-5472.CAN-14-1855

[94] Jain RK. Normalizing tumor microenvironment to treat cancer: bench to bedside to biomarkers. Journal of Clinical Oncology. 2013;**31**(17):2205–18. DOI: 10.1200/JCO.2012.46.3653

[95] Jain RK, Duda DG, Willett CG, et al. Biomarkers of response and resistance to antiangiogenic therapy. Nature Reviews Clinical Oncology. 2009;**6**(6):327–38. DOI: 10.1038/nrclinonc.2009.63

[96] Rini BI, et al. Association of diastolic blood pressure (dBP) $\geq$ 90 mmHg with overall survival (OS) in patients treated with axitinib (AG-013736). Journal Clinical Oncology (Meeting Abstracts). 2008;**26**(90150):3543. DOI: 10.1200/jco.2008.26.90150.3543

[97] Robinson ES, Khankin EV, Karumanchi SA, Humphreys BD. Hypertension induced by VEGF signaling pathway inhibition: mechanisms and potential use as a biomarker. Seminars in Nephrology. 2010;**30**(6):591–601. DOI: 10.1016/j.semnephrol.2010.09.007

[98] Kim JJ. VEGF single nucleotide polymorphisms (SNPs) and correlation to sunitinib-induced hypertension (HTN) in metastatic renal cell carcinoma (mRCC) patients (pts). Journal of Clinical Oncology. 2009;**27**(15):15S 5005.

[99] Hegde PS, Jubb AM, Chen D, et al. Predictive impact of circulating vascular endothelial growth factor in four phase III trials evaluating bevacizumab. Clinical Cancer Research. 2013;**19**:929–37. DOI: 10.1158/1078-0432.CCR-12-2535

[100] Harmon CS, DePrimo SE, Figlin RA, et al. Circulating proteins as potential biomarkers of sunitinib and interferon-α efficacy in treatment-naïve patients with metastatic renal cell carcinoma. Cancer Chemotherapy and Pharmacology. 2014;**73**(1):151–61. DOI: 10.1007/s00280-013-2333-4

[101] Motzer RJ, Hutson TE, Hudes GR, et al. Investigation of novel circulating proteins, germ line single-nucleotide polymorphisms, and molecular tumor markers as potential efficacy biomarkers of first-line sunitinib therapy for advanced renal cell carcinoma. Cancer Chemotherapy and Pharmacology. 2014;**74**(4):739–750. DOI: 10.1007/s00280-014-2539-0

[102] Wehland M, Bauer J, Magnusson NE, Infanger M, Grimm D. Biomarkers for anti-angiogenic therapy in cancer. International Journal of Molecular Sciences. 2013;**14**(5):9338–64. DOI: 10.3390/ijms14059338

[103] Ellingson BM, Sahebjam S, Kim HJ, Pope WB, Harris RJ, Woodworth DC, Lai A, Nghiemphu PL, Mason WP, Cloughesy TF. Pretreatment ADC histogram analysis is a predictive imaging biomarker for bevacizumab treatment but not chemotherapy in recurrent glioblastoma. American Journal of Neuroradiology. 2014;**35**:673–9. DOI: 10.3174/ajnr.A3748

[104] Sharan S, Woo S. Systems pharmacology approaches for optimization of antiangiogenic therapies: challenges and opportunities. Frontiers in Pharmacology. 2015;**6**:33. DOI: 10.3389/fphar.2015.00033

[105] Kim ST, Park KH, Shin SW, Kim YH. Dose KRAS mutation status affect on the effect of VEGF therapy in metastatic colon cancer patients? Cancer Research and Treatment: Official Journal of Korean Cancer Association. 2014;**46**(1):48–54. DOI: 10.4143/crt.2014.46.1.48

[106] Goel S, Wong AH-K, Jain RK. Vascular normalization as a therapeutic strategy for malignant and nonmalignant disease. Cold Spring Harbor Perspectives in Medicine. 2012;**2**(3):a006486. DOI: 10.1101/cshperspect.a006486

[107] Bennouna J, Sastre J, Arnold D, et al. Continuation of bevacizumab after first progression in metastatic colorectal cancer (ML18147): a randomised phase 3 trial. *The Lancet Oncology.* 2013;**14**(1):29–37. DOI: 10.1016/S1470-2045(12)70477-1

[108] Wong R, Cunningham D, Barbachano Y, Saffery C, Valle J, Hickish T. A multicentre study of capecitabine, oxaliplatin plus bevacizumab as perioperative treatment of patients with poor-risk colorectal liver-only metastases not selected for upfront resection. Annals of Oncology. 2011;**22**(9):2042–8. DOI: 10.1093/annonc/mdq714

[109] Ebos JM, Mastri M, Lee CR, et al. Neoadjuvant antiangiogenic therapy reveals contrasts in primary and metastatic tumor efficacy. EMBO Molecular Medicine. 2014;**6**(12):1561–76. DOI: 10.15252/emmm.201403989

[110] National Cancer Institute: FDA Approval for Ramucirumab [Internet]. 2015. Available from: http://www.cancer.gov/about-cancer/treatment/drugs/fda-ramucirumab [Accessed 2016-06-12].

[111] Fuchs, Charles S, et al. Ramucirumab monotherapy for previously treated advanced gastric or gastro-oesophageal junction adenocarcinoma (REGARD): an international, randomised, multicentre, placebo-controlled, phase 3 trial. The Lancet. 2014;**383**:31–9. DOI: 10.1016/S0140-6736(13)61719-5

[112] Garen, EB. Ramucirumab plus docetaxel versus placebo plus docetaxel for second-line treatment of stage IV non-small-cell lung cancer after disease progression on platinum-based therapy (REVEL): a multicentre, double-blind, randomised phase 3 trial. The Lancet 2014;**384**(9944):665–73. DOI: 10.1016/S0140-6736(14)60845-X

[113] Li J, et al. Randomized, double-blind, placebo-controlled phase III trial of apatinib in patients with chemotherapy-refractory advanced or metastatic adenocarcinoma of the stomach or gastroesophageal junction. Journal of Clinical Oncology. 2016;**34**(13):1448–54. DOI: 10.1200/JCO.2015.63.5995.

[114] Fontanella C, Ongaro E, Bolzonello S, Guardascione M, Fasola G, Aprile G. Clinical advances in the development of novel VEGFR2 inhibitors. Annals of Translational Medicine. 2014;**2**(12):123.

[115] U.S. Food and Drug Administration. Cabozantinib (CABOMETYX) [Internet]. 2016. Available from: http://www.fda.gov/Drugs/InformationOnDrugs/ApprovedDrugs/ucm497483.htm [Accessed 2016-06-09].

[116] Duong T, Koopman P, Francois M. Tumor lymphangiogenesis as a potential therapeutic target. Journal of Oncology. 2012, Article ID 204946, 2012, 23 p. DOI:10.1155/2012/204946

[117] Chen H-M, Tsai C-H, Hung W-C. Foretinib inhibits angiogenesis, lymphangiogenesis and tumor growth of pancreatic cancer in vivo by decreasing VEGFR-2/3 and TIE-2 signaling. Oncotarget. 2015;**6**(17):14940–52. DOI: 10.18632/oncotarget.3613

[118] Yoo K-H, Park J-H, Lee D-Y, et al. Corosolic acid exhibits anti-angiogenic and anti-lymphangiogenic effects on *in vitro* endothelial cells and on an *in vivo* CT-26 colon carcinoma animal model. Phytotherapy Research. 2015;**29**(5):714–23. DOI: 10.1002/ptr.5306

[119] Dewerchin M, Carmeliet P. Placental growth factor in cancer. Expert Opinion on Therapeutic Targets. 2014;**18**(11):1339–54. DOI: 10.1517/14728222.2014.948420

[120] Lou, K-J. PlGF point-counterpoint. Science–Business eXchange. [Internet]. 2010;**3**(16). DOI: 10.1038/scibx.2010.484

[121] Bessho H, et al. Inhibition of placental growth factor in renal cell carcinoma. Anticancer Research. 2015;**35**(1):531–41.

[122] Jayson G, Kerbel R, et al. Antiangiogenic therapy in oncology: current status and future directions. The Lancet. 2016;388 (10046):518-529. DOI: 10.1016/S0140-6736(15)01088-0

[123] Morserle L, Jimenez-Valerio G, Casanovas O. Antiangiogenic therapies: going beyond their limits. Cancer Discovery. 2014;**4**(1):31–41. DOI: 10.1158/2159-8290.CD-13-0199

[124] Ma J, Waxman D. Combination of anti-angiogenesis with chemotherapy for more effective cancer treatment. Molecular Cancer Therapeutics. 2008;**7**(12):3670–84. DOI: 10.1158/1535-7163.MCT-08-0715

[125] National Cancer Institute: FDA Approval for Bevacizumab [Internet]. 2014. Available from: http://www.cancer.gov/about-cancer/treatment/drugs/fda-bevacizumab [Accessed 2016-04-14].

[126] National Cancer Institute: FDA Approval for Pazopanib [Internet]. 2013. Available from: http://www.cancer.gov/about-cancer/treatment/drugs/fda-pazopanibhydrochloride [Accessed 2016-04-14].

[127] National Cancer Institute: FDA Approval for Ziv-Aflibercept [Internet]. 2013. Available from: update. http://www.cancer.gov/about-cancer/treatment/drugs/fda-ziv-aflibercept [Accessed 2016-04-14].

8

Role of Notch, SDF-1 and Mononuclear Cells Recruitment in Angiogenesis

Ivanka Dimova and Valentin Djonov

Abstract

Intussusceptive angiogenesis (IA) known also as splitting angiogenesis is a recently described mechanism of vascular growth alternative to sprouting. It plays an essential role in the vascular remodeling and adaptation of vessels during normal and pathological angiogenesis. It is an "escape" mechanism during and after irradiation and anti-VEGF therapy, both inducing angiogenic switch from sprouting to IA by formation of multiple transluminal tissue pillars. Our recently published data revealed the significant induction of IA after inhibition of Notch signaling associated with an increased capillary density by more than 50%. The induced IA was accompanied by detachment of pericytes from basement membrane, increased vessel permeability and recruitment of mononuclear cells toward the pillars; the process was dramatically enhanced after injection of bone marrow-derived mononuclear cells. The extravasation of mononuclear cells with eventual bone marrow origin was associated with upregulation of chemotaxis factors SDF-1 and CXCR4. In addition, SDF-1 expression was upregulated in the endothelium of liver sinusoids in Notch1 knockout mouse, together with vascular remodeling by intussusception. In this chapter, we discuss this important mechanism of angiogenesis, as well as the role of Notch signaling, SDF-1 signaling and mononuclear cells in the complex process of angiogenesis.

Keywords: intussusceptive angiogenesis, Notch signaling, mononuclear cells, SDF-1/CXCR4 signaling

1. Introduction: intussusceptive angiogenesis

Angiogenesis is essential for normal embryonic development and reproductive cycle and plays a key role in pathological conditions such as tumor growth and ischemic cardiovascular diseases. This is a complex process involving essential signaling pathways for instance VEGF, bFGF, and Notch, etc., in vasculature, as well as additional players such as bone marrow-derived endothelial progenitor cells. Better understanding the role of the different pathways and the crosstalk between different cells during angiogenesis is a crucial factor for developing more effective proangiogenic and antiangiogenic anticancer therapy.

Angiogenesis involves the formation of new blood vessels from a preexisting vascular plexus, and based on morphological characteristics two main distinct processes have been identified, sprouting and intussusceptive angiogenesis (IA) [1–3]. Sprouting angiogenesis has been well described since more than 150 years. Recent publications indicated that sprouting involves tip/stalk cell differentiation and crosstalk process which is tightly controlled by the VEGF and Notch/Dll4 signaling pathway [4, 5]. Intussusceptive angiogenesis (IA) is a particular form of vascular growth and remodeling in which endothelial cells make invagination intraluminally instead of extraluminally like it is in the sprouting. The cells form protrusions toward the vessel lumen resulting in the appearance of transluminal endothelial pillars–the hallmarks of intussusception. The arising pillars afterward are successively reshaped and fused and lead to "splitting" of the preexisting vessel in two segments, thus doing remodeling and organization of the vasculature. The effect is the formation of hierarchically organized vessels with supplying and draining function, pruning of arteries, and veins, and finally development of the primitive capillary plexuses into the functional vascular system. IA is a process with several consecutive steps, including intussusceptive microvascular growth, intussusceptive arborization, and intussusceptive remodeling [2, 3, 6, 7]. These processes end in the formation of mature vascular networks. In comparison to sprouting angiogenesis, intussusception is a quite fast process, enabling the vascular system to swift adaptation in unfavorable conditions. IA has been identified as the leading mode of vascular growth in animal models of liver regeneration and in alveolar angiogenesis following pneumonectomy. Intussusception appears to be predominant above sprouting in extra-embryonic vasculatures including the vitelline circulation as well [8-10]. The intensive work of our group in the past few decades clearly documented the morphological features of this specific angiogenic mode and demonstrated its definite presence during development and tumorigenesis as a complementary to sprouting vessel growth. Surprisingly, the cellular and molecular regulation of intussusception is less well known but recent evidence suggests that it might involve a component regulated by blood flow and Notch signaling [7, 9]. We provided with evidence showing that Notch regulates intussusception involving interaction with circulating mononuclear cells in developing vascular networks [11].

Intussusceptive angiogenesis (IA) is a well-documented and widely spread mode of angiogenesis, occurring during both normal development and in pathological conditions. In contrast to sprouting angiogenesis, whereby abluminal sprouts outgrow and subsequently merge with the existing capillaries, intussusceptive angiogenesis is elaborated by intraluminal growth of endothelial cell processes. The last protrude from the opposing sides of the vessel wall and form transluminal tissue pillar, representing endothelial bilayer, which is afterward perforated and stabilized from outside by collagen bindles. Repetitive formation of pillars and their subsequent fusion leads to the splitting of vessels and vascular expansion. Another way of intussusceptive angiogenesis is to increase the size of the pillar and form meshes, thus splitting the vessel. Intussusceptive angiogenesis is a process linked to both blood vessel replication and remodeling in development. It is present within the regions of increased vascular density in alveolar angiogenesis during compensatory growth after pneumonectomy in a murine model of postpneumonectomy lung growth [8]. The remodeling of the retiform meshworks in the avian lung was essentially accomplished by intussusceptive angiogenesis as well [12].

In addition to its developmental role, intussusceptive angiogenesis is well documented as a mechanism of vascular adaptation in response to different environmental stimuli. In the adult mouse retina, it was reported as a main adaptive mechanism to chronic systemic hypoxia [13]. These investigations contribute to our understanding of hypoxia-induced angiogenesis and microvascular remodeling. The process of intraluminal division participates in the inflammation-induced neovascularization associated with chemically induced murine colitis [14]. *Scanning electron microscopy* (SEM) of vascular corrosion casts demonstrated replication of the mucosal plexus without significant evidence of sprouting angiogenesis, whereas pillar formation and septation were present within days of the onset of inflammation. The authors conclude that intussusceptive angiogenesis is a fundamental mechanism of microvascular adaptation to prolonged inflammation. It is also a mechanism of compensation for vascular growth. In a capillary regression model of inflamed murine corneas, the abrupt termination of capillary sprouting is followed by an intussusceptive response [15]. The capillary repair during kidney recovery in Thy1.1 nephritis was done by intussusceptive angiogenesis [16]. Inhibitors of angiogenesis and radiation induce compensatory changes in the tumor vasculature both during and after cessation of treatment. There is a switch from sprouting to intussusceptive angiogenesis, which may be an adaptive response of tumor vasculature to cancer therapy that allows the vasculature to maintain its functional properties [17–19]. Potential candidates for molecular targeting of this angioadaptive mechanism are yet to be elucidated in order to improve the currently poor efficacy of contemporary antiangiogenic therapies. Important is the involvement of intussusceptive angiogenesis in pathological conditions. Vascular remodeling of the hepatic sinusoidal microvasculature in the course of liver nodular hyperplasia is a result of intussusceptive growth [9]. This angiogenic mode is widely involved in tumor development. By using electron and confocal microscopy, Paku et al. [20] observed intraluminal nascent pillars that contain a collagen bundle covered by endothelial cells (ECs) in the vasculature of experimental tumors. Tumor angiogenesis in liver metastasis from colon carcinoma is a controversial subject. Ceauşu et al. [21] concluded that in liver metastasis principal mechanism of neovascularization formation is based on intussusception. In metastatic tumors of the brain there was intussusceptive angiogenesis, whereby the fibrosarcoma cells were attached to the vessel, filled the developing pillars, and caused lumen splitting [22]. Branching angiogenesis was not observed either in the tumors or in control cerebral wounds. These data suggest that sprouting angiogenesis is not needed for the incipient growth of cerebral metastases and that tumor growth in this model is a result of incorporation of host vessels. Prolactin was found to directly stimulate angiogenesis in breast cancer progression, enhancing vessel density and the tortuosity of the vasculature by pillar formation, which are hallmarks of intussusceptive angiogenesis [23]. It is a preferred mode of angiogenesis in oral squamous cell carcinoma [24] and in hepatocellular carcinoma [25, 26].

Despite this variety of intussusceptive angiogenic roles, most of the current research is focused on the mechanism of sprouting angiogenesis because this mechanism was first described and most existing experimental models are related to sprouting angiogenesis. Consequently, the mechanism of intussusceptive angiogenesis is often overlooked in angiogenesis research [27]. Intussusception is an alternative to the sprouting mode of angiogenesis. The advantage of this mechanism of vascular growth is that blood vessels are generated more rapidly and the capillaries thereby formed are less leaky [1]. The regulation of intussusceptive angiogenesis is still to be elucidated. There are some hypotheses about the possible drivers of intussusception. In the sprouting type of angiogenesis related to hypoxia, there is no blood flow in the rising capillary sprout. In contrast, it has been shown that an increase of wall shear stress initiates the splitting type of angiogenesis in skeletal muscle [7]. Inflammation-associated intussusceptive angiogenesis in adult mice was associated with vessel angle remodeling and the morphometry of the vessel angles suggests the influence of blood flow on the location and orientation of remodeled vessels [28]. Regarding molecular regulation, very little is known for the molecular factors with potential significance. Application of the essential angiogenic factors VEGF and bFGF in an arteriovenous loop model demonstrated advanced neovascularization in the phase of remodeling by a higher incidence of intussusception, compared to control without these factors [29]. It was shown in Ewing sarcomas and rhabdomyosarcomas that treatment suppressing IGF-1 signaling decreases intussusceptive angiogenesis [30].

The main factors for maturation and hierarchical organization of vessels, especially arterial ones, are Notch, angiopoietin, and ephrin. In addition, it was shown that SDF-1 (CXCL12) is a crucial maturation factor in coronary arterial vasculature, since its mutants have immature capillary plexus and selective failure in arterial maturation, particularly with the onset of coronary perfusion [31].

Our preliminary results suggest that intussusception is most probably synchronized by chemokine factors since intussusceptive growth was associated with the recruitment of mononuclear cells [11]. After injection of bone marrow-derived mononuclear cells, we observed robust induction of intussusception in Notch inhibited samples. Notably, the chemotactic factors SDF-1/CXCR4 were upregulated only due to the Notch inhibition. Our hypothesis is that Notch inhibition disturbed vessel stability and led to pericyte detachment followed by extravasation of mononuclear cells due to the activation of the SDF-1/CXCR4 axis. The stromal cell-derived factor SDF-1 is binding to its receptor CXCR4 and directs migration of progenitor cells into the appropriate sites. The mononuclear cells contributed to the formation of transluminal pillars with sustained IA resulting in a dense vascular plexus.

2. Notch signaling and intussusceptive angiogenesis

The crucial role for Notch/DLL4 signaling in regulating vascular development was established based on findings from the analysis of targeted mouse and zebrafish mutants in Notch pathway components [32–35]. The common characteristics of the most of these mutants were the absence of angiogenic vascular remodeling, lack of arterial markers, and arteriovenous malformations. Mouse embryos deficient for Notch-ligand Jagged1 (Jag1), Notch1, Notch1/Notch4, or the presenilins, die between E9.5 and 10.5 and have severely disorganized vasculature [36]. Transgenic mice with inappropriate activation of Notch4 also display similar defects and die, which suggests that the appropriate Notch expression pattern (in levels, sites, and time) is critical for embryonic vascular development [37]. It was found out that Notch1, Notch2, and Notch4 are expressed predominantly in endothelial cells of aorta and arteries, whereas Notch3 was in VSMCs of arteries [38].

Recently, we have established that Notch inhibition disturbs vessel stability and induces intussusceptive neo-angiogenesis, triggering in this way the augmentation of the capillary plexus but without the accompanying vascular maturation and remodeling. It was associated with extravasation of mononuclear cells of bone marrow origin possibly by upregulation SDF-1/CXCR4 chemotactic factors.

Using the chick area vasculosa (and inhibiting Notch signaling by the γ-secretase inhibitor–GSI) and a mouse model of Notch inhibition (MxCre Notch1lox/lox mice), we have demonstrated that in already existing vascular beds disruption of Notch-signaling triggers rapid augmentation of the vasculature predominantly by intussusceptive angiogenesis [11]. The process is initiated by pericyte detachment followed by extravasation of mononuclear cells (**Figure 1**). The latter cells contributed to formation of transluminal pillars [11]. The sustained IA results in a very dense vascular plexus but without the usual concomitant vascular remodeling or maturation.

The genetic approach in mice substantiated by pharmacological studies for developing vascular networks in chicken embryo enabled us to show that Notch is critical for intussusceptive angiogenesis. In both models we demonstrated considerable changes in vascular morphogenesis, resulting in massive induction of intussusception. Inhibition of DLL4/Notch signaling by novel therapeutic antibody against DLL4, performed in a recently published study [39], was associated with threefold increase in vessel density and stimulation of vessel formation. At the same time, marked reduction in the number of smooth muscle actin (SMA)-positive mural cells was noted. Two-dimensional appearance of the blood vessels in the described phenotype highly resembles the data in our chicken and mouse models. Similar phenotypes were observed after Notch inhibition during developmental angiogenesis, in skeletal muscle and in tumor models, showing increased vessel number and increased vascular permeability [40–43]. The terminology for the resultant vascular pattern, used by authors in these studies, was "abnormal vessels" or "excessive, nonproductive angiogenesis." They focused mainly on the front of sprouting invasion after blocking Notch signaling, thus describing only newly developing, nonperfused vasculature. Along with the observed significantly increased vessel density under Notch inhibition, there was evidently demonstrated reduced mural cell coverage. The authors reported positivity for endothelial markers in the endothelial protrusions toward the vessel lumen and in the intraluminal vessel occlusions [44], but they did not attribute this phenomenon to the induced intussusceptive angiogenesis. The detailed investigation of this vascular pattern behind the sprouting mode of vessels invasion demonstrated that Notch inhibition led to IA in already perfused vascular bed and this is a complementary mechanism of angiogenesis. In fact, the authors above mentioned here nicely described the characteristic features of intussusceptive microvascular growth even though they did not use the terminology.

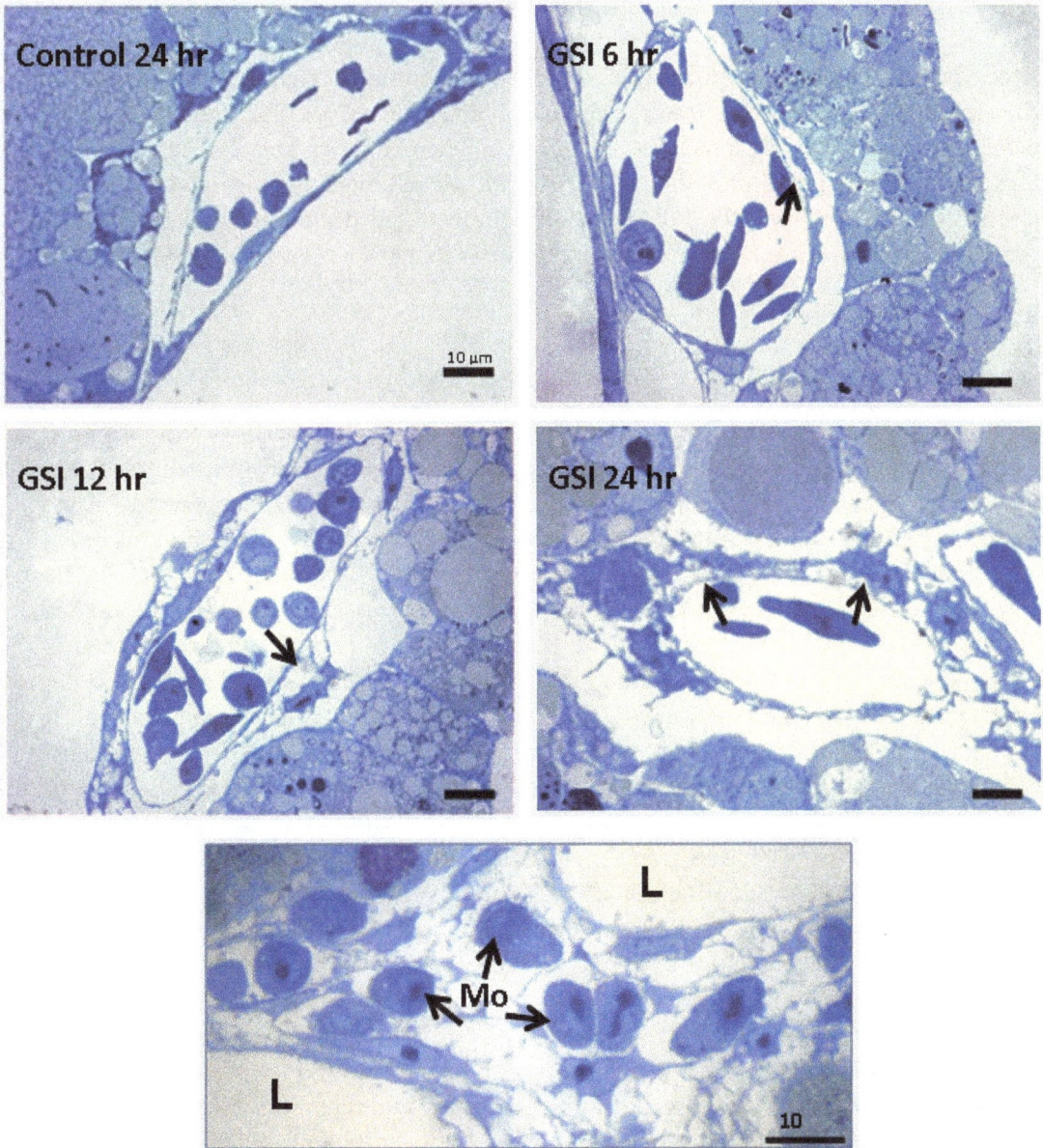

Figure 1. Inhibition of Notch signaling led to detachment of pericytes from endothelium (indicated by arrows), as it is shown at different time points after the application of GSI; it is followed by the extravasation of mononuclear cells (Mo); L–vessel lumen.

3. Role of mononuclear cells in angiogenesis

To test the role of bone marrow cells in the process of intussusception, in our previous study we isolated bone marrow mononuclear cells (BMMNC) from E14 chicken embryos and/or 4-week-old mice, labeled them with a fluorescent cell tracker (TAMRA) and injected them into the Notch inhibited (by GSI) and control samples 3 hours prior to time point 24 hours at which time the samples were visualized by FITC injection [11]. About 3–4 hours after BMMNCs injection, we observed a significant induction of intussusception in the GSI-treated area as we detected high increase in the pillar number (4.2-fold) in inhibited samples as compared to controls. Injection of BMMNCs in the area vasculosa after Notch inhibition dramatically induced increase in microvascular density by onset of IA. Microvascular area density increases significantly by 80% after injection of BMD cells in Notch-inhibited samples in comparison with injection of BMD cells in PBS. Pillar density demonstrated dramatic augmentation by 63% compared to the Notch inhibition alone and more than 400% as compared to PBS.

We have largely expanded our knowledge about the role of bone marrow-derived cells in stimulating angiogenesis after their discovery in 1997 [45] and now their capability to promote vessel formation is intensively investigated. There are large clinical perspectives for their use in many diseases, connected to angiogenesis.

With the tendency of aging, the elderly will account for a great part of population world wide. This aging will be accompanied by chronic vascular dementia, due to chronic cerebral hypoperfusion. Cellular therapy is an emerging investigational approach for cerebral ischemia. The most attractive source for such therapy is bone marrow-derived mononuclear cells (BMMNC), since they consist of different types of stem cells. Several independent studies report the significant effects of BMMNC in ischemic repair after acute and chronic ischemic disorders. The intravenous infusion of BMMNC into rat brain ischemic model reduced neurologic impairments, increased angiogenesis and cognitive function in rodent [46]. Mononuclear cells from blood have therapeutic potential as well. The neuroprotective potential of CD34+ human cord blood cells was demonstrated in regard to Parkinson's disease [47]. These cells did not differentiate into neural phenotypes, but they rather exerted their effect by stimulating the production of new neuroblasts and angiogenesis. CD34+ stem cell therapy was enrolled in 2011 for 37 patients with longstanding dilated cardiomyopathy (DCM) by cell mobilization with colony stimulating factor (G-SCF) and apheresis collection [48]. Clinical response and stem cells retention were evaluated. About half of the patients (51%) were responders to the stem cells therapy, whereby the clinical response was predefined as an increase in left ventricle ejection fraction (LVEF) of >5% in 3 months. Looking for biomarkers, which can be instrumental in prediction which patients will be responders, the authors suggested some baseline factors, positively associated with both clinical response and retention, such as G-CSF, SDF-1, LIF, MCP-1, and MCP-3. The most recent study described the significant effect of human cord blood mononuclear cells (CB-MNCs) injection for cardiac repair in ischemic heart disease, mainly by promotion of angiogenesis in the infarcted region [49].

The mechanisms of action for mononuclear cells in angiogenesis have been intensively studied. The domain comes to be multifaceted and contradictory data were sometimes arising.

First, it was proposed and evidence was provided that myeloid cells can turn into endothelial cells in hypoxic tissue demand. Asahara et al. reported that purified CD34+ hematopoietic progenitor cells in adults can differentiate *ex vivo* to an endothelial phenotype [45]. The cells were at the same time positive for VEGFR2, a specific endothelial marker and they were named endothelial progenitor cells (EPC). Thus, EPC expresses both hematopoietic stem cell and endothelial cell markers on their surface [50]. The intensive studies in the past few years allowed distinguishing subpopulations of mononuclear cells existing in the adult bone marrow and circulating in peripheral blood which support angiogenesis without incorporating permanently into the newly formed vessel–circulating angiogenic cells (CAC) [51]. Currently, bone marrow-derived (BMD) cellular populations with angiogenic properties are classified according to their phenotypic markers in the following groups: (i) EPC, which express VEGFR2, Tie2, CXCR4, CD31, CD34, CD133 (for immature progenitor cells) and they are negative for CD14; (ii) monocytes, which express CD14 and have different subclasses such as positive for Tie2, CXCR4, VEGFR2, or VEGFR1; and (iii) macrophages, mostly positive for CXCR4 and VEGFR1 [52].

Several clinical studies have shown a correlation between a high number of tumor-associated macrophages and increased microvessel density, suggesting that these cells might promote tumor angiogenesis, particularly due to production of proangiogenic and angiogenesis modulating factors [53]. A number of functional *in vitro* and *in vivo* studies demonstrate that tumors stimulate neutrophils to promote angiogenesis and immunosuppression, as well as migration, invasion, and metastasis of the tumor cells [54]. In inflammation, the SDF-1/CXCR4 signaling pathway plays an important role in the modulation of neutrophil activity, not only by promoting chemotaxis but also by suppressing cell death [55]. Although limited, there is evidence to suggest that tumor-infiltrating eosinophils can influence angiogenesis [53]. Freshly isolated human blood eosinophils or supernatants from cultured eosinophils induce endothelial cell proliferation *in vitro* and angiogenesis in the rat aortic ring assay, suggesting that eosinophils can directly influence angiogenesis. The high number of mast cells (MC) has been observed in various tumors where increased MC density positively correlates with increased microvessel density [53]. Dendritic cells (DC) promote tumor angiogenesis both by their secretion of pro-angiogenic cytokines (vascular endothelial growth factor (VEGF), interleukin (IL)-8, tumor necrosis factor (TNF)-alpha) and their ability to serve as a local supply of endothelial progenitors [56]. Natural killer (NK) cells control both local tumor growth and metastasis and participate in cancer elimination by inhibiting cellular proliferation and angiogenesis [57]. T helper (Th) cell-mediated immunity has traditionally been viewed as favoring tumor growth, both by promoting angiogenesis and by inhibiting cell-mediated immunity and subsequent tumor cell killing, there are also many studies demonstrating the antitumor activity of CD4+ Th2 cells, particularly in their collaboration with tumor-infiltrating eosinophils or due to direct antiangiogenic effects of IL-4 [58]. T regulatory cells (Tregs) are potent immunosuppressive cells that promote progression of cancer through their ability to limit antitumor immunity and promote angiogenesis. The accumulation of Tregs in tumors correlates with biomarkers of accelerated angiogenesis such as VEGF overexpression and increased microvessel density, providing clinical cues for an association between Tregs and angiogenesis [59].

Mononuclear cells, derived from bone marrow or umbilical cord, yielded in culture two types of cells with angiogenic properties, distinguished by morphology–late endothelial progenitor cells (EPC) and mesenchymal stem cells (MSC). Quantitative PCR analyses revealed high expression levels of Ang-1, FGF-2, SDF1α, and VEGF-A in the MSC, whereas late EPC had higher expression of PDGF-B, PlGF, KDR, CD31, VE-cadherin, and Ang-2 [60]. After transplantation of EPC and MSC in the ischemic hearts, mRNA levels of Ang-1, FGF2, SDF1α, and IGF-1 were significantly increased in tissues collected from the peri-infarct zones; notably the upregulated factors were the same in both cell types transplanted. The data demonstrate that these cells upregulate a number of paracrine factors connected to angiogenesis and cell survival during the critical period of heart repair.

Although the role of bone marrow and peripheral blood mononuclear cells in neovascularization has been convincingly shown, the question remains: how do these cells improve neovascularization? The discovery that mononuclear cells can home to sites of hypoxia and enhance neoangiogenesis has faced the possibility for using the isolated hematopoietic stem cells or EPC for therapeutic vasculogenesis [61]. Remarkably, infusion of terminally differentiated mature endothelial cells did not improve neovascularization [62, 63] suggesting that a not-yet-defined functional characteristic (e.g., chemokine or integrin receptors mediating homing) is essential for EPC-mediated vascular augmentation after ischemia [64]. Monocytic cells may play a crucial role also in collateral growth by adherence to the vascular wall during both arteriogenesis and tumor angiogenesis [53]. These data suggest that monocytic cells are necessary for arteriogenesis and possibly neovascularization. For therapeutic application, the local enhancement of monocyte recruitment might be better suited than systemic infusion of monocytic cells, which only leads to a relatively minor increase in the number of circulating monocytes. During endothelial repair after vascular injury and during tumor angiogenesis BMMNC do not seem to be involved in reendothelialization stressing rather their supportive role over trans-differentiation [65, 66].

The hypothesis for endothelial trans-differentiation of EPC and MSC was tested in the experiment with CM-Dil-labeled (red fluorescent dye) mononuclear cells and subsequent transplantation in infarcted hearts. Interestingly, both EPC and MSC were detected in the pericytic or perivascular areas with minimal and negligible endothelial trans-differentiation effects (<1%). It was suggested that these cells function mainly by paracrine action and vessel stabilization in the perivascular area. The efficiency of neovascularization therefore may not solely be attributable to the incorporation of these cells in newly formed vessels, but may also be influenced by the release of proangiogenic factors in a paracrine manner [67]. It was recently shown that secreting factors from peripheral blood mononuclear cells enhance neoangiogenesis [68]. The capacity of EPC to physically contribute to vessel-like structures may contribute to their potent capacity to improve neovascularization as well [69]. Further studies are in demand to be designed to elucidate the contribution of physical incorporation, paracrine effects and possible effects on vessel remodeling and facilitating vessel branching in EPC-mediated improvement of neovascularization. Likely, paracrine effects contribute in addition to the physical incorporation of EPC into newly formed capillaries. The influence of the incorporation of a rather small number of circulating cells on remodeling and vessel maturation has to be further elucidated.

Only recently the bone marrow-derived monocytes have been related to VEGF-independent angiogenesis [70]. An open question is what drives BMD and PBM cells recruitment to the sites of angiogenesis? Ischemia is believed to upregulate VEGF or SDF-1 [71], which in turn are released to the circulation and induce mobilization of progenitor cells from the bone marrow via a MMP-9–dependent mechanism [72, 73]. Indeed, SDF-1 has been proven to stimulate recruitment of progenitor cells to the ischemic tissue [74]. SDF-1 protein levels were increased during the first day after induction of myocardial infarction [75]. Moreover, over-expression of SDF-1 augmented stem cell homing and incorporation into ischemic tissues [74, 75]. Interestingly, hematopoietic stem cells were shown to be exquisitely sensitive to SDF-1 and did not react to G-CSF or other chemokines (e.g., IL-8 and RANTES) [76]. The migratory capacity of EPC or bone marrow cells toward VEGF and SDF-1, respectively, determined the functional improvement of patients after stem cell therapy [77].

SDF-1/CXCR4 axis is crucial in the homing mechanisms of hematopoietic cells and the metas-tasis of solid tumors. In the past few years, numerous studies have focused on studying the role of this signaling in angiogenesis and proved its angiogenic activity in organ repair and tumor development. However, the precise mechanisms by which SDF-1 exerts its proangio-genic effects are not fully elucidated. Since it is supposed to be an angiogenic growth factor, it is a good candidate for pro- and antiangiogenic therapy. It was reported that transient dis-ruption of the SDF-1/CXCR4 axis using CXCR4 blocking antibody blocked the recruitment of bone marrow-derived cells into the angiogenic sites of tumor tissue, and resulted in complete inhibition of accelerated tumor growth after chemotherapy in mouse [78]. SDF-1 is constitu-tively expressed in the bone marrow and various tissues, which enables it to regulate the traf-ficking, localization, and function of immature and mature leukocytes, including monocytes, neutrophils, dendritic cells, and T lymphocytes [79]. All these immune cells play an important role in tumor angiogenesis and vascularization. However, the precise role of SDF-1/CXCR4 axis on function of monocytes/macrophages, neutrophils, DC, T lymphocytes in the process of angiogenesis is still known and is worthy to be investigated.

4. SDF-1 as a key regulator of vessel development

Global mouse knockouts of SDF-1 (CXCL12) or of its receptor CXCR4 die shortly before birth with vascular deficiency in gut, kidney, and skin and with multiple hematopoietic and neural defects [80-82]. Disrupted CXCL12 signaling led to defective coronary vessel organization in mouse embryos. This signaling was connected to perfusion of the coronary arteries and respectively to embryo growth [31].

SDF-1–positive endothelium was found lining the newly formed intraluminal vessels in lob-ular capillary hemangiomas [83], possibly these were sites of pillar formation. Wrag et al. demonstrated that transplantation of rat bone marrow-derived progenitor cells, positive for VEGFR1, and CXCR4, in ischemic hind limbs increased capillary density by an SDF-1–depen-dent manner, but did not differentiate into vascular structures like endothelial cells or smooth muscle cells [84]. In our previous study, we observed upregulation of SDF-1 and CXCR4 after Notch inhibition being in association with intussusceptive angiogenesis. These chemokine factors are most probably essential for the recruitment of mononuclear cells, participating in the formation of pillars.

It is well known that blocking of SDF-1/CXCR4 axis results in prevention or delay of tumor recurrence after irradiation by inhibiting the recruitment of CD11b+ monocytes/macrophages that participate in tumor revascularization [85]. It was shown that CXCR4 is expressed on eosinophils [86] and concentrations of SDF-1 correlates with eosinophil recruitment [87]. It is known that SDF-1/CXCR4 signaling has pivotal role in mast cell (MC) recruitment in tumor tissue [88] and that MC produce proangiogenic chemokines in response to SDF-1 [89]. CXCR4+ dendritic cells (DC) promote angiogenesis during embryo implantation in mice [90] and CXCR4 is known as a critical chemokine receptor for migration of plasmacytoid DC [91]. CXCR4 is expressed on both NK and NKT cells and regulates their migration in inflamed and tumor tissues in response to SDF-1 as well [92, 93]. SDF-1/CXCR4 signaling is important for migration and activation of T cells [94]. However, the role of SDF-1/CXCR4 signaling in T cell–mediated angiogenesis is unknown. B cells promote tumor progression through STAT-3 regulated angiogenesis [95] and SDF-1/CXCR4 axis is essential for B-lymphocyte production [96] and maintenance of B-cell homeostasis [97].

SDF-1 is the key regulator for homing of stem and progenitor cells to the ischemic injury and its gradient is the major determinant of these cells' recruitment. It has been shown that SDF-1 expression levels are increased in ischemic cardiomyopathy and this was accompanied by the improvement of cardiac function. In addition, SDF-1 high circulation levels were detected in patients with heart failure. Using the ELISA method, Liu et al. [98] proved significantly higher circulating SDF-1 levels in HF patients (5101 ± 1977 pg/ml) compared to controls (1879 ± 1417 pg/ml). Platelet-bound SDF-1 was correlated with acute coronary syndrome and congestive heart failure as well. It was associated with the number of circulating CD34+ progenitor cells. CD34 is coexpressed with CXCR4, which is the ultimate SDF-1 receptor, in progenitor cells, originated from bone marrow, cord blood, and fetal liver. SDF-1 levels were measured in 3359 Framingham Heart Study participants and was suggested as a biomarker of heart failure and all-cause mortality risk. In this study, CD34+ cell frequency was inversely related to SDF-1, in contrast to above-mentioned direct associations. The study has several limitations as the SDF-1 measurement at one time point. There is evidence for modulation of SDF-1 levels in humans and its effect is rather cumulative and chronic than acute.

The crucial role of SDF-1 for cardiac repair in chronic ischemic heart failure was the reason for conducting clinical trial using SDF-1 nonviral gene therapy via its endomyocardial administration [99]. This blinded placebo-controlled STOP-HF trial demonstrated improvement of clinical status based on composite endpoint of six MWD (6-min walk distance) and MLWHFQ (Minnesota Living with Heart Failure Quality of life Questionnaire). Another clinical trial–MARVEL was announced in 2015 to advance into US FDA Phase 3 clinical evaluation of regenerative/cellular therapy of chronic heart failure, planned to be combined with SDF-1.

What trigger the SDF-1 upregulation is still elusive. Some authors postulate it is induced by HIF1α in response to hypoxia. However, other mechanisms of induction are also possible such as inflammation and subsequent release of mediators like interleukin-1 or tumor necrosis factor-α into circulation. It is evident by its induction not only in ischemic, but also in nonischemic cardiomyopathy. SDF-1 circulating levels were not influenced by the local heart hypoxia, but showed positive correlation with CRP, which is a marker for inflammation.

Recently, we have demonstrated the endothelial expression of SDF-1 in liver of Notch1 knockout mouse, whereby it was associated with intussusception (**Figure 2**).

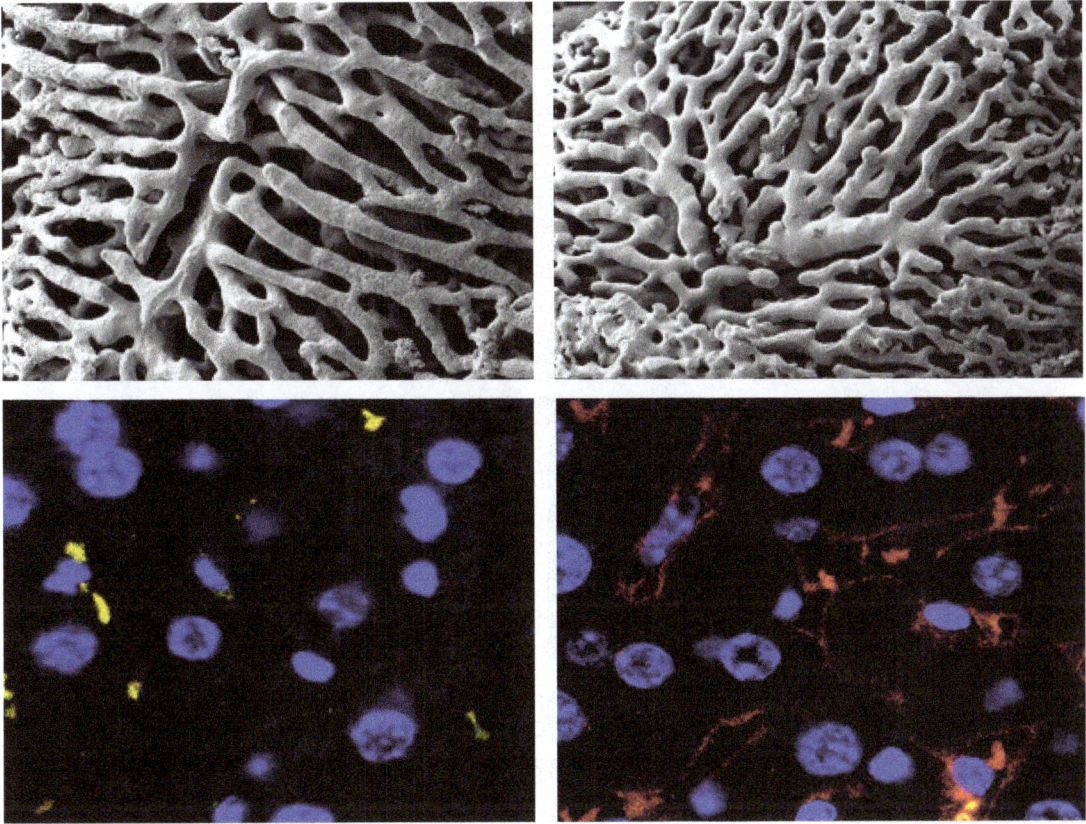

Figure 2. Vascular casts revealed predominant mode of intussusceptive angiogenesis in liver nodular regeneration after Notch1 knockout (B) compared to wild type mouse (A). Immunofluorescence for SDF-1 demonstrated strong sinusoidal positivity for this marker only in Notch1 knockout mouse (D) but not in the wild type (C).

Connecting our observations for SDF-1 positivity and mononuclear cells (MNCs) partici-pation in intussusceptive angiogenesis, we hypothesize that both processes are involved in vessel remodeling. Using our model of chicken area vasculosa, we performed detailed ultrastructural vessel study after application of recombinant SDF-1. A specific behavior of mononuclear cells was detected during this experiment. They were involved in a step-wise process of recruitment and extravasation (**Figure 3**). We determined five distinguished states: 1, MNCs are free in the circulation; 2, MNCs are recruited to the endothelium and rolling under the blood flow; 3, MNCs are bound to the endothelium; 4, MNCs are extravasating; 5, MNCs are localized in the perivascular space.

1. MC free in circulation–nonadhesive to endothelial cells

2. MC tethered to endothelium and rolling under force of blood flow

3. MC bound to endothelium and migrating

4. Extravasation of MC from blood vessel

5. MC in perivascular space–stabilizing function

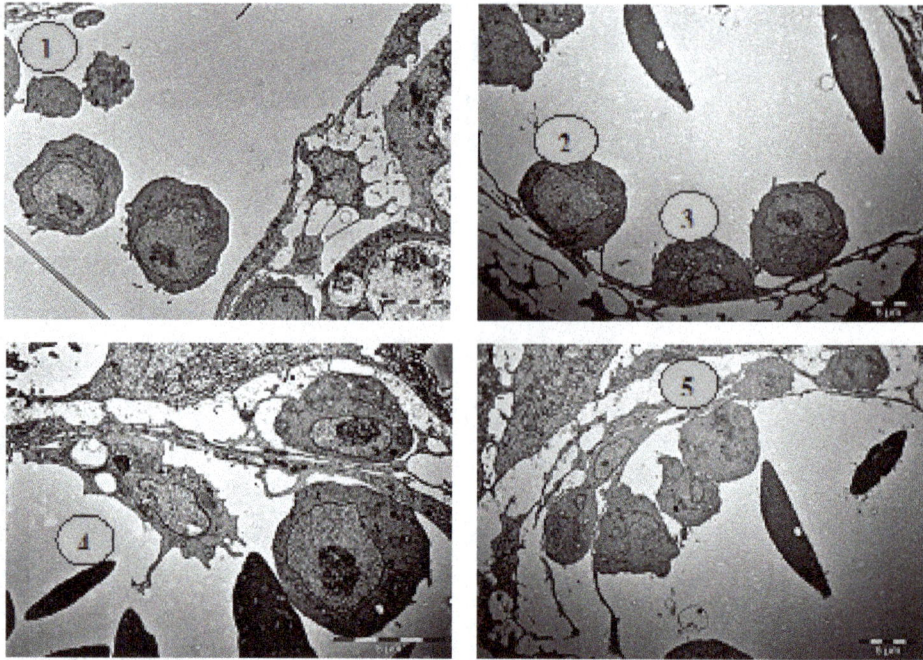

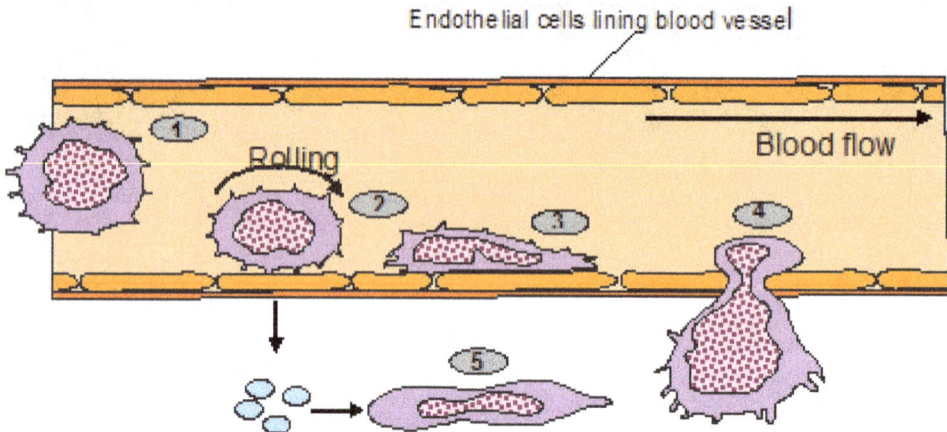

Figure 3. Transmission electron microscopy of chicken area vasculosa after the application of recombinant SDF-1 and the proposed model for mononuclear cells (MC) extravasation.

5. Summary

- Angiogenesis is a complex process involving essential signaling pathways (for instance VEGF, bFGF, Notch, etc.) in vasculature, as well as additional players such as bone marrow-derived mononuclear cells.

- Intussusceptive angiogenesis (IA) is a well-documented and widely spread mode of angiogenesis, occurring both during normal development and in pathological conditions.

- Our preliminary results suggest that IA is most probably synchronized by chemokine factors since intussusceptive growth was associated with the recruitment of mononuclear cells.

- The intensive studies in the past few years allowed distinguishing subpopulations of mononuclear cells existing in the adult bone marrow and circulating in peripheral blood which support angiogenesis.

- During endothelial repair after vascular injury and during tumor angiogenesis mononuclear cells do not seem to be involved in reendothelialization stressing rather their supportive role over trans-differentiation.

- We have demonstrated the endothelial expression of SDF-1 in liver of Notch1 knockout mouse, whereby it was associated with intussusceptive angiogenesis.

- We suggest that this chemokine factor is most probably essential for the recruitment of mononuclear cells, participating in step-wise process of extravasation and stabilizing the formation of intussusceptive pillars.

Acknowledgement

This work was supported by Contract No IZ73Z0_152454 of SNSF, Switzerland.

Author details

Ivanka Dimova[1]* and Valentin Djonov[2]

*Address all correspondence to: ivanka.i.dimova@gmail.com

1 Department of Medical genetics, Medical University Sofia, Sofia, Bulgaria

2 Institute of Anatomy, University of Bern, Bern, Switzerland

References

[1] Ribatti D, Crivellato E: "Sprouting angiogenesis", a reappraisal. Dev Biol. 2012;372(2):157–65.

[2] Djonov V, Baum O, Burri PH: Vascular remodeling by intussusceptive angiogenesis. Cell Tissue Res. 2003;314(1):107–17.

[3] Djonov V, Schmid M, Tschanz SA, Burri PH: Intussusceptive angiogenesis: its role in embryonic vascular network formation. Circ Res. 2000;86(3):286–92.

[4] Jakobsson L, Franco CA, Bentley K, Collins RT, Ponsioen B, Aspalter IM, Rosewell I, Busse M, Thurston G, Medvinsky A, Schulte-Merker S, Gerhardt H: Endothelial cells dynamically compete for the tip cell position during angiogenic sprouting. Nat Cell Biol. 2010;12(10):943–53.

[5] Blanco R, Gerhardt H: VEGF and Notch in tip and stalk cell selection. Cold Spring Harb Perspect Med. 2013 Jan 1;3(1):a006569.

[6] Makanya AN, Hlushchuk R, Djonov VG: Intussusceptive angiogenesis and its role in vascular morphogenesis, patterning, and remodeling. Angiogenesis. 2009;12(2):113–23.

[7] Styp-Rekowska B, Hlushchuk R, Pries AR, Djonov V: Intussusceptive angiogenesis: pillars against the blood flow. Acta Physiol (Oxf). 2011;202(3):213–23.

[8] Konerding MA, Gibney BC, Houdek JP, Chamoto K, Ackermann M, Lee GS, Lin M, Tsuda A, Mentzer SJ: Spatial dependence of alveolar angiogenesis in post-pneumonectomy lung growth. Angiogenesis. 2012;15(1):23–32.

[9] Dill MT, Rothweiler S, Djonov V, Hlushchuk R, Tornillo L, Terracciano L, Meili-Butz S, Radtke F, Heim MH, Semela D: Disruption of Notch1 induces vascular remodeling, intussusceptive angiogenesis, and angiosarcomas in livers of mice. Gastroenterology. 2012;142(4):967–77.

[10] Baum O, Suter F, Gerber B, Tschanz SA, Buergy R, Blank F, Hlushchuk R, Djonov V: VEGF-A promotes intussusceptive angiogenesis in the developing chicken chorioallantoic membrane. Microcirculation. 2010;17(6):447–57.

[11] Dimova I, Hlushchuk R, Makanya A, Styp-Rekowska B, Ceausu A, Flueckiger S, Lang S, Semela D, Le Noble F, Chatterjee S, Djonov V: Inhibition of Notch signaling induces extensive intussusceptive neo-angiogenesis by recruitment of mononuclear cells. Angiogenesis. 2013 Oct;16(4):921–37.

[12] Makanya AN, Hlushchuk R, Djonov V: The pulmonary blood-gas barrier in the avian embryo: inauguration, development and refinement. Respir Physiol Neurobiol. 2011 Aug 31;178(1):30–8.

[13] Taylor AC, Seltz LM, Yates PA, Peirce SM: Chronic whole-body hypoxia induces intussusceptive angiogenesis and microvascular remodeling in the mouse retina. Microvasc Res. 2010 Mar;79(2):93–101.

[14] Konerding MA, Turhan A, Ravnic DJ, Lin M, Fuchs C, Secomb TW, Tsuda A, Mentzer SJ: Inflammation-induced intussusceptive angiogenesis in murine colitis. Anat Rec (Hoboken). 2010 May;293(5):849–57.

[15] Peebo BB, Fagerholm P, Traneus-Röckert C, Lagali N: Cellular level characterization of capillary regression in inflammatory angiogenesis using an in vivo corneal model. Angiogenesis. 2011 Sep;14(3):393–405.

[16] Wnuk M, Hlushchuk R, Janot M, Tuffin G, Martiny-Baron G, Holzer P, Imbach-Weese P, Djonov V, Huynh-Do U: Podocyte EphB4 signaling helps recovery from glomerular injury. Kidney Int. 2012 Jun;81(12):1212–25.

[17] Hlushchuk R, Makanya AN, Djonov V: Escape mechanisms after antiangiogenic treatment, or why are the tumors growing again? Int J Dev Biol. 2011;55(4–5):563–67.

[18] Hlushchuk R, Riesterer O, Baum O, Wood J, Gruber G, Pruschy M, Djonov V: Tumor recovery by angiogenic switch from sprouting to intussusceptive angiogenesis after treatment with PTK787/ZK222584 or ionizing radiation. Am J Pathol. 2008 Oct;173(4):1173–85.

[19] Abdullah SE, Perez-Soler R: Mechanisms of resistance to vascular endothelial growth factor blockade. Cancer. 2012 Jul 15;118(14):3455–67.

[20] Paku S, Dezso K, Bugyik E, Tóvári J, Tímár J, Nagy P, Laszlo V, Klepetko W, Döme B: A new mechanism for pillar formation during tumor-induced intussusceptive angiogenesis: inverse sprouting. Am J Pathol. 2011 Sep;179(3):1573–85.

[21] Ceauşu RA, Cîmpean AM, Gaje P, Gurzu S, Jung I, Raica M: CD105/Ki67 double immunostaining expression in liver metastasis from colon carcinoma. Rom J Morphol Embryol. 2011;52(2):613–16.

[22] Bugyik E, Dezso K, Reiniger L, László V, Tóvári J, Tímár J, Nagy P, Klepetko W, Döme B, Paku S : Lack of angiogenesis in experimental brain metastases. J Neuropathol Exp Neurol. 2011 Nov;70(11):979–91.

[23] Reuwer AQ, Nowak-Sliwinska P, Mans LA, van der Loos CM, von der Thüsen JH, Twickler MT, Spek CA, Goffin V, Griffioen AW, Borensztajn KS: Functional consequences of prolactin signalling in endothelial cells: a potential link with angiogenesis in pathophysiology? J Cell Mol Med. 2012 Sep;16(9):2035–48.

[24] Oliveira de Oliveira LB, Faccin Bampi V, Ferreira Gomes C, Braga da Silva JL, Encarnação Fiala Rechsteiner SM: Morphological characterization of sprouting and intussusceptive angiogenesis by SEM in oral squamous cell carcinoma. Scanning. 2014 May-Jun;36(3):293-300. doi: 10.1002/sca.21104.

[25] Géraud C, Mogler C, Runge A, Evdokimov K, Lu S, Schledzewski K, Arnold B, Hämmerling G, Koch PS, Breuhahn K, Longerich T, Marx A, Weiss C, Damm F, Schmieder A, Schirmacher P, Augustin HG, Goerdt S: Endothelial transdifferentiation in hepatocellular carcinoma: loss of Stabilin-2 expression in peri-tumourous liver correlates with increased survival. Liver Int. 2013 Oct;33(9):1428–40.

[26] Piguet AC, Saar B, Hlushchuk R, St-Pierre MV, McSheehy PM, Radojevic V, Afthinos M, Terracciano L, Djonov V, Dufour JF: Everolimus augments the effects of sorafenib in a syngeneic orthotopic model of hepatocellular carcinoma. Mol Cancer Ther. 2011 Jun;10(6):1007–17.

[27] De Spiegelaere W, Casteleyn C, Van den Broeck W, Plendl J, Bahramsoltani M, Simoens P, Djonov V, Cornillie P: Intussusceptive angiogenesis: a biologically relevant form of angiogenesis. J Vasc Res. 2012;49(5):390–404.

[28] Ackermann M, Tsuda A, Secomb TW, Mentzer SJ, Konerding MA: Intussusceptive remodeling of vascular branch angles in chemically-induced murine colitis. Microvasc Res. 2013 May;87:75–82.

[29] Polykandriotis E, Arkudas A, Beier JP, Dragu A, Rath S, Pryymachuk G, Schmidt VJ, Lametschwandtner A, Horch RE, Kneser U: The impact of VEGF and bFGF on vascular stereomorphology in the context of angiogenic neo-arborisation after vascular induction. J Electron Microsc (Tokyo). 2011;60(4):267–74.

[30] Ackermann M, Morse BA, Delventhal V, Carvajal IM, Konerding MA: Anti-VEGFR2 and anti-IGF-1R-Adnectins inhibit Ewing's sarcoma A673-xenograft growth and normalize tumor vascular architecture. Angiogenesis. 2012 Dec;15(4):685–95.

[31] Cavallero S., Shen H., Yi Ch., Lien C., Ram Kumar S., Sucov H: CXCL12 signaling is essential for maturation of the ventricular coronary endothelial plexus and establishment of functional coronary circulation. Dev Cell. 2015 May 26;33(4):469–477.

[32] Kovall RA: Structures of CSL, Notch and Mastermind proteins: piecing together an active transcription complex. Curr Opin Struct Biol. 2007;17(1):117–27.

[33] Parks AL, Stout JR, Shepard SB, Klueg KM, Dos Santos AA, Parody TR, Vaskova M, Muskavitch MA: Structure-function analysis of delta trafficking, receptor binding and signalling in Drosophila. Genetics. 2006;174(4):1947–61.

[34] Seo S, Kume T: Forkhead transcription factors, Forkhead box C1 (Foxc1) and Forkhead box C2 (Foxc2), are required for the morphogenesis of the cardiac outflow tract. Dev Biol. 2006;296(2):421–36.

[35] Domenga V, Fardoux P, Lacombe P, Monet M, Maciazek J, Krebs L, Klonjkowski B, berrou E, Mericskay M, Li Z, et al: Notch3 is required for arterial identity and maturation of vascular smooth muscle cells. Genes Dev. 2004;18:2730–2735

[36] Krebs LT, et al: Notch-signalling is essential for vascular morphogenesis in mice. Genes Dev. 2000;14:1343–1352.

[37] Uyttendaele H, Ho J, Rossant J, Kitajewski J: Vascular patterning defects associated with expression of activated Notch4 in embryonic endothelium. Proc Natl Acad Sci USA. 2001;98:5643–5648.

[38] Villa N, Walker L, Lindcell CE, Gasson J, Iruela-Arispe ML, Weinmaster G: Vascular expression of Notch pathway receptors and ligands is restricted to arterial vessels. Mech Dev. 2001;108:161–164.

[39] Jenkins DW, Ross S, Veldman-Jones M, Foltz IN, Clavette BC, Manchulenko K, Eberlein C, Kendrew J, Petteruti P, Cho S, Damschroder M, Peng L, Baker D, Smith NR, Weir HM, Blakey DC, Bedian V, Barry ST: MEDI0639: a novel therapeutic antibody targeting Dll4 modulates endothelial cell function and angiogenesis in vivo. Mol Cancer Ther. 2012;11(8):1650–60.

[40] Noguera-Troise I, Daly C, Papadopoulos NJ, Coetzee S, Boland P, Gale NW, Lin HC, Yancopoulos GD, Thurston G: Blockade of Dll4 inhibits tumour growth by promoting non-productive angiogenesis. Novartis Found Symp. 2007;283:106–20.

[41] Ridgway J, Zhang G, Wu Y, Stawicki S, Liang WC, Chanthery Y, Kowalski J, Watts RJ, Callahan C, Kasman I, Singh M, Chien M, Tan C, Hongo JA, de SF, Plowman G, Yan M: Inhibition of Dll4 signalling inhibits tumour growth by deregulating angiogenesis. Nature. 2006;444(7122):1083–87.

[42] Thurston G, Noguera-Troise I, Yancopoulos GD: The Delta paradox: DLL4 blockade leads to more tumour vessels but less tumour growth. Nat Rev Cancer. 2007;7(5):327–31.

[43] Al Haj ZA, Oikawa A, Bazan-Peregrino M, Meloni M, Emanueli C, Madeddu P: Inhibition of delta-like-4-mediated signaling impairs reparative angiogenesis after ischemia. Circ Res. 2010;107(2):283–93.

[44] Kalen M, Heikura T, Karvinen H, Nitzsche A, Weber H, Esser N, Yla-Herttuala S, Hellstrom M: Gamma-secretase inhibitor treatment promotes VEGF-A-driven blood vessel growth and vascular leakage but disrupts neovascular perfusion. PLoS One. 2011;6(4):e18709.

[45] Asahara T, Murohara T, Sullivan A, Silver M, van der Zee R, Li T, Witzenbichler B, Schatteman G, Isner JM: Isolation of putative progenitor endothelial cells for angiogenesis. Science. 1997 Feb 14;275(5302):964–67.

[46] Wang J, Fu X, Yu L, Li N, Wang M, Liu X, Zhang D, Han W, Zhou C, Wang J: Preconditioning with VEGF enhances angiogenic and neuroprotective effects of bone marrow mononuclear cell transplantation in a rat model of chronic cerebral hypoperfusion. Mol Neurobiol. 2016 Nov;53(9):6057–6068.

[47] Corenblum MJ, Flores AJ, Badowski M, Harris DT, Madhavan L: Systemic human CD34(+) cells populate the brain and activate host mechanisms to counteract nigrostriatal degeneration. Regen Med. 2015;10(5):563–77.

[48] Haddad F, Sever M, Poglajen G, Lezaic L, Yang P, Maecker H, Davis M, Kuznetsova T, Wu JC, Vrtovec B: Immunologic network and response to intramyocardial CD34+ stem cell therapy in patients with dilated cardiomyopathy. J Card Fail. 2015 Jul;21(7):572–82.

[49] Chang MY, Huang TT, Chen CH, Cheng B, Hwang SM, Hsieh PC: Injection of human cord blood cells with hyaluronan improves postinfarction cardiac repair in pigs. Stem Cells Transl Med. 2016 Jan;5(1):56–66.

[50] Zhao YH, Yuan B, Chen J, Feng DH, Zhao B, Qin C, Chen YF: Endothelial progenitor cells: therapeutic perspective for ischemic stroke. CNS Neurosci Ther. 2013 Feb;19(2):67–75.

[51] Fang S, Salven P: Stem cells in tumor angiogenesis. J Mol Cell Cardiol. 2011 Feb;50(2):290–95.

[52] Favre J, Terborg N, Horrevoets AJ: The diverse identity of angiogenic monocytes. Eur J Clin Invest. 2013 Jan;43(1):100–7.

[53] Murdoch C, Muthana M, Coffelt SB, Lewis CE: The role of myeloid cells in the promotion of tumour angiogenesis. Nat Rev Cancer. 2008 Aug;8(8):618–31.

[54] Dumitru CA, Lang S, Brandau S: Modulation of neutrophil granulocytes in the tumor microenvironment: mechanisms and consequences for tumor progression. Semin Cancer Biol. 2013 Jun;23(3):141–48.

[55] Yamada M, Kubo H, Kobayashi S, Ishizawa K, He M, Suzuki T, Fujino N, Kunishima H, Hatta M, Nishimaki K, Aoyagi T, Tokuda K, Kitagawa M, Yano H, Tamamura H, Fujii N, Kaku M: The increase in surface CXCR4 expression on lung extravascular neutrophils and its effects onneutrophils during endotoxin-induced lung injury. Cell Mol Immunol. 2011 Jul;8(4):305–14.

[56] Strioga M, Schijns V, Powell DJ Jr, Pasukoniene V, Dobrovolskiene N, Michalek J: Dendritic cells and their role in tumor immunosurveillance. Innate Immun. 2013 Feb;19(1):98–111.

[57] Levy EM, Roberti MP, Mordoh J: Natural killer cells in human cancer: from biological functions to clinical applications. J Biomed Biotechnol. 2011;2011:676198.

[58] Ellyard JI, Simson L, Parish CR: Th2-mediated anti-tumour immunity: friend or foe? Tissue Antigens. 2007 Jul;70(1):1–11.

[59] Facciabene A, Motz GT, Coukos G: T-regulatory cells: key players in tumor immune escape and angiogenesis. Cancer Res. 2012 May 1;72(9):2162–71.

[60] Kim SW, Jin HL, Kang SM, Kim S, Yoo KJ, Jang Y, Kim HO, Yoon YS: Therapeutic effects of late outgrowth endothelial progenitor cells or mesenchymal stem cells derived from human umbilical cord blood on infarct repair. Int J Cardiol. 2016 Jan 15;203:498–507.

[61] Wara AK, Croce K, Foo S, Sun X, Icli B, Tesmenitsky Y, Esen F, Rosenzweig A, Feinberg MW: Bone marrow-derived CMPs and GMPs represent highly functional proangiogenic cells: implications for ischemic cardiovascular disease. Blood. 2011 Dec 8;118(24):6461–64.

[62] Kocher AA, Schuster MD, Szabolcs MJ, Takuma S, Burkhoff D, Wang J, Homma S, Edwards NM, Itescu S: Neovascularization of ischemic myocardium by human bone-marrow-derived angioblasts prevents cardiomyocyte apoptosis, reduces remodeling and improves cardiac function. Nat Med. 2001 Apr;7(4):430–36.

[63] Hur J, Yoon CH, Kim HS, Choi JH, Kang HJ, Hwang KK, Oh BH, Lee MM, Park YB: Characterization of two types of endothelial progenitor cells and their different contributions to neovasculogenesis. Arterioscler Thromb Vasc Biol. 2004 Feb;24(2):288–93.

[64] Cochain C, Rodero MP, Vilar J, Récalde A, Richart AL, Loinard C, Zouggari Y, Guérin C, Duriez M, Combadière B, Poupel L, Lévy BI, Mallat Z, Combadière C, Silvestre JS: Regulation of monocyte subset systemic levels by distinct chemokine receptors controls post-ischaemic neovascularization. Cardiovasc Res. 2010 Oct 1;88(1):186–95.

[65] Dudley AC, Udagawa T, Melero-Martin JM, Shih SC, Curatolo A, Moses MA, Klagsbrun M: Bone marrow is a reservoir for proangiogenic myelomonocytic cells but not endothelial cells in spontaneous tumors. Blood. 2010 Oct 28;116(17):3367–71.

[66] Hagensen MK, Raarup MK, Mortensen MB, Thim T, Nyengaard JR, Falk E, Bentzon JF: Circulating endothelial progenitor cells do not contribute to regeneration of endothelium after murine arterial injury. Cardiovasc Res. 2012 Feb 1;93(2):223–31.

[67] Ribatti D, Crivellato E: Immune cells and angiogenesis. J Cell Mol Med. 2009 Sep;13(9A):2822–33.

[68] Mildner M, Hacker S, Haider T, Gschwandtner M, Werba G, Barresi C, Zimmermann M, Golabi B, Tschachler E, Ankersmit HJ: Secretome of peripheral blood mononuclear cells enhances wound healing. PLoS One. 2013;8(3):e60103.

[69] Urbich C, Heeschen C, Aicher A, Dernbach E, Zeiher AM, Dimmeler S: Relevance of monocytic features for neovascularization capacity of circulating endothelial progenitor cells. Circulation. 2003 Nov 18;108(20):2511–16.

[70] Botta C, Barbieri V, Ciliberto D, Rossi A, Rocco D, Addeo R, Staropoli N, Pastina P, Marvaso G, Martellucci I, Guglielmo A, Pirtoli L, Sperlongano P, Gridelli C, Caraglia M, Tassone P, Tagliaferri P, Correale P: Systemic inflammatory status at baseline predicts bevacizumab benefit in advanced non-small cell lung cancer patients. Cancer Biol Ther. 2013 Jun;14(6):469–75.

[71] Lee SH, Wolf PL, Escudero R, Deutsch R, Jamieson SW, Thistlethwaite PA: Early expression of angiogenesis factors in acute myocardial ischemia and infarction. N Engl J Med. 2000 Mar 2;342(9):626–33.

[72] Heissig B, Hattori K, Dias S, Friedrich M, Ferris B, Hackett NR, Crystal RG, Besmer P, Lyden D, Moore MA, Werb Z, Rafii S: Recruitment of stem and progenitor cells from the bone marrow niche requires MMP-9 mediated release of kit-ligand. Cell. 2002 May 31;109(5):625–37.

[73] Shintani S, Murohara T, Ikeda H, Ueno T, Honma T, Katoh A, Sasaki K, Shimada T, Oike Y, Imaizumi T: Mobilization of endothelial progenitor cells in patients with acute myocardial infarction. Circulation. 2001 Jun 12;103(23):2776–79.

[74] Yamaguchi J, Kusano KF, Masuo O, Kawamoto A, Silver M, Murasawa S, Bosch-Marce M, Masuda H, Losordo DW, Isner JM, Asahara T: Stromal cell-derived factor-1 effects on ex vivo expanded endothelial progenitor cell recruitment for ischemic neovascularization. Circulation. 2003 Mar 11;107(9):1322–28.

[75] Askari AT, Unzek S, Popovic ZB, Goldman CK, Forudi F, Kiedrowski M, Rovner A, Ellis SG, Thomas JD, DiCorleto PE, Topol EJ, Penn MS: Effect of stromal-cell-derived factor 1 on stem-cell homing and tissue regeneration in ischaemic cardiomyopathy. Lancet. 2003 Aug 30;362(9385):697–703.

[76] Wright DE, Bowman EP, Wagers AJ, Butcher EC, Weissman IL: Hematopoietic stem cells are uniquely selective in their migratory response to chemokines. J Exp Med. 2002 May 6;195(9):1145–54.

[77] Britten MB, Abolmaali ND, Assmus B, Lehmann R, Honold J, Schmitt J, Vogl TJ, Martin H, Schächinger V, Dimmeler S, Zeiher AM: Infarct remodeling after intracoronary progenitor cell treatment in patients with acute myocardial infarction (TOPCARE-AMI): mechanistic insights from serial contrast-enhanced magnetic resonance imaging. Circulation. 2003 Nov 4;108(18):2212–28.

[78] Murakami J, Li TS, Ueda K, Tanaka T, Hamano K: Inhibition of accelerated tumor growth by blocking the recruitment of mobilized endothelial progenitor cells after chemotherapy. Int J Cancer. 2009;124(7):1685–1692.

[79] Karin N: The multiple faces of CXCL12 (SDF-1alpha) in the regulation of immunity during health and disease. J Leukoc Biol. 2010 Sep;88(3):463–73.

[80] Ma Q, Jones D, Borghesani PR, Segal RA, Nagasawa T, Kishimoto T, Bronson RT, Springer TA: Impaired B-lymphopoiesis, myelopoiesis, and derailed cerebellar neuron migration in CXCR4- and SDF-1-deficient mice. Proc Natl Acad Sci U S A. 1998 Aug 4;95(16):9448–53.

[81] Nagasawa T, Hirota S, Tachibana K, Takakura N, Nishikawa S, Kitamura Y, Yoshida N, Kikutani H, Kishimoto T: Defects of B-cell lymphopoiesis and bone-marrow myelopoiesis in mice lacking the CXC chemokine PBSF/SDF-Nature. 1996 Aug 15;382(6592):635–38.

[82] Tachibana K, Hirota S, Iizasa H, Yoshida H, Kawabata K, Kataoka Y, Kitamura Y, Matsushima K, Yoshida N, Nishikawa S, Kishimoto T, Nagasawa T: The chemokine receptor CXCR4 is essential for vascularization of the gastrointestinal tract. Nature. 1998 Jun 11;393(6685):591–94.

[83] Morrow D, Cullen JP, Cahill PA, Redmond EM: Cyclic strain regulates the Notch/CBF-1 signaling pathway in endothelial cells: role in angiogenic activity. Arterioscler Thromb Vasc Biol. 2007;27(6):1289–96.

[84] Williams CK, Segarra M, Sierra ML, Sainson RC, Tosato G, Harris AL: Regulation of CXCR4 by the Notch ligand delta-like 4 in endothelial cells. Cancer Res. 2008;68(6):1889–95.

[85] Tseng D, Vasquez-Medrano DA, Brown JM: Targeting SDF-1/CXCR4 to inhibit tumour vasculature for treatment of glioblastomas. Br J Cancer. 2011 Jun 7;104(12):1805–9.

[86] Dulkys Y, Buschermöhle T, Escher SE, Kapp A, Elsner J: T-helper 2 cytokines attenuate senescent eosinophil activation by the CXCR4 ligand stromal-derived factor-1alpha (CXCL12). Clin Exp Allergy. 2004 Oct;34(10):1610–20.

[87] Negrete-García MC, Velazquez JR, Popoca-Coyotl A, Montes-Vizuet AR, Juárez-Carvajal E, Teran LM: Chemokine (C-X-C motif) ligand 12/stromal cell-derived factor-1 is associated with leukocyte recruitment in asthma. Chest. 2010 Jul;138(1):100–doi: 10.1378/chest.09-Epub 2010 Mar 18.

[88] Põlajeva J1, Sjösten AM, Lager N, Kastemar M, Waern I, Alafuzoff I, Smits A, Westermark B, Pejler G, Uhrbom L, Tchougounova E: Mast cell accumulation in glioblastoma with a potential role for stem cell factor and chemokine CXCLPLoS One. 2011;6(9):edoi: 10.1371/journal.pone.0025222.

[89] Lin TJ, Issekutz TB, Marshall JS: SDF-1 induces IL-8 production and transendothelial migration of human cord blood-derived mast cells. Int Arch Allergy Immunol. 2001 Jan–Mar;124(1–3):142–45.

[90] Barrientos G, Tirado-González I, Freitag N, Kobelt P, Moschansky P, Klapp BF, Thijssen VL, Blois SM: CXCR4(+) dendritic cells promote angiogenesis during embryo implantation in mice. Angiogenesis. 2013 Apr;16(2):417–27.

[91] Umemoto E1, Otani K, Ikeno T, Verjan Garcia N, Hayasaka H, Bai Z, Jang MH, Tanaka T, Nagasawa T, Ueda K, Miyasaka M: Constitutive plasmacytoid dendritic cell migration

to the splenic white pulp is cooperatively regulated by CCR7- and CXCR4-mediated signaling. J Immunol. 2012 Jul 1;189(1):191–doi: 10.4049/jimmunol.1200802.

[92]   Robertson MJ: Role of chemokines in the biology of natural killer cells. J Leukoc Biol. 2002 Feb;71(2):173–83.

[93]   Lindau D, Gielen P, Kroesen M, Wesseling P, Adema GJ: The immunosuppressive tumour network: myeloid-derived suppressor cells, regulatory T cells and natural killer T cells. Immunology. 2013 Feb;138(2):105–15.

[94]   Patrussi L1, Baldari CT: Intracellular mediators of CXCR4-dependent signaling in T cells. Immunol Lett. 2008 Jan 29;115(2):75–82.

[95]   Yang C1, Lee H, Pal S, Jove V, Deng J, Zhang W, Hoon DS, Wakabayashi M, Forman S, Yu H: B cells promote tumor progression via STAT3 regulated-angiogenesis. PLoS One. 2013 May 29;8(5):edoi: 10.1371/journal.pone.0064159.

[96]   Nagasawa T: A chemokine, SDF-1/PBSF, and its receptor, CXC chemokine receptor 4, as mediators of hematopoiesis. Int J Hematol. 2000 Dec;72(4):408–11.

[97]   Mountz JD, Wang JH, Xie S, Hsu HC: Cytokine regulation of B-cell migratory behavior favors formation of germinal centers in autoimmune disease. Discov Med. 2011 Jan;11(56):76–85.

[98]   Liu K, Yang S, Hou M, Chen T, Liu J, Yu B: Increase of circulating stromal cell-derived factor-1 in heart failure patients. Herz. 2015 Mar;40(Suppl 1):70–doi: 10.1007/s00059-014-4169-z.

[99]   Chung ES, Miller L, Patel AN, et al: Changes in ventricular remodelling and clinical status during the year following a single administration of stromal cell-derived factor-1 non-viral gene therapy in chronic ischaemic heart failure patients: the STOP-HF randomized Phase II trial. European Heart Journal. 2015;36(33):2228–doi:10.1093/eurheartj/ehv254.

9

Angiogenesis Meets Skeletogenesis: The Cross-Talk between Two Dynamic Systems

Tamara A. Franz-Odendaal, Daniel Andrews and Shruti Kumar

Abstract

In this chapter, we describe the complex relationship between angiogenesis and skeletogenesis. While much is known about the interactions of these two dynamic systems for bones that ossify via a cartilage template, comparatively little is known about directly ossifying bones. Most of the bones of the head develop from osteogenic condensations and undergo intramembranous (direct) ossification during development. Our understanding of the relationship between osteogenic cell condensations (in particular) and angiogenesis is currently inadequate and prevents a comprehensive understanding of vertebrate head development. This chapter highlights our understanding of both direct and indirectly ossifying bones shedding light on where there are important gaps in our understanding.

Keywords: avascular, skeletogenic condensation, osteoblasts, chondrocytes, cell culture, VEGF, HIF

1. Introduction

The coordinated development of tissues is critical for proper development. Bone is a highly vascularized tissue that also houses the hematopoetic cell niche, which provides a lifelong supply of blood cells (in humans and most other vertebrates). In this chapter, we will explore the role angiogenesis plays during the development of bones. Bones that ossify endochondrally (from cartilage) versus bones that ossify intramembranously (without cartilage) have different relationships with vasculature and hence with the process of angiogenesis. These bones start development by forming a skeletogenic condensation, however, the molecular signals within these condensations differ [1]. We begin with a discussion of bones that develop from a cartilage precursor (endochondral ossification) since more is known about this process than about directly ossifying bones (intramembranous ossification). We also discuss data from cell culture and bone grafts that shed light on the cross talk between these two dynamic processes, angiogenesis and skeletogenesis. Some pathological implications are also included.

2. Bones that ossify via endochondral ossification

2.1. Angiogenesis during formation of the cartilage template

Endochondrally ossifying bones are bones that form via a cartilage template. The process of endochondral ossification begins with stem cells originating from the mesenchyme in the future area of bone development. These stem cells aggregate to form a chondrogenic condensation. Once this cell aggregation reaches a critical size, cells begin to differentiate into chondrocytes (chondroblasts) that will then secrete extracellular matrix (ECM), collagen type II. This matrix matures into the cartilage template that will eventually ossify (e.g., long bones). Cartilage itself is avascular when first deposited, however, differentiated chondrocytes secrete anti-angiogenic factors (inhibitors) to maintain the avascular nature of the cartilage. These early chondrocytes are typically referred to as pre-hypertrophic chondrocytes. As these chondrocytes mature, they gradually become hypertrophic and begin to secrete a number of pro-angiogenic factors. Vascular endothelial-derived growth factor (VEGF), a protein which is important for angiogenesis and the subsequent ossification of the cartilage, is a key angiogenic factor during bone development. Hypoxia-inducible factor is one of the key upstream regulators of VEGF, and changes in the level of HIF can alter the level of VEGF thus dramatically changing bone mass (discussed later).

During the maturation of hypertrophic chondrocytes, these cells release VEGF into the extracellular matrix and into the area surrounding the perichondrium layer of the cartilage. The hypertrophic chondrocytes also secrete fibroblast growth factor (FGF), bone morphogenetic protein (BMP) and connective tissue growth factor (CTGF) [2, 3]. With the arrival of these factors to the site of bone formation, angiogenesis in the bone can now occur. There is a complex cross talk between bone-forming cells (osteoblasts), the angiogenic factors present, and the invading vasculature. These growth factors, in particular VEGF, recruit osteo/chondro-clasts, osteoprogenitors and other bone precursors to the area in order to initiate the primary ossification center, the first site of bone formation within the cartilage template [2, 4].

Osteoclasts are bone matrix resorbing cells, and once recruited, they secrete multiple factors that contribute to the initiation of vascularization, including the release of more VEGF and FGFs [2, 5]. Among these factors are matrix metalloproteinases (MMPs) and hypoxia-inducible factors (HIFs) which, along with VEGF, are other key proteins important in the development of vasculature in bone. The MMPs break down the ECM and release matrix-bound VEGF that allows for the resorption of cartilage so that osteoblasts can infiltrate and deposit bone. MMPs, primarily MMP9 and MMP13, also function to recruit osteoclasts and osteoprogenitors, further aiding in the subsequent deposition of bone [2, 4]. The matrix-bound VEGF that is released is a key player in the formation of bone vasculature. HIFs regulate VEGF expression in bone, which has an effect on angiogenesis [2]. Thus VEGF, MMPs and HIFs play a central role in angiogenesis during endochondral ossification.

2.2. Vascular invasion of the cartilage

Vascular invasion of the cartilage template is the first major step in angiogenesis in the developing bone. The vasculature from the perichondrium penetrates the previously avascular cartilage and begins to invade the rest of the cartilage. Vascular invasion is coupled to a number of events in the cartilage, the degradation of the extracellular matrix by MMPs, which releases matrix-bound VEGF and favors the invasion of the cartilage, as well as apoptosis of the hypertrophic chondrocytes which were responsible for secreting many of the growth factors that resulted in the invasion [2, 4, 6]. As vasculature penetrates the cartilage and the hypertrophic chondrocytes undergo apoptosis, they are promptly replaced by osteoblasts in the resulting bone cavity (i.e., by the osteoblasts previously recruited by factors such as VEGF). These osteoblasts then secrete collagen type I to initiate ossification to form the bone matrix in the primary ossification center. The same growth factors in and around the growth plate of the bone will allow the vasculature to continue its invasion of the bone to the secondary ossification centers located at either ends of the long bone, in the same way that the primary ossification centers were formed [2].

Angiogenesis during endochondral ossification is heavily dependent on the cellular components of the skeleton, namely osteoblasts and chondrocytes. Without these cells, the valuable pro-angiogenic factors would not be properly secreted and will not be able to induce vascular invasion. However, the reverse is also true. In order for bone to continue to form properly, efficient and effective vascular invasion is required. The vasculature that invades cartilage likely also carries required factors for bone growth; the vascular epithelium is thought to carry osteoprogenitors, more VEGF, FGFs and other factors which assist with the resorption of the surrounding cartilage and the ossification of bone [6]. Without vasculature invading the cartilage, bone formation is impaired. A study on mouse long bones showed that expression of SOX9 can block the expression of VEGFA, which results in impaired vascular invasion, and as a result, the bones do not ossify [7]. (SOX9 is a key marker of chondrogenic condensations [1].) VEGF also plays a role in the ongoing maintenance of bone vasculature endogenous VEGF was shown to enhance vascularization of bone and subsequently allows more rapid healing of injured bones, indicating the role of vascularization in the formation and turnover of endochondral bone [6].

Along with VEGF, another key factor in the invasion of vasculature into bone is hypoxia. The lack of oxygen will result in the release of hypoxia-inducible factors (HIFs) which regulate the production of the extracellular matrix and VEGF expression. The matrix binds VEGF triggering vascular invasion. The HIFs expressed by osteoblasts support both the proper vascularization of bone as well as the proper functioning of osteoblasts. Increased expression of HIFs results in more vascularization and thicker bones, whereas deletion of HIFs (and the resulting reduced expression of VEGF) results in less vascularization and thinner bones [2]. Thus, VEGFs and HIFs are two major factors that couple angiogenesis to endochondral bone formation [2, 6].

Thus in summary, endochondral ossification is dependent on the interaction between pro-angiogenic factors acting on bone-forming cells (**Figure 1**), and endochondral ossification is impaired in the absence of these factors.

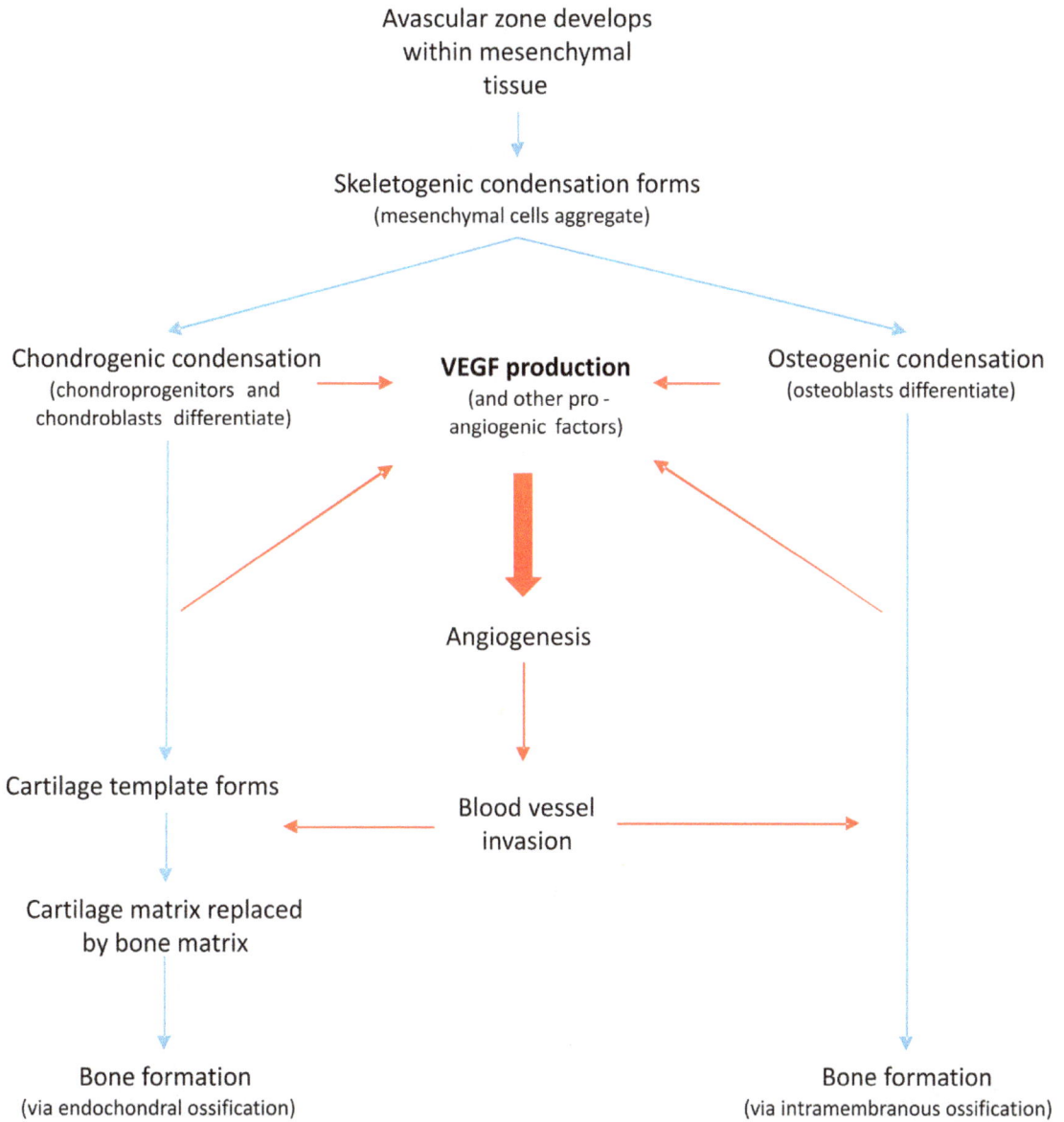

Figure 1. Schematic showing the complex cross talk between angiogenesis and skeletogenesis. Mesenchymal cells aggregate in an avascular (hypoxic) zone to form skeletogenic condensations. Differences in the molecular characteristics of these cells determine the fate of the condensation. Cells within this condensation produce VEGF and other pro-angiogenic factors, and this induces angiogenesis. Left side: Cells within the chondrogenic condensation continue to produce these angiogenic factors, and ultimately, the condensation differentiates into a cartilage template, which is still avascular. Following angiogenesis surrounding this template, blood vessels invade the cartilage perichondrium layer, and this triggers osteoblast differentiation, cartilage matrix degradation, bone matrix production and the further release of more pro-angiogenic factors. Ossification begins in the diaphysis (shaft) of long bones and spreads to the epiphyses (ends of the bone). Right side: As cells within the skeletogenic condensation differentiate, they continue to produce angiogenic factors. These factors induce angiogenesis and subsequent blood vessel invasion into the outer edges of the condensation. As more cells within the condensation differentiate, the wave of bone matrix deposition and blood vessel invasion spreads outwards.

3. Bones that ossify via intramembranous ossification

3.1. Directly ossifying bones

Intramembranously ossifying bones form without a cartilage template. Motile mesenchymal cells fated to differentiate into osteoblasts aggregate to from skeletogenic condensations at the site of the future bone. As these osteogenic aggregations enlarge and reach a critical size, the central cells begin to differentiate into osteoblasts, lose their mobility and deposit bone matrix. This process results in osteoblasts becoming embedded or trapped in bone matrix, forcing them to differentiate into osteocytes [8]. The majority of the craniofacial skeleton forms via intramembranous ossification [9]. A common example is the skull vault (the calvariae). Less common examples are the scleral ossicles (in reptiles), parts of the clavicles and scapula (in mammals), the cleithra and opercula (in fish) and sesamoid bones (e.g., the patella in humans) [9]. Although vascularization has been extensively studied in endochondral ossification as discussed above, comparatively little research has been conducted to understand the relationship between angiogenesis and intramembranous ossification.

3.2. Angiogenesis during formation of the initial phase of directly ossifying bones

The most studied intramembranous bones are the calvariae (or skull vault). Cells in the osteogenic condensations proliferate resulting in growth of the condensations until a critical size is reached. Ossification begins at the center of the condensation and expanding outwards toward the apex of the head [10]. Once this has occurred, cells at the osteogenic front proliferate, and the bones grow toward one another [11]. Areas that ossified first form a trabecular bone structure that later becomes woven bone [10]. Interestingly, the frontal and parietal bones in humans each develop two condensations, each with their own ossification centers; these centers then fuse as ossification progresses [12].

There is a significant difference in the gene expression patterns in prechondrogenic and preosteogenic condensations [1]. Avascularity within condensations may be necessary for the formation of the condensations themselves and/or to provide positional cues [10, 13]. Indeed, in scleral ossicles, an avascular zone develops surrounding the condensation [14, 15]. Manipulating the size of this avascular zone has a direct effect on subsequent bone development [15]. Although not much is known about the process of vascularization during intramembranous ossification, it is thought that similar to endochondral bones, hypoxic conditions are important to induce angiogenesis. Avascular zones likely surround all preosteogenic condensations in mammals and avians, however, the mechanism by which these zones are established is not known [10]. Percival and colleagues [10] postulate that this avascularity may be important for condensation growth, and subsequent intramembranous ossification (as in the case for prechondrogenic condensations of endochondrally ossifying bones, **Figure 1**).

A single study describes in detail, the association of angiogenesis and intramembranous bones [16]. This study of the development of the chick frontal bone showed that small capillaries invade the thin avascular layer of loose mesenchymal cells of the condensation prior to invading the condensation at/near the site of initial ossification [16]. This association between vascular invasion and ossification continues and cascades as the bone expands in all directions. As the bone mineralizes in the wake of this vascular invasion front, the internal and external vasculature is remodeled.

Based on studies of endochondral ossification and distraction osteogenesis, Percival and colleagues [10] recently developed a model of angiogenesis during intramembranous ossification. They propose that prior to the onset of mineralization, small capillaries begin to invade the surrounding avascular loose mesenchymal tissue due to the presence of pro-angiogenic factors. At around the time of mineralization onset, these capillaries invade the osteogenic condensations and branch outwards from the ossification center (**Figure 1**). These capillaries branch toward regions of pro-angiogenic factor expression and thus support the proliferating mesenchymal cells of the condensation. Mineralization thus first occurs at sites closest to the capillaries and then at sites progressively further away. Once the osteogenic condensation stops expanding, the capillaries along with the mineralization front continue to moves toward the presumptive sutures (i.e., the edges of the future bone), thus allowing continued calvarial growth.

Interestingly, while osteoblasts in endochondrally ossifying bones express both HIF1α and HIF2α, only HIF2α is detected in the osteoblasts of directly ossifying bones (i.e., those that undergo intramembranous ossification) [17]. This altered expression pattern of the HIFα subunits could suggest that alternative regulatory pathways trigger angiogenesis in these distinct types of ossification [17]. Percival and Richtsmeier [10] provide a comprehensive list of hypotheses relating to intramembranous osteogenesis and angiogenesis that require testing. The cross talk between these two dynamic processes is summarized in **Figure 1**.

4. Insights from cell culture and bone graft studies

VEGF is a chemoattractant for primary osteoblasts and mesenchymal progenitor cells [18] and can directly promote differentiation of primary human osteoblasts in culture in a dose-dependent manner [19]. Osteoblasts and mesenchymal stem cells are the two cell types most often used in bone tissue engineering. Interestingly, the type of cell used can influence the mode of ossification that occurs and the organization of blood vessels [20]. Implantation of osteoblasts leads to the formation of fibrous tissue and disorganized blood vessels. The osteoblasts become trapped in the secreted bone matrix (i.e., intramembranous ossification occurs). In contrast, implantation of stem cells leads to the formation of cartilaginous tissue (i.e., endochondral ossification) and well-organized blood vessels.

Basic fibroblast growth factor (bFGF) is another important pro-angiogenic factor. When bone mesenchymal stem cells were transfected with bFGF and then implanted into rats with calvarial defects, an increase in vascularization and osteogenesis was observed [21]. Similarly, the addition of sonic hedgehog (Shh) in engineered bone grafts *in vitro* also promotes vascularization of the grafts [22]. Shh is expressed during fracture healing and neovascularization after trauma and has been used *in vitro* to promote the organization of blood vessels in artificial tissue grafts similarly to VEGF [22, 23]. Furthermore, when these grafts were implanted subcutaneously in mice, there was increased bone formation of both directly and indirectly ossifying bone types [22]. For large defects, supplementing the graft with platelet-rich plasma results in increased bone formation [24].

5. Pathological implications

The role of growth factors like VEGF, FGF, CTGFs and others in both bone growth and angiogenesis has been demonstrated in a number of recent studies investigating the growth and healing of bones. For example, FGF9$^{+/-}$ mice exhibit a reduction in the healing of bones accompanied by a lack of VEGF expression in the area of injury, suggesting that FGF9 is required for angiogenesis and for healing long bones [25]. Hypomorphic VEGF$^{120/120}$ mice have reduced mineralization of the calvarial bones and consequently reduced bone thickness. This has been attributed to a reduction and delay in vascular invasion [26]. Additionally, conditional deletion of VEGFA in mice cranial neural crest cells causes cleft palate with reduced ossification of the mandibular bone due to reduced endothelial cell proliferation and decreased angiogenesis [27]. Mice with a VEGF-deficient osteoblastic lineage exhibit age-dependent loss of bone mass and increased bone marrow fat, similar to the changes associated with osteoporosis in humans [28].

6. Conclusions and summary

VEGF mediates angiogenesis, chondrocyte differentiation, osteoblast differentiation and osteoclast recruitment [29], and thus, its role during osteogenesis is complex ([10], **Figure 1**). Yang et al. [30] provide a useful tabulation of the effects of VEGF on intramembranous and endochondral ossification. Importantly, this chapter highlights that the relationship between angiogenesis and intramembranous ossification is not well understood. For example, only one study describes the detailed relationship between these two dynamic systems [16], and a very recent study provides a model of this process [10]. This model should be examined in several directly ossifying bones in the skeleton in order to confirm whether all directly ossifying bones follow the model or whether subtle differences exist depending perhaps on the location of the bone or the origin of the bone cells. This lack of a fundamental understanding about the developmental interactions between angiogenesis and skeletogenic condensations (particularly with respect to directly ossifying bones) contributes to our inadequate understanding of skull formation [10].

It should be noted that bones that ossify from the perichondrium of a cartilage template can be considered endochondral or intramembranous (since the perichondrium is a membrane of the cartilage). An example is Meckel's cartilage. The relationship between angiogenesis and bones that develop via the perichondrium has not been studied.

Acknowledgements

The authors acknowledge funding from the Natural Sciences and Engineering Research Council of Canada. We also acknowledge M. Bhade who collated literature for this book chapter.

Author details

Tamara A. Franz-Odendaal[1,2]*, Daniel Andrews[1] and Shruti Kumar[1,2]

*Address all correspondence to: tamara.franz-odendaal@msvu.ca

1 Mount Saint Vincent University, Nova Scotia, Canada

2 Saint Mary's University, Nova Scotia, Canada

References

[1] Eames BF, Helms JA: Conserved molecular program regulating cranial and appendicular skeletogenesis. Developmental Dynamics. 2004;231:4–13.

[2] Silvaraj KK, Adams RH: Blood vessel formation and function in bone. Development. 2016;513:2706–2715. doi:10.1242/dev.136861

[3] Liu ES, Raimann A, Chae BT, Martins JS, Baccarini M, Demay MB: C-Raf promotes angiogenesis during normal growth plate maturation. Development. 2016;143:348–355. doi:10.1242/dev.127142

[4] Ortega N, Wang K, Ferrara N, Werb Z, Vu TH: Complementary interplay between matrix metalloproteinase-9, vascular endothelial growth factor and osteoclast function drives endochondral bone formation. Disease Models and Mechanisms. 2010;3:224–235. doi:10.1242/dmm004226

[5] Berendsen AD, Olsen BR: How vascular endothelial growth factor-A (VEGF) regulated differentiation of mesenchymal stem cells. Journal of Histochemistry & Cytochemistry. 2014;62:103–108. doi:10.1369/0022155413516347

[6] Maes C: Role and regulation of vascularization processes in endochondral bones. Calcified Tissue International. 2013;92:307–323. doi:10.1007/s00223-012-9689-z

[7] Hattori T, Muller C, Gebhard S, Bauer E, Pausch F, Schlund B, Bosl MR, Hess A, Surmann-Schmitt C, von der Mark H, de Crombrugghe B, von der Mark K: SOX9 is a major negative regulator of cartilage vascularization, bone marrow formation and endochondral ossification. Development. 2010;137:901–911. doi:10.1242/dev.045203

[8] Franz-Odendaal TA, Hall BK, Witten PE: Buried alive: how osteoblasts become osteocytes. Developmental Dynamics. 2006;235:176–190.

[9] Franz-Odendaal, TA: Induction and patterning of intramembranous bone. (Special Issue – Signaling Mechanisms in Development) Frontiers in Biosciences. 2011;16: 2734–2746.

[10] Percival CJ, Richtsmeier JT: Angiogenesis and intramembranous osteogenesis. Developmental Dynamics. 2013;242(8):909–22.

[11] Rice R, Rice DP, Olsen BR, Thesleff I: Progression of calvarial bone development requires Foxc1 regulation of Msx2 and Alx4. Developmental Biology. 2003;262(1):75–87.

[12] Lemier RJ: Embryology of the skull. In Craniosynostosis: Diagnosis, Evaluation and Management. Cohen MM Jr. ed. Raven Press, New York, Chapter 5; 1986.

[13] Yin M, Pacifici M: Vascular regression is required for mesenchymal condensation and chondrogenesis in the developing limb. Devlopmental Dynamics. 2001;222:5–533.

[14] Jourdeuil K, Franz-Odendaal TA: Vasculogenesis and the induction of skeletogenic condensations in the avian eye. The Anatomical Record. 2012;285:691–698.

[15] Jabalee J, Franz-Odendaal TA: Vascular endothelial growth factor signaling regulates angiogenesis and osteogenesis during the development of scleral ossicles. Developmental Biology 2015:406:52–62.

[16] Thompson TJ, Owens PD, Wilson DJ: Intramembranous osteogenesis and angiogenesis in the chick embryo. Journal of Anatomy. 1989;166:55–65.

[17] De Spiegelaere W, Cornillie P, Casteleyn C, Burvenich C, Van Den Broeck W: Detection of hypoxia inducible factors and angiogenic growth factors during foetal endo-chondral and intramembranous ossification. Anatomia, Histologia, Embryologia. 2010;39(4):376–384.

[18] Fiedler J, Leucht F, Waltenberger J. et al.: VEGF-A and PIGF-1 stimulate chemotactic migration of human mesenchymal progenitor cells. Biochemical and Biophysical Research Communications. 2005;334(2):561–568.

[19] Street J, Bao M, deGuzman L. et al.: Vascular endothelial growth factor stimulates bone repair by promoting angiogenesis and bone turnover. Proceedings of the National Academy of Sciences of the United States of America. 2002;99(15):9656–9661.

[20] Tortelli F, Tasso R, Loiacono F, Cancedda R: The development of tissue-engineered bone of different origin through endochondral and intramembranous ossification following the implantation of mesenchymal stem cells and osteoblasts in a murine model. Biomaterials. 2010;31(2):242–249.

[21] Qu D, Li J, Li Y, Gao Y, Zuo Y, Hsu Y, Hu J: Angiogenesis and osteogenesis enhanced by bFGF ex vivo gene therapy for bone tissue engineering in reconstruction of calvarial defects. Journal of Biomedical Materials Research Part A. 2011;96(3):543–551.

[22] Rivron NC, Raiss CC, Liu J, Nandakumar A, Sticht C, Gretz N, Truckenmüller R, Rouwkema J, van Blitterswijk CA: Sonic Hedgehog-activated engineered blood ves-

sels enhance bone tissue formation. Proceedings of the National Academy of Sciences. 2012;109(12):4413–4418.

[23] Correia C, Grayson WL, Park M, Hutton D, Zhou B, Guo XE, Niklason L, Sousa RA, Reis RL, Vunjak-Novakovic G: In vitro model of vascularized bone: synergizing vascular development and osteogenesis. PLoS One. 2011;6(12):e28352.

[24] Dong Z, Li B, Liu B, Bai S, Li G, Ding A, Zhao J, Liu Y: Platelet-rich plasma promotes angiogenesis of prefabricated vascularized bone graft. Journal of Oral and Maxillofacial Surgery. 2012;70(9):2191–2197.

[25] Behr B, Leucht P, Longaker MT, Quarto N: *Fgf-9* is required for angiogenesis and osteogenesis in long bone repair. PNAS. 2010;107:11853–11858. doi:10.1073/pnas.100331710.

[26] Zelzer E, McLean W, Ng YS, Fukai N, Reginato AM, Lovejoy S, D'Amore PA, Olsen BR: Skeletal defects in VEGF120/120 mice reveal multiple roles for VEGF in skeletogenesis. Development. 2002;129(8):1893–1904.

[27] Hill C, Jacobs B, Kennedy L, Rohde S, Zhou B, Baldwin S, Goudy S: Cranial neural crest deletion of VEGFa causes cleft palate with aberrant vascular and bone development. Cell and Tissue Research. 2015;361(3):711–722.

[28] Lui Y, Olsen BR: Distinct VEGF functions during bone development and homeostasis. Archivum Immunologiae et Therapiae Experimentalis. 2014;62:363–368.

[29] Zelzer E, Olsen BR: Multiple roles of vascular endothelial growth factor (VEGF) in skeletal development, growth, and repair. Current Topics in Developmental Biology. 2004;65:169–187.

[30] Yang Y, Tan Y, Wong R, Wenden A, Zhang L, Rabie ABM: The role of vascular endothelial growth factor in ossification. International Journal of Oral Science. 2012;4:64–68. doi:10.1038/ijos.2012.33

10

Novel Methods to Study Angiogenesis Using Tissue Explants

Tomoko Takahashi, Keiko Fujita and Masumi Akita

Abstract

Tissue explants of skeletal muscles, brain, kidney, liver and spleen from mice were cultured using collagen gel. Electron microscopic observation revealed that formation of capillary tubes with pericyte-like cells occurred only from the tissue explant of skeletal muscles. The capillary tubes formed in the collagen gel were positive for tomato lectin and platelet/endothelial cell adhesion molecule (PCAM)-1 antibody. Formation of capillary tubes in the rat was more predominant than in the mouse. Plasmalemmal vesicles were clearly observed in the capillary tubes from rat tissue explant. Muscle fiber-type differences were also observed. In the soleus muscle, the formation of capillary tubes was predominant than the tibialis anterior muscle. Using this culture model from the rat soleus muscle, effects of α-isoproterenol (β-adrenergic receptor agonist) and low-frequency electrical stimulation were examined on the formation of capillary tubes and fine structures of skeletal muscle explant. The formation of capillary tubes was promoted by α-isoproterenol administration. At low-frequency electrical stimulation, the formation of capillary tubes was inhibited. Both α-isoproterenol and electrical stimulation reduced the degeneration of skeletal muscles. This culture method of skeletal muscles may provide a useful model that can examine the effects of various drugs and physical stimulations.

Keywords: angiogenesis, skeletal muscles, collagen gel culture, α-isoproterenol, low-frequency electrical stimulation

1. Introduction

To study the process of angiogenesis and test new agents with angiogenic or anti-angiogenic potential, suitable assays are essential [1]. For in vitro studies of angiogenesis, several culture techniques have been developed. The most commonly used in vivo assays are the chorioallantoic membrane (CAM) assay, the corneal micropocket assay and the dorsal skin-fold assay [2–5]. The corneal micropocket assay, an analysis conducted within an avascular environment, is often used to study the efficacy of angiogenic compounds. The efficacy of anti-angiogenic compounds in inhibiting growth factor-induced vascularization and spontaneous vascularization is usually studied in vascular environments such as the CAM assay or the dorsal skin-fold assay. These assays have proven useful and have dramatically advanced our knowledge of angiogenesis. However, they are also limited in several respects (for a detailed review see Refs. [6, 7]) : (a) complicated surgical techniques are required; (b) only a limited number of test compounds can be assayed (e.g., in the case of the micropocket assay); and (c) simultaneous assessment of both angiogenic and anti-angiogenic compounds in the same assay is not feasible without the addition of exogenous growth factors. Fortunately, the method using collagen gel is free from these limitations. Collagen gel culture has been widely used for analyzing the biological process of angiogenesis [8–11]. Using the collagen gel culture, we have conducted electron microscopic studies and immunohistochemical studies during angiogenesis. In the collagen gel culture of aortic explants, capillary tubes with pericyte-like cells were observed [12]. As a source of angiogenesis, however, aortic explants were generally used in the collagen gel culture. Capillary permeability varies greatly among tissues, and this can be correlated partly with the type of endothelium. For simulation of angiogenesis, establishment of suitable in vitro model of capillaries might be effective. The endothelial cells of some capillaries have fenestrations or pores. For instance, fenestrated capillaries occur in renal glomeruli. Capillaries without fenestrations in the brain and skeletal muscle are known as continuous capillaries. As discontinuous capillaries, there are sinusoids. Sinusoids occur in large numbers in the liver and spleen [13].

In this study, we report the formation of capillary tubes from tissue explants of skeletal muscle, brain, kidney, liver and spleen from mice was cultured using collagen gel. Electron microscopic observation revealed that the formation of capillary tubes with pericyte-like cells occurred only from the skeletal muscle explant. Lectin and immunohistochemical studies showed that the capillary tubes formed in the collagen gel have architecture of capillary in vivo. There were some differences regarding the formation of capillary tubes among animal species and fiber types. We demonstrated that the soleus muscle from rats was most suitable model to study angiogenesis. Using tissue explant from the rat soleus muscle, effects of α-isoproterenol and low-frequency electrical stimulation were examined.

2. Materials and methods

2.1. Collagen gel culture

This collagen culture technique is a modification of our previous works [14, 15]. Samples (soleus muscles, cerebral cortex of frontal lobe, liver, cortex of kidney and spleen) were obtained from 1-month-old ICR male mice ($n = 5$). The samples were cut into small pieces (2 $\times$ 2 $\times$ 2 mm) under a stereoscopic microscope. The small pieces were placed at the bottom of tissue culture dish (35 mm; $n = 25$). Each tissue culture dish consists four pieces. An even layer of reconstituted collagen solution (0.3% Cellmatrix type IA, Nitta Gelatin, Tokyo, Japan) was

overlaid and gelled at 37°C for about 10 min. After gelation, Ham's F-12 medium (Invitrogen Corp., Carlsbad, CA, USA) containing 20% fetal bovine serum (FBS), 1% nonessential amino acids, 100 units/ml of penicillin and 100 mg/ml of streptomycin (Invitrogen Corp., Carlsbad, CA, USA) was added. Cultures were performed for 14 days in an incubator (95% air/5% CO_2). During the culture period, a phase contrast microscope was used to observe the capillary tube formation. These experiments were made three times. To examine the differences in animal species and fiber type, explants from skeletal muscles (soleus and tibialis anterior muscles) from rats were cultured as described above. All animal experiments were approved by the Committee on Animal Experimentation, Saitama Medical University (Permission No. 851 for mice and No. 934 for rats) and carried out in accordance with the "Guidelines for Animal Experimentation at Saitama Medical University."

2.2. Electron microscopy

The cultured materials were fixed with 2.5% glutaraldehyde in 0.1 M phosphate buffer (pH 7.2) for 1 h and then fixed with 1% OsO_4 in 0.1 M phosphate buffer (pH 7.2) for another hour. After dehydration with ethanol, samples were embedded in epoxy resin. After preparation of ultrathin sections, ultrathin sections were stained with uranyl acetate and lead citrate. Kajikawa's tannic acid stain was also used for demonstrating of elastic fibers [16]. The stained ultrathin sections were observed under a transmission electron microscope (JEOL JEM-1010, Tokyo, Japan). When capillary-like structures were observed, following lectin and immuno-histochemistry were performed.

2.3. Lectin and immunohistochemistry

After fixation with cold 80% ethanol, capillary tubes were observed with FITC-conjugated endothelial cell-specific tomato lectin (*Lycopersicon esculentum*; EY Labo, CA, USA), a lectin that selectively binds to fucose residues on the endothelial cell surface [17]. Cold 80% ethanol-fixed, collagen gel-embedded specimens were stained by streptavidin/peroxidase immuno-histochemistry technique for intercellular adhesion molecule-1 (ICAM-1), platelet/endothelial cell adhesion molecule-1 (PCAM-1) and integrin β_2 detection. The specimens were treated with 0.3% H_2O_2 in methanol to block endogenous peroxide activity and then incubated with the polyclonal rabbit anti-rat ICAM-1, PCAM-1 or integrin β_2 antibody (Santa Cruz Biotechnology, Inc. California, USA). Biotinylated anti-rabbit immunoglobulin was added as a secondary antibody. The horseradish peroxidase labeled streptavidin-biotin complex was then used to detect the second antibody. Finally, the specimens were stained with 3,3'-diaminobenzidine, which was used as a chromogen. The brown or dark brown stained cells were considered as positive. Some specimens were stained with Giemsa before being examined under a light microscope.

2.4. Effects of α-isoproterenol and low-frequency electrical stimulation

Excised material was divided into three groups as follows:

a. α-isoproterenol administration group (n = 48): To the culture medium, 10 μM α- isoproterenol was added [18].

b. low-frequency electrical stimulation group (n = 24): Using C-Dish (ION Optix, Milton, MA, USA), electrical stimulation (50 Hz, 2 h at 1.0 V; [19]) was performed by Ohm Pulser LFP-4000 A (Zen Iryoki corp, Fukuoka, Japan).

c. control group (n = 48): without α-isoproterenol and low-frequency electrical stimulation.

2.5. Semiquantitative enzyme-linked immunosorbent assay (ELISA)

Eight different cytokines involved in angiogenesis in the culture medium were semiquantified by ELISA (Signosis; Angiogenesis ELISA Strip, Santa Clara, CA, USA). Tumor necrosis factor (TNF)-α, vascular endothelial growth factor (VEGF), interleukin (IL)-6, fibroblast growth factor (FGF)-2, interferon (IFN)-γ, leptin, insulin-like growth factor (IGF)-1 and epidermal growth factor (EGF) were tested. ELISA was carried out according to the manufacturer's instructions. Outline is as follows. Eight wells were coated with eight different primary antibodies against a specific angiogenesis cytokine. The test sample was sandwiched between the primary antibody and enzyme-linked antibody. After incubation, unbound-labeled antibodies were washed out. TMB (3,3',5,5'-tetramethylbenzidine) is added, and the color developed. After addition of stop solution, absorbance is measured spectrophotometrically at 450 nm. The concentrations of the test samples are directly proportional to the color intensity. Data were shown as fold change relative control group.

2.6. Measurement of the length of the capillary tubes

Digital photography equipment (FUJIX DIGITAL CAMERA HC-2500, 3CCD, FUJI PHOTO FILM, Tokyo, Japan) was used with an optical microscope (objective lens ×5). Because capillary tubes were overlapped in the vicinity of the explant, it is impossible to identify each other. Length of capillary tubes was measured from a distance of 200 μm of the outer edge of the explant. Using six culture dishes (four pieces of the explant per dish), capillary tubes captured by the objective lens ×5 (1262 × 991 pixel). It was taken four places of one explant.

2.7. Statistical analysis

Tube formation from the soleus and tibialis anterior muscles of rats is quantified by measuring the length of these capillary tubes in two-dimensional microscope images of six culture dishes. Data were shown as means ± standard error of the mean. Statistical analysis for the data represented was conducted using two samples, with Mann–Whitney U test. A particular result was considered significant if the p value was <0.01 for a two-tailed test.

3. Results

3.1. Collagen gel culture

3.1.1. Skeletal muscles

After 2 days, some cells were migrating in the collagen gel in the vicinity of the explants (**Figure 1a**). Spindle-shaped cells were orientated radially to the explant. After 6–7 days, the cell strands were recognized. At this time, lumen formation could not be clearly demonstrated

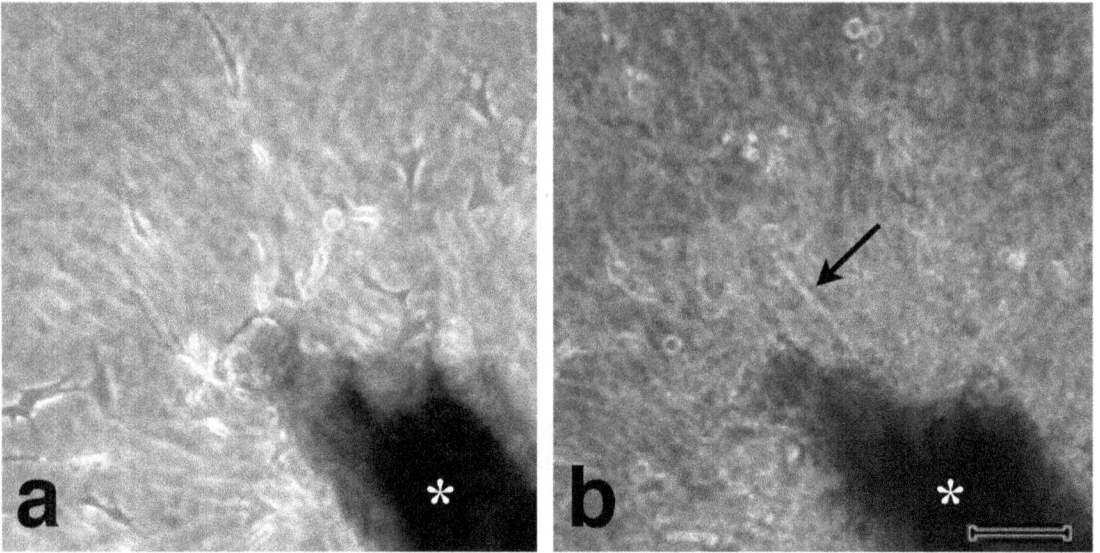

Figure 1. Mouse soleus muscle. (a) After 2 days of cultivation, phase-contrast microscopy reveals fibroblastic cells outgrown from a mouse skeletal muscle explant (*) into a three-dimensional collagen gel. (b) After 6 days of cultivation, phase-contrast microscopy shows a tubular structure protruding (arrow) from a mouse skeletal muscle explant (*) into a three-dimensional collagen gel. Scale bar:90 μm.

(**Figure 1b**). After 10 days, the capillary tube formation with lumen was well demonstrated by electron microscopic observation. As revealed by cross section, several endothelial cells with pericyte-like cells were involved in the composition of capillary tubes (**Figure 2a, b**). The structure as capillary tubes was maintained at least 2 weeks. When the culture was continued, degradation of the capillary tubes was observed.

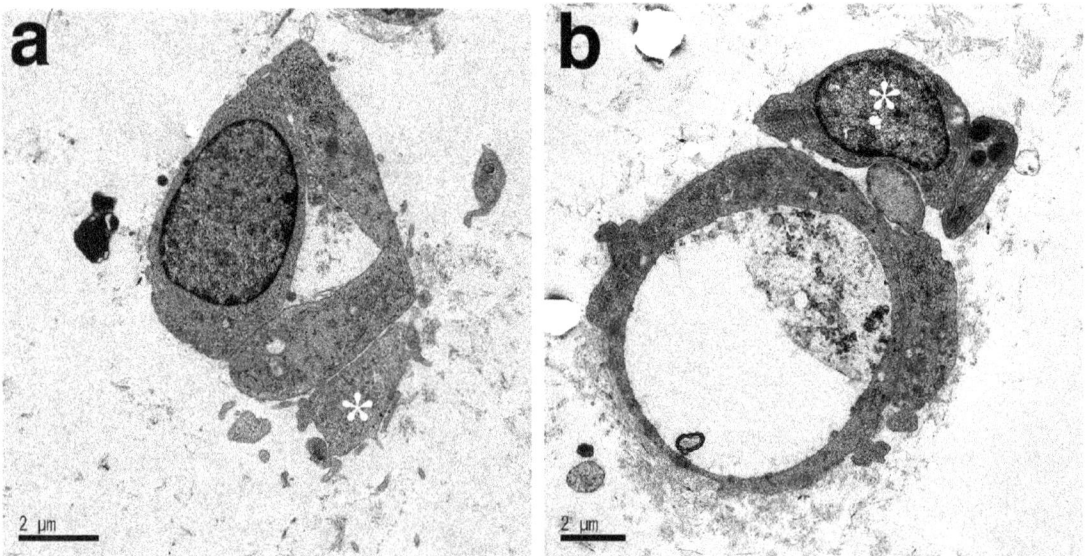

Figure 2. Mouse soleus muscle. (a, b) Electron micrographs of capillary tubes. In a cross section of capillary tube, the lumen is surrounded by two to three cells. Pericyte-like cells (*) are associated with the capillary tube. Scale bar: 2 μm.

3.1.2. Cerebral cortex of frontal lobe

After 3–4 days, spindle-shaped cells were migrated from the explants. The number was quite few. The strand of spindle-shaped cells was elongated (**Figure 3a**). The longitudinal axis was orientated radially to the stump. As revealed by cross section, several cells surrounded a cell with elastic membrane-like structure. Tube formation with lumen was not recognized (**Figure 3b**).

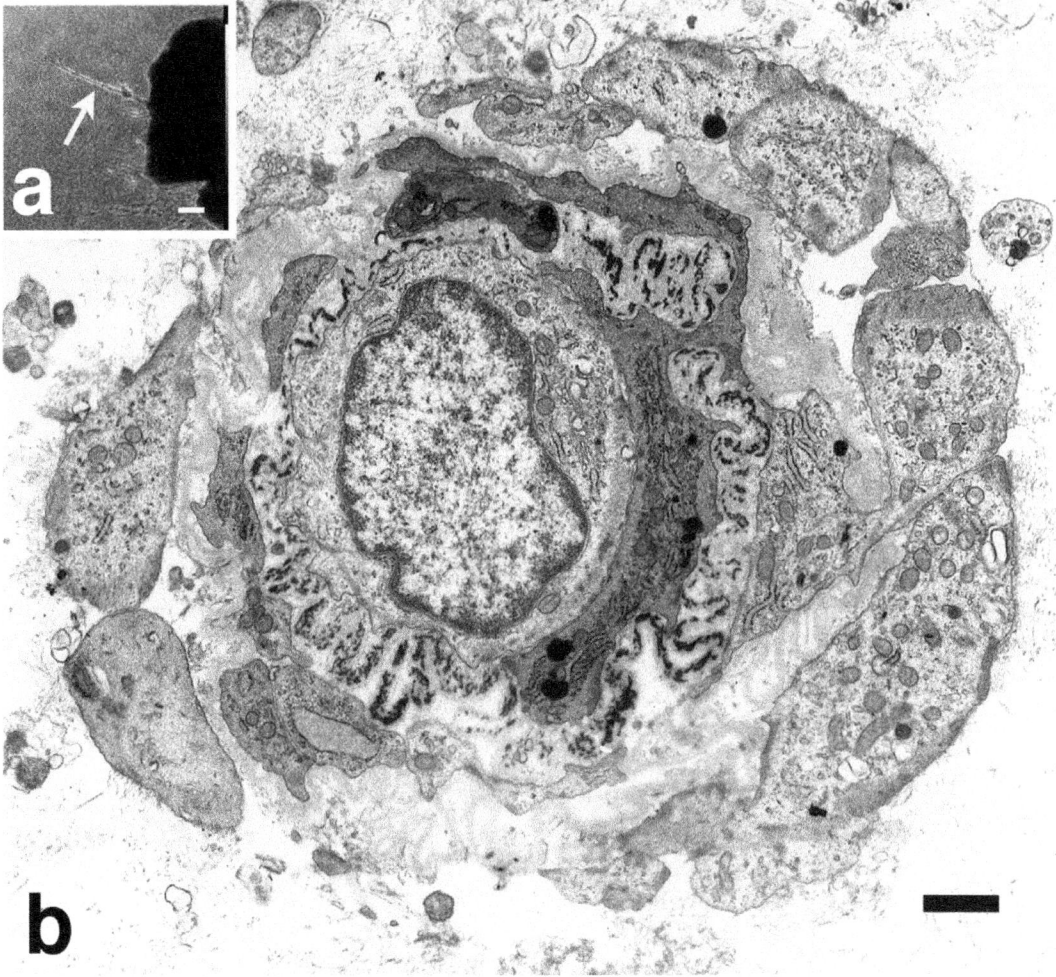

Figure 3. Mouse brain. (a) After 12 days of cultivation, a phase-contrast microphotograph shows tube formation (arrow) from mouse cortex of brain into a three-dimensional collagen gel. Scale bar: 50 μm. (b) An electron microphotograph of the collagen gel-induced tube formation. A cross section shows no lumen. Kajikawa's tannic acid stain for elastic fibers. Electron dense materials are defined among cells. Scale bar:1 μm.

3.1.3. Cortex of kidney

After 3–4 days, spindle- and cobblestone-shaped cells were migrated from the explants. The strands of spindle-shaped cells were elongated (**Figure 4a**). As revealed by cross section, several cells were attached each other and formed cellular mass (**Figure 4b**). Some area, a single cell, formed the outline of a tube with a lumen. A cell of the wall was consisted of microvilli (**Figure 4c**).

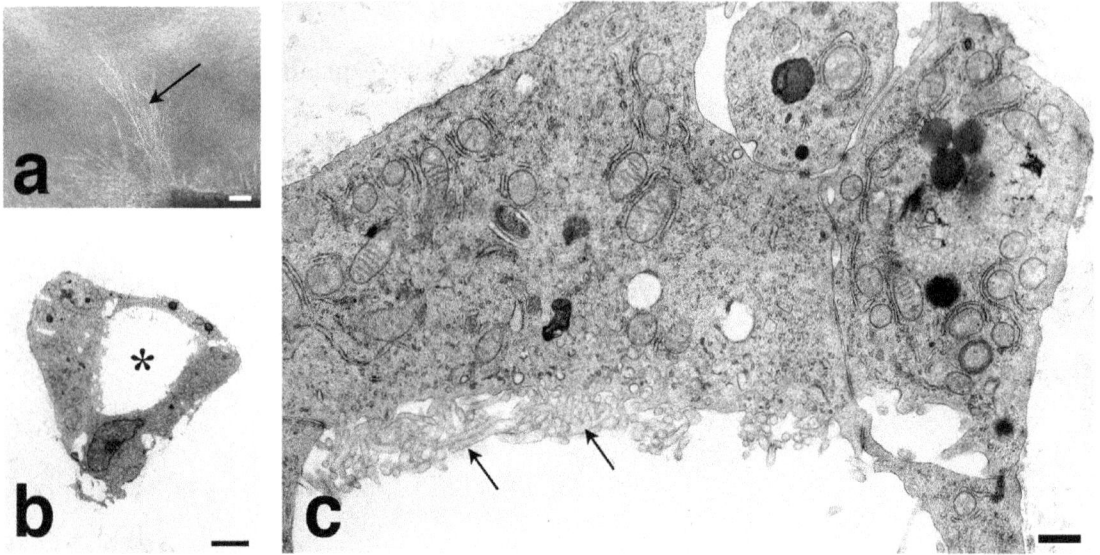

Figure 4. Mouse kidney. (a) After 7 days of cultivation, a phase-contrast microphotograph shows tube-like structure (arrow) from mouse cortex of kidney into a three-dimensional collagen gel. Scale bar: 50 μm. (b) An electron microphotograph of the collagen gel-induced tube-like structure. A cross section shows lumen (*). Scale bar: 2 μm. (c) Enlarged electron microphotograph of the cells showed in (b). Arrows indicate microvilli. Scale bar: 500 nm.

3.1.4. Liver

After 3–4 days, spindle-shaped cells were migrated from the explants. The strands of spindle-shaped cells were elongated (**Figure 5a**). As revealed by cross section, several cells were attached each other and formed cellular mass (**Figure 5b**).

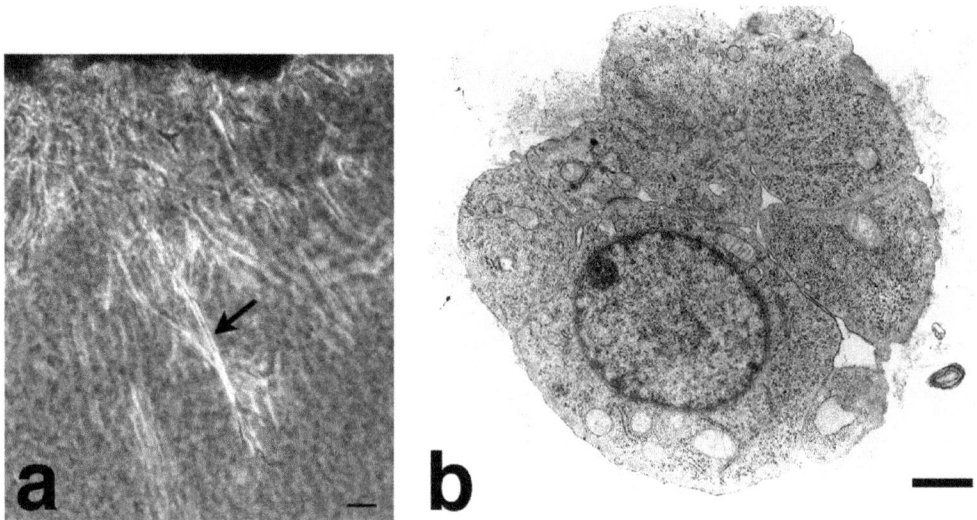

Figure 5. Mouse liver. (a) After 10 days of cultivation, a phase-contrast microphotograph shows tube-like structure (arrow) from mouse liver into a three-dimensional collagen gel. Scale bar: 50 μm. (b) An electron microphotograph of the collagen gel-induced tube-like structure. A cross section shows tightly connected cells. Scale bar: 1 μm.

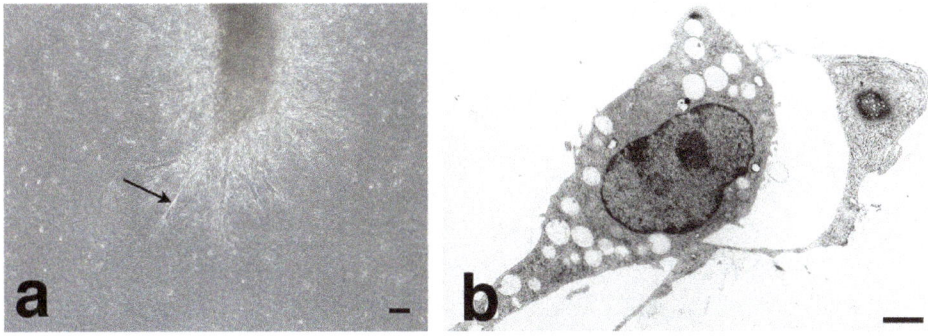

Figure 6. Mouse spleen. (a) After 7 days of cultivation, a phase-contrast microphotograph shows tube-like structure (arrow) from mouse spleen into a three-dimensional collagen gel. Scale bar: 50 μm. (b) An electron microphotograph of the collagen gel-induced tube-like structure. A cross section shows loosely contacted cells. Scale bar: 1 μm.

3.1.5. Spleen

After 2 days, numerous cells were migrated from the explants. Numerous cell strands of spindle-shaped cells were elongated (**Figure 6a**). Some cells were partly contacted, but distinct lumen was not observed (**Figure 6b**).

3.2. Lectin and immunohistochemistry

Since capillary tubes were observed only from the skeletal muscle explants, lectin and immunohistochemistry with antibodies were performed only for the cultured materials from skeletal muscle explants. Capillary tubes formed in the collagen gel were strongly positive for tomato lectin (**Figure 7**). Capillary tubes formed from the explants of muscles showed clearly

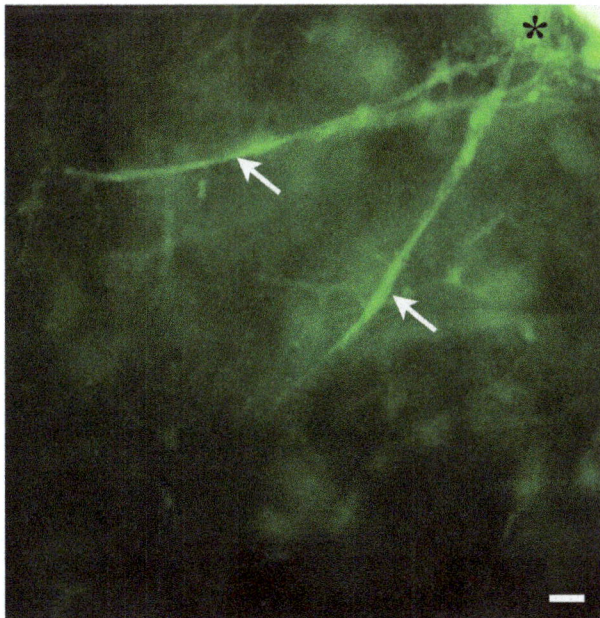

Figure 7. Mouse soleus muscle. After 11 days of cultivation, a fluorescent microphotograph of capillary tube (arrows). Capillary tube is strongly positive for FITC-conjugated endothelial cell-specific tomato lectin. Asterisk shows a muscle tissue explant. Scale bar: 50 μm.

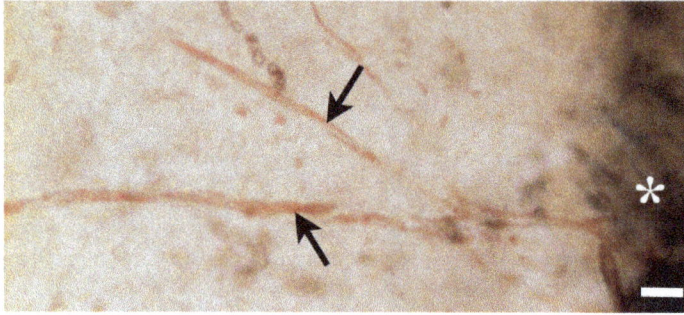

Figure 8. Mouse soleus muscle. Capillary tubes (arrows) showed clearly immunoreactivity of PCAM-1. Asterisk shows a muscle tissue explant. Scale bar: 50 μm.

immunoreactivity of PCAM-1 (**Figure 8**). ICAM-1 and integrin β_2 positive cells were sparsely distributed, but capillary tubes were almost negative (figure not shown).

3.3. Species difference in capillary tube formation from the skeletal muscle explant

In rats, numerous and long capillary tubes were observed from an explant. In mice, capillary tubes were few in number and short. Even without the statistical analysis, the difference is apparent (**Figure 9a, b**). Capillary tubes from rats were also positive for tomato lectin (**Figure 9c**) and PCAM-1 antibody (figure not shown). By electron microscopic observation, plasmalemmal vesicles or caveolae were clearly observed (**Figure 10a, b**). Typical gap junctions and tight junctions were not observed. Larger capillary tubes were also observed (**Figure 11**).

3.4. Difference in capillary tube formation between the soleus and tibialis anterior muscles

In the soleus muscle containing a large amount of red muscle fibers, the formation of capillary tube was predominant than the tibialis anterior muscle containing a large amount of white muscle fibers (**Figure 12a, b**). **Figure 13** indicates the results of statistical analysis.

3.5. Effects of α-isoproterenol and low-frequency electrical stimulation

3.5.1. α-Isoproterenol

Fine structures of explant: compared with the control group, the α-isoproterenol administration group was kept striated pattern (**Figure 14a, b**).

Formation of capillary tubes: in the α-isoproterenol administration group was seen promoting effect on the formation of capillary tubes (**Figure 15a, b**).

3.5.2. Low-frequency electrical stimulation

Fine structures of explant: compared with the control group, the low-frequency electrical stimulation group was kept striated pattern (**Figure 14a, c**).

Formation of capillary tubes: compared with the control group, the formation of capillary tubes was suppressed. Also, it appeared to have led to damage to the migratory cells (**Figure 15a, c**). **Figure 16** indicates the results of statistical analysis.

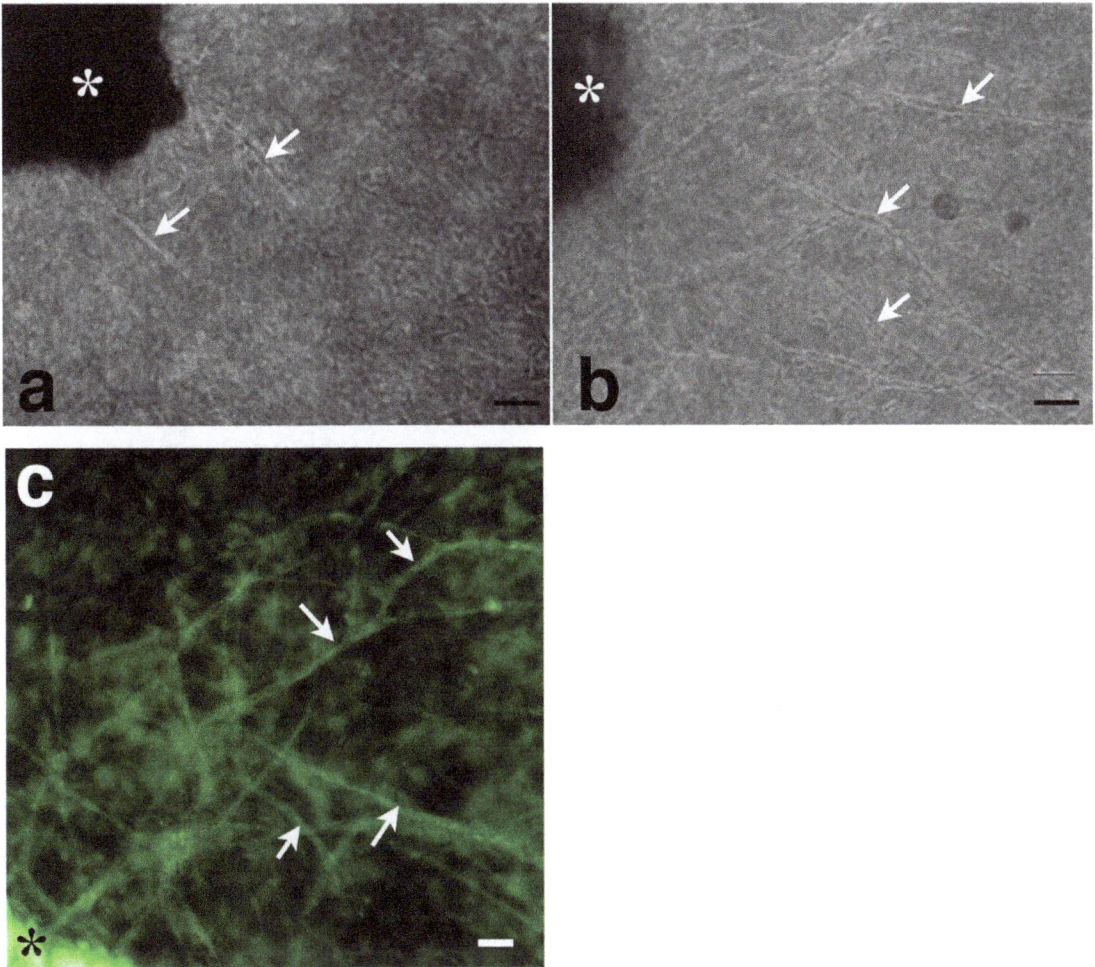

Figure 9. After 10 days of cultivation of soleus muscles. (a) Mouse soleus muscle, (b) rat soleus muscle. Phase-contrast microphotographs. Arrows indicate numerous and long capillary tubes. Scale bar: 90 μm. (c) Rat soleus muscle, tomato lectin staining. Arrows indicate numerous and long capillary tubes (cf. **Figure 7**). Scale bar: 50 μm. Asterisks show a muscle tissue explant.

3.6. ELISA

Compared with the culture medium, significant difference ($p < 0.01$) was observed only in the concentration of FGF-2 in the culture medium of the mouse soleus muscle. In the rat, no significant difference was observed. No significant difference in the concentration of eight kinds of angiogenic factor was observed between the soleus and tibialis anterior muscles from the rat and mouse (data not shown). In the α-isoproterenol administration group, increase in leptin was observed in the rat soleus muscle. However, no significant difference was observed. In the electrical stimulation group, increase in angiogenic factors except for the TNF-alpha was observed. Significant difference ($p < 0.01$) was seen in the concentration of the VEGF, FGF-2 and EGF (**Table 1**).

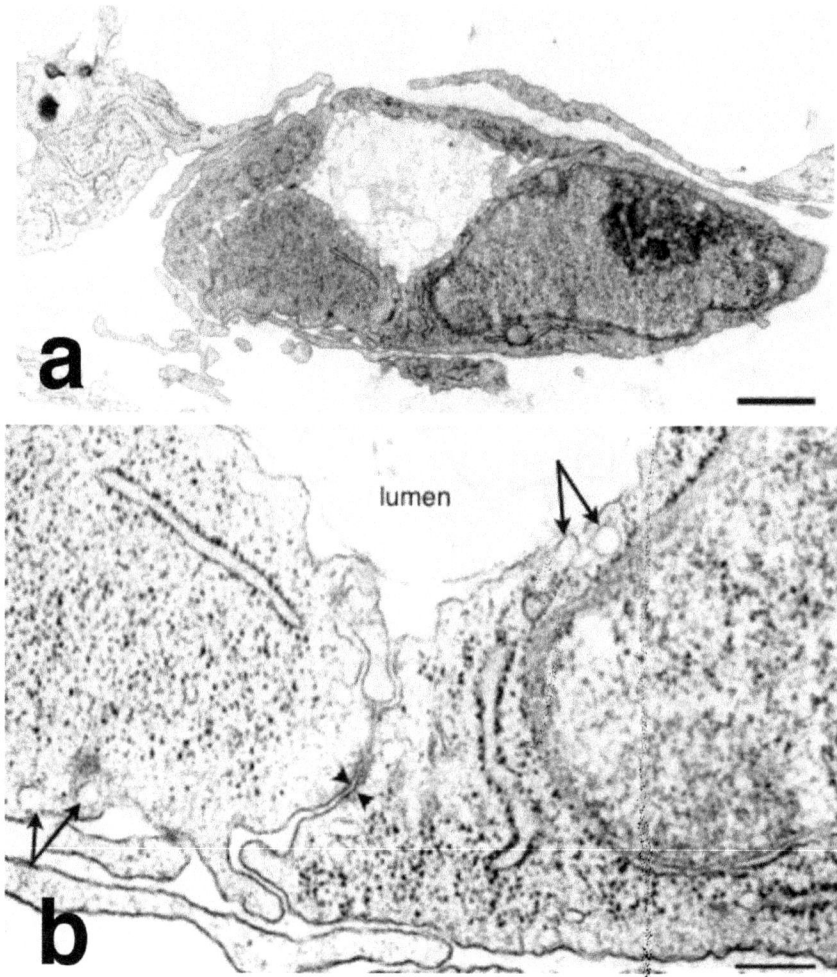

Figure 10. Rat soleus muscle. (a) Electron micrograph of capillary tube from rat soleus muscle. In a cross section of capillary tube, the lumen is surrounded by two to three cells. Scale bar: 1 μm. (b) Higher magnification of a part of (a). Arrowheads indicate a focal adhesion or an adherens junction. Arrows indicate plasmalemmal vesicles or caveolae. Scale bar: 200 nm.

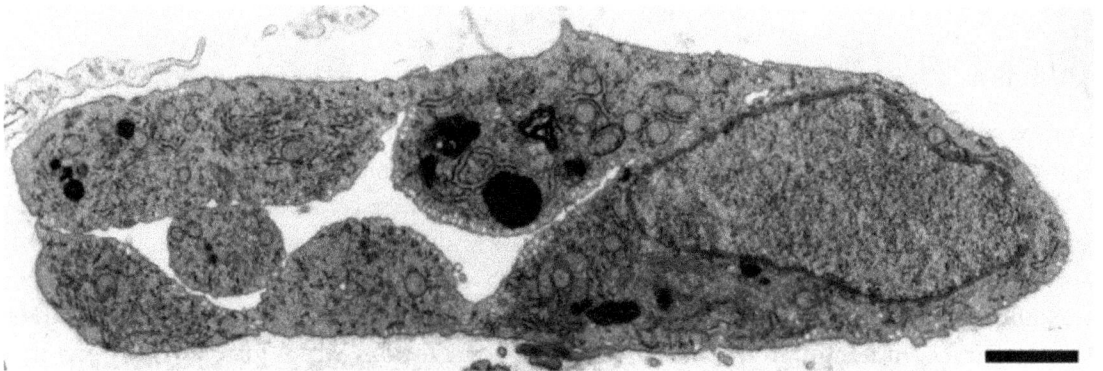

Figure 11. Rat soleus muscle. Electron micrograph of a large capillary tube. The wall is made up by five cells. Scale bar: 1 μm.

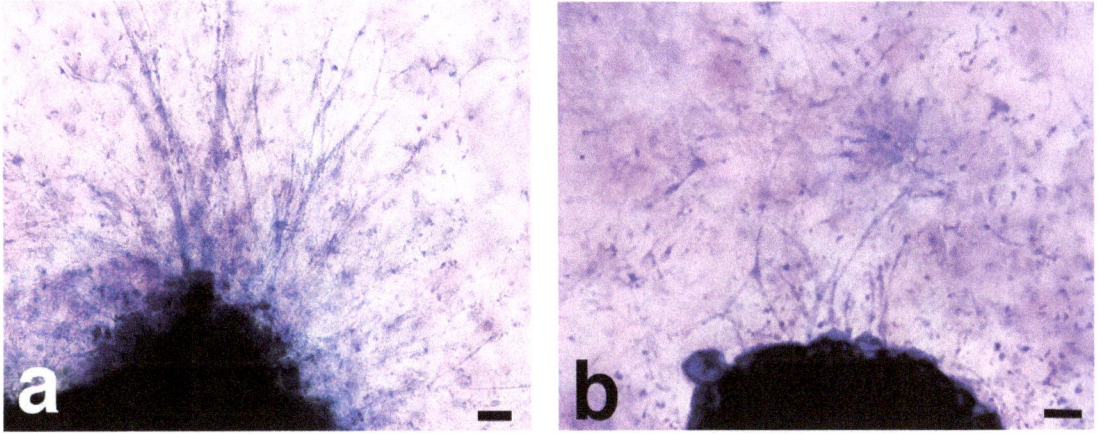

Figur 12. Capillary density of rat soleus and tibialis anterior muscles. (a) Rat soleus muscle, (b) rat tibialis anterior muscle. Capillary tubes were stained by Giemsa solution. Scale bar: 50 μm.

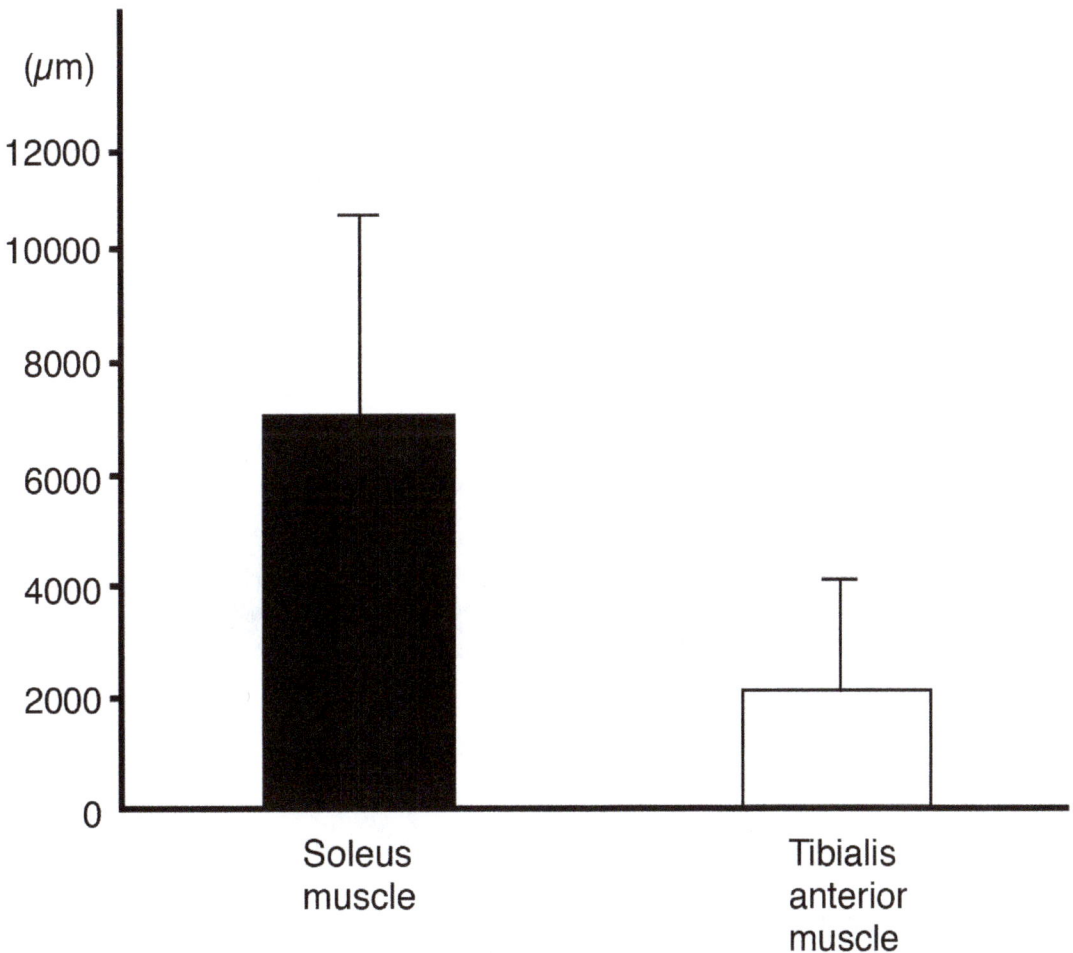

Figure 13. Statistical analysis of length of capillary tubes. Capillary density of soleus muscles had significantly greater than tibialis anterior muscles at $p < 0.01$.

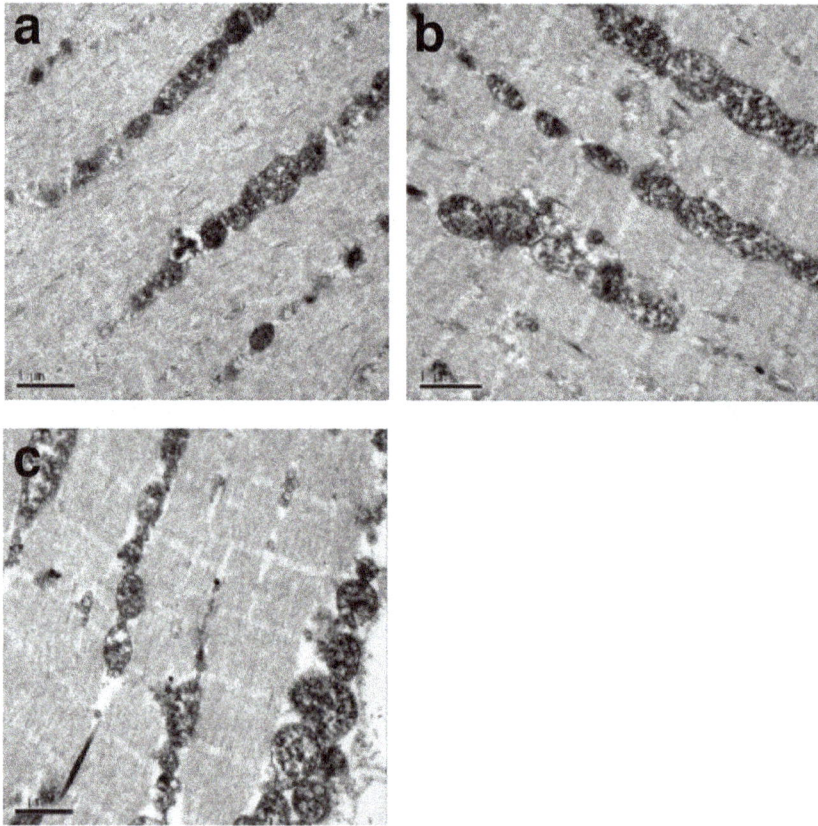

Figure 14. Electron micrographs of tissue explants of rat soleus muscle. (a) Control, (b) α-isoproterenol administration, (c) electrical stimulation. Both α-isoproterenol and electrical stimulation reduced the degeneration of skeletal muscles. Banding pattern of skeletal muscles is maintained when compared to the control. Scale bar: 1 μm.

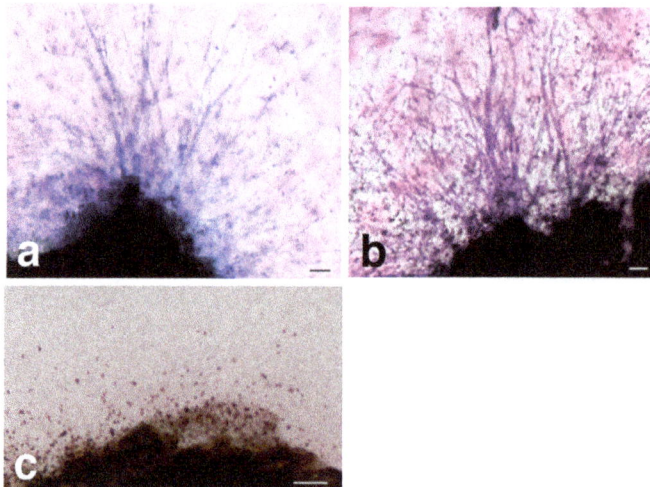

Figure 15. Rat soleus muscle. Effects of α-isoproterenol administration and electrical stimulation. Numerous capillary tubes were observed both control and α-isoproterenol administration groups. No capillary tubes were observed in the electrical stimulation group. (a) Control, rat soleus muscle. (b) α-Isoproterenol administration. (c) Electrical stimulation. Capillary tubes were stained by Giemsa solution. Numerous capillary tubes were observed both control and α-isoproterenol administration groups. No capillary tubes were observed in the electrical stimulation group. Scale bar: 100 μm.

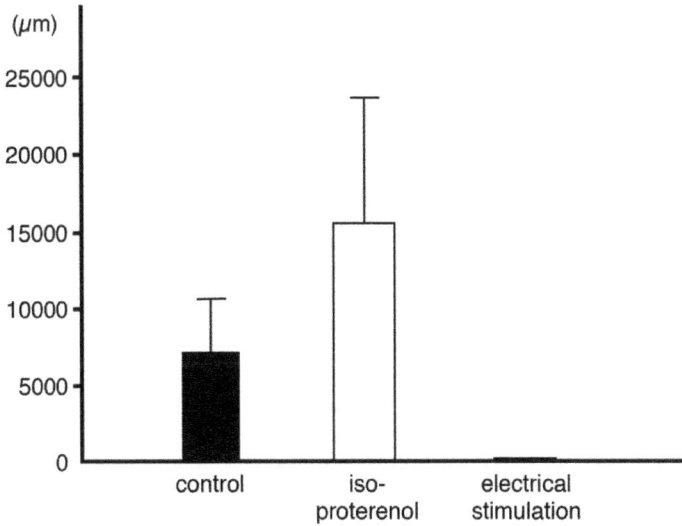

Figure 16. Statistical analysis of length of capillary tubes. Control: rat soleus muscle. The formation of capillary tubes was promoted by α-isoproterenol administration. At low-frequency electrical stimulation, the formation of capillary tubes was inhibited. Capillary density of α-isoproterenol administration group had significantly greater than control group at $p < 0.01$.

	Control	α-Isoproterenol	Electric stimulation
TNF-α	1	1.040	1.016
VEGF	1	0.843	1.542*
IL-6	1	0.980	1.350
FGF-2	1	0.912	1.335*
IFN-γ	1	0.969	1.286
Leptin	1	1.232	1.446
IGF-1	1	0.913	1.003
EGF	1	1.027	1.313*

Data were shown as fold change relative control. In the α-isoproterenol administration group, no significant difference was observed. In the electrical stimulation group, significant difference (*$p < 0.01$) was seen in the concentration of the VEGF, FGF-2 and EGF.

Table 1. ELISA of eight angiogenic factors.

4. Discussion

4.1. Formation of capillary tube from tissue explant of skeletal muscles

In this study, we tested tissue explants of skeletal muscles, brain, kidney, liver and spleen. In the light microscopic level, tubular structures are newly formed from all tissue explants tested. By electron microscopic observation, tubular structures with a lumen were observed only from the tissue explant of skeletal muscles and kidney cortex. By further detail electron microscopic observation, tubular structures from the kidney cortex have microvilli. The capillary tubes had quite similar architecture observed in the collagen gel culture of aortic explant [12]. Plasmalemmal vesicles or caveolae were also observed. Plasmalemmal vesicles are plasma membrane invaginations. They are particularly numerous in the continuous endothelium of microvascular beds such as skeletal muscles in which they have been identified as transcytotic vesicular carriers [20, 21].

In the present study, we demonstrated that capillary tubes have architecture of capillary by tomato lectin, as we have previously shown [22]. Cell adhesion molecules are a family of closely related cell surface glycoproteins involved in cell-cell interactions during growth and are thought to play an important role in embryogenesis and development. PECAM-1, also referred to as CD31, is a glycoprotein expressed on the cell surfaces of endothelial cells, as well as platelets and mononuclear cells. PECAM-1 positive cells were clearly demonstrated as a capillary-like structure. ICAM-1, also referred to as CD54, is an integral membrane protein of the immunoglobulin superfamily and recognizes the $\beta2\alpha1$ and $\beta2\alpha M$ integrins. In the present study, ICAM-1 positive cells were sparse. It may accord with $\beta2$ integrin which was not detected. We have reported that pericyte-like cells were observed in the aortic explant culture (for a detailed review see Ref. [12]). Pericyte-like cells were positive for actin [12, 23]. In this study, pericyte-like cells were also observed around the capillary tubes, as shown in the aortic explant culture. Pericytes were reported to stimulate angiogenesis through the secretion of growth factors such as fibroblast growth factor (FGF) [24], VEGF and placenta growth factor [25]. In addition, pericytes appear to promote endothelial cell (EC) survival [26] and affect EC behavior such as sprouting [27]. It is strongly suggested that pericytes play an important role in angiogenesis. VEGF is a key promoter of angiogenesis. VEGF acts as a chemoattractant and directs capillary growth. VEGF concentration gradients are important for activation and chemotactic guidance of capillary sprouting [28, 29]. Zhang et al. [30] reported that a variety of cells in the body, including myocyte (skeletal muscle fibers), secrete VEGF at different rates. Ji et al. [31] also reported that VEGF is secreted by myocytes and binds VEGF receptors and neuropilin-1 on endothelial cell surface. Further studies are needed to understand the angiogenic factors.

It should be noted that, when compared with mice and rats, capillary tubes formation was predominant in rats than mice. We could not demonstrate the difference in angiogenic factors between rats and mice. It is widely accepted that endothelial cells derived from different species display different morphological, biochemical and phenotypical heterogeneity [32, 33]. For instance, FGF1 or collagen-coated dish is not required for culturing endothelial cells from the bovine and pig, unlike the rabbit and rat [34]. Difference in the properties of endothelial cells by species is considered in angiogenesis. It should be also noted that there is difference between red and white muscles. The number of capillaries in the soleus muscle of rat is 2.8/ muscle fiber. The corresponding value for the tibialis anterior muscle is 1.2–2.0 [35]. The density of capillaries in the soleus muscle is greater than the tibialis anterior muscle. The difference in the capillary density may relate the formation of capillary tubes.

4.2. Effects of α-isoproterenol

Isoproterenol (β-adrenergic receptor agonist) promotes skeletal muscle hypertrophy in several animals, including rats and mice [36, 37]. The hypertrophy by isoproterenol induces through the stimulation of β_2-adrenergic receptor [38], and β-adrenergic receptor is involved in skeletal muscle growth and regeneration [39]. Expression of β-adrenergic receptor and its coupling to cAMP are important components of the signaling mechanism that controls atrophy and hypertrophy of skeletal muscle [40]. We have reported that α-isoproterenol reduced the degeneration of muscle after the facial nerve crush [41]. In this study, the direct effect of α-isoproterenol was confirmed even in vitro.

There are a number of reports about the increase in skeletal muscle capillary density with exercise. Exercise such as endurance training increases the capillary network to adapt to oxygen demand, particularly arteriolar portion of capillaries to favor the oxygen supply [42, 43]. When the endurance training was loaded in normal rats, angiogenesis of the soleus muscle is promoted, and arteriolar portion of capillaries is increased significantly [44]. Increase in arteriolar portion of capillaries is believed to be caused by "arteriolarization of capillaries" promoted by an increase in wall tension [44–46]. From the fact that circulating catecholamines (adrenalin and noradrenalin) are concerned with contraction/expansion of the blood vessels, catecholamines are expected to be associated with an increase in capillary density. Circulating catecholamines, which are adrenergic receptor agonist, are the main hormones whose concentrations increase markedly during exercise [47]. Many researchers have worked on the effect of exercise on these catecholamines and reported 1.5 to >20 times basal concentrations depending on exercise characteristics (e.g., duration and intensity) [48]. The increase in circulating catecholamines results in stimulating of β-adrenergic receptor activity and, consequently, increased intercellular concentration of cyclic AMP [49]. However, we have no direct effect that catecholamines associate with an increase in capillary density. Although an experiment in culture, in the brown fat precursor cells, noradrenalin encourages the growth of capillaries [50]. In the soleus muscle in the present study, α-isoproterenol, which is also an adrenergic receptor agonist, encourages the growth of capillary tubes. Although we could not detect the angiogenic factors, it has become possible to study the direct effect of α-isoproterenol on the skeletal muscle and formation of capillary tubes.

4.3. Effects of low-frequency electrical stimulation

From the results of the electrical stimulation, the effect of suppressing the denaturation of the muscle was observed. Young et al. [39] reported that electrical stimulation increased the number of β-receptors and promoted the synthesis of cAMP.

In this study, we could demonstrate that electrical stimulation also reduced the degeneration of skeletal muscles.

For angiogenesis in skeletal muscle in vivo, Cotter et al. [51] showed an increase in capillary density by the low-frequency electrical stimulation. After that, angiogenesis by skeletal muscle has been made under the various conditions of electrical stimulation [52–54].

For electrical stimulation in vitro, studies using myoblast cell line have been reported [55–57]. However, in vitro study of skeletal muscles capillaries is very few. Endothelial cells isolated from skeletal muscle capillaries are studied to make physical and chemical stress to the cells [58]. A number of angiogenic factors involve in angiogenesis by electrical stimulation [59, 60]. VEGF can be mentioned as the most important proteins. VEGF encourages the growth of vascular endothelial cells. VEGF played a central role in angiogenesis [59, 60].

As the mechanism, skeletal muscle contraction due to electrical stimulation has been considered to induce hypoxia [61, 62] and shear stress [63]. However, Kanno et al. [19] applied the electrical stimulation (50 Hz) without muscle contraction to the skeletal muscle and showed the increase in VEGF protein in vitro, and they showed the increased in capillary density in the rat model of hindlimb ischemia. In this study, the condition (50 Hz) according to the report of Kanno et al. [19] was adopted.

Electrical stimulation upregulated FGF-2 and EGF protein levels in the brains of stroke rats [64]. In this study, VEGF, FGF-2 and EGF protein levels are increased. However, under the condition used in this study, it was harmful to the migrating cells. The effect of promoting angiogenesis was not observed. On the contrary, angiogenesis was inhibited. Further studies including the setting of the condition are necessary.

4.4. The usefulness of this in vitro model

Endothelial progenitor cells derived from bone marrow are present in the peripheral blood. These cells reach the ischemic site, and angiogenesis occurs by proliferation and differentiation. However, it is difficult to collect a large amount of bone marrow stem cells for treatment of ischemia. Transplantation of CD133-positive endothelial precursor cells to the damaged muscle tissue has been studied [65]. In this report, angiogenesis is promoted, and the damaged muscle tissue is expected to recover. Recently, cardiac tissue sheets from human iPS cells have been shown to be effective in engraftment and transplantation in the rat model of myocardial infarction [66]. This cardiac tissue sheets include vascular cells (vascular endothelial cells and pericytes), in addition to the cardiomyocytes. Higher survival rate than the sheet of only cardiomyocytes has been shown. Transplantation including vascular cells may become research to increase the possibility of therapeutic angiogenesis.

In this study, we propose the possibility of autologous transplantation using tissue explants of skeletal muscle in cardiovascular disease including critical hind limb ischemia.

4.5. The drawback of this in vitro model

Clearly, those capillary tubes that emanate from the muscle explants are very similar to capillaries in vivo. However, the capillary tubes are not filled with flowing blood. Although the structure as capillary tubes is maintained at least 2 weeks, further studies are needed for long-term culture.

Author details

Tomoko Takahashi[1], Keiko Fujita[1] and Masumi Akita[2,*]

*Address all correspondence to: makita@saitama-med.ac.jp

1 Department of Anatomy, Saitama Medical University, Saitama, Japan

2 Division of Morphological Science, Biomedical Research Center, Saitama Medical University, Saitama, Japan

References

[1] Deckers M, van der Pluijm G, Dooijewaard S, Kroon M, van Hinsbergh V, Papapoulos S, Lowik C: Effect of angiogenic and antiangiogenic compounds on the outgrowth of capillary structures from fetal mouse bone explants. Lab Invest. 2001; 81:5–15.

[2] Jakob W, Jentzsch KD, Mauersberger B, Heder G: The chick embryo choriallantoic membrane as a bioassay for angiogenesis factors: reactions induced by carrier materials. Exp Pathol (Jena). 1978; 15:241–249.

[3] Fournier GA, Lutty GA, Watt S, Fenselau A, Patz A: A corneal micropocket assay for angiogenesis in the rat eye. Invest Ophthalmol Vis Sci. 1981; 21:351–354.

[4] Kenyon BM, Voest EE, Chen CC, Flynn E, Folkman J, D'Amato RJ: A model of angiogenesis in the mouse cornea. Invest Ophthalmol Vis Sci. 1996; 37:1625–1632.

[5] Lehr HA, Leunig M, Menger MD, Nolte D, Messmer K: Dorsal skinfold chamber technique for intravital microscopy in nude mice. Am J Pathol. 1993; 143:1055–1062.

[6] Jain RK, Schlenger K, Hockel M, Yuan F: Quantitative angiogenesis assays: progress and problems. Nat Med. 1997; 3:1203–1208.

[7] Staton CA, Stribbling SM, Tazzyman S, Hughes R, Brown NJ, Lewis CE: Current methods for assaying angiogenesis in vitro and in vivo. Int J Exp Pathol. 2004; 85:233–248.

[8] Montesano R, Mouron P, Orci L: Vascular outgrowths from tissue explants embedded in fibrin or collagen gels: a simple in vitro model of angiogenesis. Cell Biol Int Rep. 1985; 9:869–875.

[9] Mori M, Sadahira Y, Kawasaki S, Hayashi T, Notohara K, Awai M: Capillary growth from reversed rat aortic segments cultured in collagen gel. Acta Pathol Jpn. 1988; 38:1503–1512.

[10] Nicosia RF, Ottinetti A: Growth of microvessels in serum-free matrix culture of rat aorta. A quantitative assay of angiogenesis in vitro. Lab Invest. 1990; 63:115–122.

[11] Artym VV, Matsumoto K: Imaging Cells in Three-Dimensional Collagen Matrix. Curr Protoc Cell Biol. 2010; Chapter 10: Unit–10.1820. doi:10.1002/0471143030.cb1018s48.

[12] Akita M: Development of in vitro method for assaying anti angiogenic effect of drugs. In: Atta-ur-Rahman, M.Iqbal Choudhary, editors. Anti-Angiogenesis Drug Discovery and Development, Vol. 2. Sharjah: Bentham Science Publishers; 2014, pp. 63-111. doi:10 .2174/9781608058666211140201

[13] Standring S: Smooth muscle and the cardiovascular and lymphatic systems. In: Standring S, editor-in-chief. Gray's Anatomy 39th ed. Churchill Livingstone, London: Elsevier; 2005. p.143.

[14] Akita M, Murata E, Merker HJ, Kaneko K: Formation of new capillary-like tubes in a three-dimensional in vitro model (aorta/collagen gel). Ann Anat. 1997; 179:137–147.

[15] Akita M, Murata E, Merker HJ, Kaneko K: Morphology of capillary-like structures in a three-dimensional aorta/collagen gel culture. Ann Anat. 1997; 179:127–136.

[16] Kajikawa K, Yamaguchi T, Katsuda S, Miwa A: An improved electron stain for elastic fibers using tannic acid. J Electron Microsc (Tokyo). 1975; 24:287–289.

[17] Hoffmann S, Spee C, Murata T, Cui JZ, Ryan SJ, Hinton DR: Rapid isolation of chorio-capillary endothelial cells by Lycopersicon esculentum-coated Dynabeads. Graefes Arch Clin Exp Ophthalmol. 1998; 236:779–784.

[18] Inomata T, Murata E, Akita M: Effects of α-isoproterenol on the atrophy of soleus and tibialis anterior muscles after sciatic nerve crush injury, and on microstructure of submandibular gland. J Saitama Medical University. 2001; 28:171–178.

[19] Kanno S, Oda N, Abe M, Saito S, Hori K, Handa Y, Tabayashi K, Sato Y: Establishment of a simple and practical procedure applicable to therapeutic angiogenesis. Circulation. 1999; 99:2682–2687.

[20] Fawcett DW: Surface specializations of absorbing cells. J Histochem Cytochem. 1965; 13:75–91.

[21] Stan RV, Roberts WG, Predescu D, Ihida K, Saucan L, Ghitescu L, Palade GE: Immunoisolation and partial characterization of endothelial plasmalemmal vesicles (caveolae). Mol Biol Cell. 1997; 8:595–605.

[22] Fujita K, Komatsu K, Tanaka K, Ohshima S, Asami Y, Murata E, Akita M: An in vitro model for studying vascular injury after laser microdissection. Histochem Cell Biol. 2006; 125:509–514.

[23] Fujita K, Asami Y, Tanaka K, Akita M, Merker HJ: Anti-angiogenic effects of thalido-mide: expression of apoptosis-inducible active-caspase-3 in a three-dimensional colla-gen gel culture of aorta. Histochem Cell Biol. 2004; 122:27–33.

[24] Watanabe S, Morisaki N, Tezuka M, Fukuda K, Ueda S, Koyama N, Yokote K, Kanzaki T, Yoshida S, Saito Y: Cultured retinal pericytes stimulate in vitro angiogenesis of endothe-lial cells through secretion of a fibroblast growth factor-like molecule. Atherosclerosis. 1997; 130:101–107.

[25] Yonekura H, Sakurai S, Liu X, Migita H, Wang H, Yamagishi S, Nomura M, Abedin MJ, Unoki H, Yamamoto Y, Yamamoto H: Placenta growth factor and vascular endothe-lial growth factor B and C expression in microvascular endothelial cells and pericytes. Implication in autocrine and paracrine regulation of angiogenesis. J Biol Chem. 1999; 274:35172–35178.

[26] Benjamin LE, Hemo I, Keshet E: A plasticity window for blood vessel remodeling is defined by pericyte coverage of the preformed endothelial network and is regulated by PDGF-B and VEGF. Development. 1998; 125:1591–1598.

[27] Nehls V, Denzer K, Drenckhahn D: Pericyte involvement in capillary sprouting during angiogenesis in situ. Cell Tissue Res. 1992. 270:469–474.

[28] Gerhardt H, Golding M, Fruttiger M, Ruhrberg C, Lundkvist A, Abramsson A, Jeltsch M, Mitchell C, Alitalo K, Shima D, Betsholtz C: VEGF guides angiogenic sprouting utilizing endothelial tip cell filopodia. J Cell Biol. 2003; 161:1163–1177.

[29] Helm CL, Fleury ME, Zisch AH, Boschetti F, Swartz MA: Synergy between interstitial flow and VEGF directs capillary morphogenesis in vitro through a gradient amplification mechanism. Proc Natl Acad Sci USA. 2005; 102:15779–15784.

[30] Zhang QX, Magovern CJ, Mack CA, Budenbender KT, Ko W, Rosengart TK: Vascular endothelial growth factor is the major angiogenic factor in omentum: mechanism of the omentum-mediated angiogenesis. J Surg Res. 1997; 67:147–154.

[31] Ji JW, Mac Gabhann F, Popel AS: Skeletal muscle VEGF gradients in peripheral arterial disease: simulations of rest and exercise. Am J Physiol Heart Circ Physiol. 2007; doi:10.1152/ajpheart.00009.2007

[32] Fajardo LF. The complexity of endothelial cells. A review. Am J Clin Pathol. 1989; 92:241–250.

[33] Browning AC, Gray T, Amoaku WM: Isolation, culture, and characterisation of human macular inner choroidal microvascular endothelial cells. Br J Ophthalmol. 2005; 89:1343–1347. doi:10.1136/bjo.2004.063602

[34] Yamamoto K: Methods for long-term cultivation of endothelial cells (in Japanese). Murota S Editor. Modern Chemistry 16, Tokyo: Tokyo Kagaku Dojin; 1989, pp. 151–157.

[35] Schmalbruch H, Oksche A, Vollrath L: Skeletal muscle, v.II/6, Handbook of Microscopic Anatomy. Berlin, Tokyo: Springer-Verlag; 1985. pp. 22–30.

[36] Deshaies Y, Willemot J, Leblanc J: Protein synthesis, amino acid uptake, and pools during isoproterenol-induced hypertrophy of the rat heart and tibialis muscle. Can J Physiol Pharmacol. 1981; 59:113–121.

[37] Mersmann HJ: Species variation in mechanisms for modulation of growth by beta-adrenergic receptors. J Nutr. 1995; 125:1777S–1782S.

[38] Hinkle RT, Hodge KM, Cody DB, Sheldon RJ, Kobilka BK, Isfort RJ: Skeletal muscle hypertrophy and anti-atrophy effects of clenbuterol are mediated by the 2-Adrenergic receptor. Muscle Nerve. 2002; 25:729–734.

[39] Beitzel F, Gregorevic P, Ryall JG, Plant DR, Sillence MN, Lynch GS: 2-Adrenoceptor agonist fenoterol enhances functional repair of regenerating rat skeletal muscle after injury. J Appl Physiol. 2004; 96:1385–1392.

[40] Young RB, Bridge KY, Strietzel CJ: Effect of electrical stimulation on beta-adrenergic receptor population and cyclic amp production in chicken and rat skeletal muscle cell cultures. In Vitro Cell Dev Biol Anim. 2000; 36:167–173.

[41] Ishii K, Sowa K, Zhai WG, Akita M. Effects of α-isoproterenol on denervation atrophy in orbicularis oculi muscle fibers. Histol Histopathol. 1998; 13:1015–1018.

[42] Suzuki J, Gao M, Batra S, Koyama T: Effects of treadmill training on the arteriolar and venular portions of capillary in soleus muscle of young and middle-aged rats. Acta Physiol Scand. 1997; 159:113–121.

[43] Suzuki J, Kobayashi T, Uruma T, Koyama T: Time-course changes in arteriolar and venular portions of capillary in young treadmill trained rats. Acta Physiol Scand. 2001; 171:77–86.

[44] Suzuki J: Effects of endurance training on skeletal muscle capillarity in IDDM model rats. 2004; 7:1–7. http://s-ir.sap.hokkyodai.ac.jp/dspace/handle/123456789/6776

[45] Price RJ, Owens GK, Skalak TC: Immunohistochemical identification of arteriolar development using markers of smooth muscle differentiation. Evidence that capillary arterialization proceeds from terminal arterioles. Circ Res. 1994; 75:520–527.

[46] Price RJ, Skalak TC: A circumferential stress-growth rule predicts arcade arteriole formation in a network model. Microcirculation. 1995; 2:41–51.

[47] Paroo Z, Noble EG: Isoproterenol potentiates exercise-induction of Hsp70 in cardiac and skeletal muscle. Cell Stress & Chaperones. 1999; 4:199–204.

[48] Zouhal H, Jacob C, Delamarche P, Gratas-Delamarche A: Catecholamines and the effects of exercise, training and gender. Sports Med. 2008; 38:401–423.

[49] Hoffman BB, Lefkowitz RL: Catecholamines and sympathomimeric drugs. In: Gilman AG, Rall TW, Taylor AS, editors. The Pharmacological Basis of Therapeutic drugs. New York: Pergamon Press; 1990. pp.187–219.

[50] Yamashita H, Sato N, Kizaki T, Oh-ishi S, Segawa M, Saitoh D, Ohira Y, Ohno H: Norepinephrine stimulates the expression of fibroblast growth factor 2 in rat brown adipocyte primary culture. Cell Growth Differ. 1995; 6:1457–1462.

[51] Cotter M, Hudlická O, Pette D, Staudte H, Vrbová G: Changes of capillary density and enzyme pattern in fast rabbit muscles during long-term stimulation. J Physiol. 1973; 230:34P–35P.

[52] Brown MD, Cotter MA, Hudlická O, Vrbová G: The effects of different patterns of muscle activity on capillary density, mechanical properties and structure of slow and fast rabbit muscles. Pflugers Arch. 1976; 361:241–250.

[53] Hudlicka O, Tyler KR: The effect of long-term high-frequency stimulation on capillary density and fibre types in rabbit fast muscles. J Physiol. 1984; 353:435–445.

[54] Hudlicka O: Growth of capillaries in skeletal and cardiac muscle. Circ Res. 1982; 50:451–461.

[55] Ohno Y, Yamada S, Sugiura T, Ohira Y, Yoshioka T, Goto K: Possible role of NF-κB signals in heat stress-associated increase in protein content of cultured C2C12 cells. Cells Tissues Organs. 2011; 194:363–370.

[56] Goto K, Okuyama R, Sugiyama H, Honda M, Kobayashi T, Uehara K, Akema T, Sugiura T, Yamada S, Ohira Y, Yoshioka T: Effects of heat stress and mechanical stretch on

protein expression in cultured skeletal muscle cells. Pflugers Arch. 2003; 447:247–253. doi:10.1007/s00424-003-1177-x

[57] Iwata M, Nishihama K, Tsuchida W, Suzuki S: The hypertrophic effect of electrical pulse stimulation on cultured skeletal muscle cells. J Health Sci, Nihon Fukushi Univ. 2013; 16:1–7.

[58] Milkiewicz M, Doyle JL, Fudalewski T, Ispanovic E, Aghasi M, T Haas TL: HIF-1α and HIF-2α play a central role in stretch-induced but not shear-stress-induced angiogenesis in rat skeletal muscle. J Physiol. 2007; 583:753–766.

[59] Hang J, Kong L, Gu JW, Adair TH: VEGF gene expression is upregulated in electrically stimulated rat skeletal muscle. Am J Physiol. 1995; 269(5 Pt2):H1827–1831.

[60] Annex BH, Torgan CE, Lin P, Taylor DA, Thompson MA, Peters KG, Kraus WE: Induction and maintenance of increased VEGF protein by chronic motor nerve stimulation in skeletal muscle. Am J Physiol. 1998; 274(3 Pt2):H860–867.

[61] Hudlicka O: Is physiological angiogenesis in skeletal muscle regulated by changes in microcirculation? Microcirculation. 1998; 5:7–23.

[62] Forsythe JA, Jiang BH, Iyer NV, Agani F, Leung SW, Koos RD, Semenza GL: Activation of vascular endothelial growth factor gene transcription by hypoxia-inducible factor 1. Mol Cell Biol. 1996; 16:4604–4613.

[63] Hudlicka O, Price S: The role of blood flow and muscle hypoxia in capillary growth in chronically stimulated fast muscles. Pflugers Arch. 1990; 417:67–72.

[64] Xiang Y, Liu H, Yan T, Zhuang Z, Jin D, Peng Y: Functional electrical stimulation-facilitated proliferation and regeneration of neural precursor cells in the brains of rats with cerebral infarction. Neural Regen Res. 2014; 9:243–251. doi:10.4103/1673-5374.128215

[65] Shi M, Ishikawa M, Kamei N, Nakasa T, Adachi N, Deie M, Asahara T, Ochi M: Acceleration of skeletal muscle regeneration in a rat skeletal muscle injury model by local injection of human peripheral blood-derived CD133-positive cells. Stem Cells. 2009; 27:949–960. doi:10.1002/stem.4.

[66] Masumoto H, Ikuno T, Takeda M, Fukushima H, Marui A, Katayama S, Shimizu T, Ikeda T, Okano T, Sakata R, Yamashita JK: Human iPS cell-engineered cardiac tissue sheets with cardiomyocytes and vascular cells for cardiac regeneration. Sci Rep. 2014; 4:6716. doi:10.1038/srep06716.

Permissions

All chapters in this book were first published in PPA, by InTech Open; hereby published with permission under the Creative Commons Attribution License or equivalent. Every chapter published in this book has been scrutinized by our experts. Their significance has been extensively debated. The topics covered herein carry significant findings which will fuel the growth of the discipline. They may even be implemented as practical applications or may be referred to as a beginning point for another development.

The contributors of this book come from diverse backgrounds, making this book a truly international effort. This book will bring forth new frontiers with its revolutionizing research information and detailed analysis of the nascent developments around the world.

We would like to thank all the contributing authors for lending their expertise to make the book truly unique. They have played a crucial role in the development of this book. Without their invaluable contributions this book wouldn't have been possible. They have made vital efforts to compile up to date information on the varied aspects of this subject to make this book a valuable addition to the collection of many professionals and students.

This book was conceptualized with the vision of imparting up-to-date information and advanced data in this field. To ensure the same, a matchless editorial board was set up. Every individual on the board went through rigorous rounds of assessment to prove their worth. After which they invested a large part of their time researching and compiling the most relevant data for our readers.

The editorial board has been involved in producing this book since its inception. They have spent rigorous hours researching and exploring the diverse topics which have resulted in the successful publishing of this book. They have passed on their knowledge of decades through this book. To expedite this challenging task, the publisher supported the team at every step. A small team of assistant editors was also appointed to further simplify the editing procedure and attain best results for the readers.

Apart from the editorial board, the designing team has also invested a significant amount of their time in understanding the subject and creating the most relevant covers. They scrutinized every image to scout for the most suitable representation of the subject and create an appropriate cover for the book.

The publishing team has been an ardent support to the editorial, designing and production team. Their endless efforts to recruit the best for this project, has resulted in the accomplishment of this book. They are a veteran in the field of academics and their pool of knowledge is as vast as their experience in printing. Their expertise and guidance has proved useful at every step. Their uncompromising quality standards have made this book an exceptional effort. Their encouragement from time to time has been an inspiration for everyone.

The publisher and the editorial board hope that this book will prove to be a valuable piece of knowledge for researchers, students, practitioners and scholars across the globe.

List of Contributors

Keiko Fujita and Masumi Akita
Department of Anatomy, Faculty of Medicine, Saitama Medical University, Saitama, Japan
Division of Morphological Science, Faculty of Medicine, Biomedical Research Center, Saitama Medical University, Saitama, Japan

Jimmy Stalin
Department of Pathology and Immunology, University Medical Center, Geneva University, Switzerland

Lucie Vivancos
Pediatric Hematology-Oncology Research Laboratory, Pediatric Division, University Hospital CHUV, Lausanne, Switzerland

Nathalie Bardin, Françoise Dignat-George and Marcel Blot-Chabaud
INSERM UMR-S 1076, Aix-Marseille University, UFR Pharmacy, Marseille, France

Ana Moraga, Ka Hou Lao and Lingfang Zeng
Cardiovascular Division, Faculty of Life Sciences and Medicine, King's College London, London, UK

Kosuke Kaji and Hitoshi Yoshiji
Third Department of Internal Medicine, Nara Medical University, Shijo-cho, Kashihara, Nara, Japan

Pavel Igorevich Makarevich and Yelena Viktorovna Parfyonova
Institute of Regenerative Medicine, Lomonosov Moscow State University, Moscow, Russia
Institute of Experimental Cardiology, Russian Cardiology Research and Production Complex, Russia

Cornelia Braicu
Research Center for Functional Genomics, Biomedicine and Translational Medicine, "Iuliu Hatieganu", University of Medicine and Pharmacy Iuliu Hatieganu, Cluj-Napoca, Romania

Ioana Berindan-Neagoe
Research Center for Functional Genomics, Biomedicine and Translational Medicine, "Iuliu Hatieganu", University of Medicine and Pharmacy Iuliu-Hatieganu, Cluj-Napoca, Romania
Medfuture—Research Center for Advanced Medicine, University of Medicine and Pharmacy Iuliu-Hatieganu, Cluj-Napoca, Romania
Department of Functional Genomics and Experimental Pathology, The Oncological Institute "Prof. Dr. Ion Chiricuta", Cluj-Napoca, Romania

Ciprian Tomuleasa
Research Center for Functional Genomics, Biomedicine and Translational Medicine, "Iuliu Hatieganu", University of Medicine and Pharmacy Iuliu-Hatieganu, Cluj-Napoca, Romania
Department of Hematology, The Oncological Institute "Prof. Dr. Ion Chiricuta", Cluj-Napoca, Romania

Diana Gulei
Medfuture—Research Center for Advanced Medicine, University of Medicine and Pharmacy Iuliu-Hatieganu, Cluj-Napoca, Romania

George Adrian Calin
Department of Experimental Therapeutics, The University of Texas M.D. Anderson Cancer Center, Houston, TX, USA

Victor Gardner
White Station High School, Memphis, TN, USA

Chikezie O. Madu
White Station High School, Memphis, TN, USA
Department of Pathology and Laboratory Medicine, University of Tennessee Health Science Center, Memphis, TN, USA

Yi Lu
Department of Pathology and Laboratory Medicine, University of Tennessee Health Science Center, Memphis, TN, USA

Ivanka Dimova
Department of Medical genetics, Medical University Sofia, Sofia, Bulgaria

Valentin Djonov
Institute of Anatomy, University of Bern, Bern, Switzerland

Daniel Andrews
Mount Saint Vincent University, Nova Scotia, Canada

Tamara A. Franz-Odendaal and Shruti Kumar
Mount Saint Vincent University, Nova Scotia, Canada
Saint Mary's University, Nova Scotia, Canada

Tomoko Takahashi and Keiko Fujita
Department of Anatomy, Saitama Medical University, Saitama, Japan

Masumi Akita
Division of Morphological Science, Biomedical Research Center, Saitama Medical University, Saitama, Japan

Index

www.ingramcontent.com/pod-product-compliance
Lightning Source LLC
Chambersburg PA
CBHW061951190326
41458CB00009B/2847